To Mary Powers

We appreciate your interest in
health care & medical care

&

with best wishes for your good health

Jim Hunt

Living Better
recipes for a healthy heart

Living Better
recipes for a healthy heart

Joyce Daly Margie, M.S.   Robert I. Levy, M.D.
James C. Hunt, M.D.

An HLS Press Publication

Chilton Book Company, Radnor, Pennsylvania

Published in Radnor, Pennsylvania, by Chilton Book Company
and simultaneously in Don Mills, Ontario, Canada,
by Nelson Canada Limited
Library of Congress Catalog Card No. 80-66979
ISBN 0-8019-7018-0
Manufactured in the United States of America

Production Staff
Manuscript Editor: Suzanne Smith
Recipe Copy Editor: Katherine Bergford
Photography: Don Sherwood/Ed Vitch

1 2 3 4 5 6 7 8 9 0   9 8 7 6 5 4 3 2 1 0

Contents

Foreword

CARDIOVASCULAR DISEASE, the number one cause of death in the United States today, results in part from one's interaction with the environment. As the lifestyle of Americans gradually evolved away from the hard work and plain food of earlier years, the incidence of heart disease rose. With increased automation, people did less physical work, but they continued to eat and drink as much, if not more, than before. Studies show that even among newly arrived immigrants, a life of affluence in the land of plenty, with its abundance of food, alcohol, and tobacco, is soon reflected in a rapid rise in heart disease. So although we became wealthy, we were apparently not so wise.

For many years, the stress and strain of modern life was blamed for this phenomenon. Heart disease was thought to be most prevalent among the more affluent, especially those in presumably "stressful" executive and managerial jobs. Now we have learned that the risk of heart disease is unrelated to education or income levels. Indeed, increased risk seems to relate predominantly to certain living habits— the things we eat and the way we live.

Unfortunately for all of us, the oft-quoted notion of one of my favorite American philosophers, Mae West, who said that "Too much of a good thing is wonderful," has proven incorrect. Medical research has shown us that high intakes of calories, fat, and salt result in obesity, hyperlipidemia, diabetes, and hypertension. And when such eating patterns are combined with cigarette smoking and physical inactivity, the result is arteriosclerotic heart disease.

Today we see changes taking place in the lifestyles of many Americans. A more sophisticated and informed public is taking a greater interest in and responsibility for its own health. Many of us are making earnest efforts to control those factors shown to adversely affect health and longevity. As our lifestyles have started to reflect a greater health consciousness, so have mortality rates. With more and more Americans heeding the message that eating, smoking, and activity patterns can help or hurt their health and lengthen or shorten their lives, death rates from heart disease have started to decline.

Many of the factors that can lead to cardiovascular disease are personal habits which can be changed. One of the primary challenges to the American medical profession today is to help people become healthier by influencing them to incorporate health awareness and health responsibility into their everyday lives— and an informed and interested public is the greatest resource we have to accomplish this end.

It is to their credit that the authors of this book are helping to bridge the gap between medical research and practical health and nutrition goals for the American public. This is as it should be. For unless those involved in research and education take the time to bring relevant medical findings to the attention of the public, the billions spent in research are spent in vain.

The authors of *Living Better: Recipes for a Healthy Heart* have taken an important step toward the goal of a healthier America by providing the pertinent information needed to make necessary lifestyle changes. The text is highly readable and easy to follow. The authors present background material on heart disease and risk factors in understandable language and provide practical information on how to incorporate sound medical advice into everyday eating and living.

If we in the United States are to sustain the progress we have made to date in the control of the cardiovascular diseases, we must each take a very personal responsibility for our own health. Concern for your nutrition and weight is the most practical step you can take to prevent future health problems.

Therefore, I strongly recommend this book to all Americans seeking to minimize the risks of heart disease and live full and healthy lives.

Theodore Cooper, M.D.
Dean, Cornell University Medical College
Provost for Medical Affairs, Cornell University

Preface

CARDIOVASCULAR DISEASE is the number one cause of death in the United States today. Cardiovascular diseases, such as heart attack, stroke, and heart and kidney failure, are responsible each year for more than 50% of all deaths in the United States. The economic costs are staggering, and the personal suffering of a family that loses a loved one, particularly someone in the prime of life, cannot be appraised.

During the last thirty years, remarkable progress has been made in understanding the basic processes involved in cardiovascular diseases. Numerous basic research concepts have been translated effectively into practical health care. These advances are reflected in the steadily declining mortality from cardiovascular disease. Overall, cardiovascular mortality has decreased by more than 35% in the last thirty years, and the trend has been accelerating so rapidly that 60% of the decline has occurred during the past ten years.

Despite these encouraging statistics, cardiovascular diseases still remain the primary cause of death in the United States. Since treating and alleviating these diseases exact an enormous toll in terms of resources and human suffering, the ultimate goal of our efforts must be prevention. For this reason, we undertook the writing of this book. Even though we do not yet have all the answers on the prevention of cardiovascular disease, it is our hope that by outlining what, to the best of our present knowledge, will possibly help prevent it, *you* can decide what steps can be taken in *your* life to lessen *your* risk of developing cardiovascular disease.

During the past thirty years cardiovascular epidemiologists have identified a long list of major and minor risk factors that predispose an individual to coronary heart disease. The evidence from several long-term studies also enables us to identify those individuals who are at greatest risk.

Risk factors are traits, habits, or conditions in individuals which are associated with an increased risk of developing cardiovascular disease. Risk factors can be grouped into categories of *definite, probable,* and *possible* and further into *modifiable* and *nonmodifiable.* Factors associated with increased cardiovascular risk include age, male sex, hypertension, cigarette smoking, hypercholesterolemia (elevated blood cholesterol), obesity, sedentary lifestyle, diabetes, a family history of heart attack, stroke, and/or premature death before age 65 from cardiovascular disease, and the use of oral contraceptives. Additional risk factors associated with hypertension include a high-sodium diet, heavy use of alcohol, and black race. In most cases, these risks do not appear as isolated factors. Usually a person has several risk factors, and it is important to remember that each additional risk factor greatly increases the possibility of developing cardiovascular disease.

The predictive power of the major risk factors is now firmly established. In fact, estimates based on epidemiological studies and national vital statistics suggest that two out of every three coronary events, such as acute heart attack (myocardial infarction), sudden cardiac death, or congestive heart failure, occur in high-risk subjects. A number of studies have established that control or modification of certain risk factors such as smoking and high blood pressure can lower the incidence of cardiovascular disease. Proof of the effectiveness of altering other risk factors, such as an elevated cholesterol level, is currently being sought. However, based on the presently available evidence, we recommend that people concerned with health adapt an overall risk-factor approach to help control their cardiovascular fate.

This book discusses cardiovascular disease in general, but it deals specifically with those risk factors associated with nutrition. Although the benefits of controlling all risk factors have not yet been proven conclusively, it is clear that nutrition can play an important role in the modification and reduction of risk factors. Based on this accumulating evidence, many health professionals now recommend that a nutritional approach be used (1) to help achieve and maintain ideal body weight by balancing caloric intake with activity level; (2) to limit the amount of saturated fat and cholesterol in the diet by decreasing consumption of foods rich in these nutrients and increasing the amounts of complex carbohydrates in the diet; and (3) to modify salt intake.

This book outlines specific guidelines for incorporating these recommendations into your daily life. In addition, a variety of appetizing, fully tested recipes have been provided not only to help control your risk but to provide pleasurable eating for the entire family.

The long-range goal of these measures is to enable you to live an active, fuller, longer life without cardiovascular disease. Today, it is not possible to achieve this by relying on physicians alone, since they often become involved in health care only after illness occurs. Each individual can make certain lifestyle changes in the effort to prevent premature coronary heart disease. The risk-factor approach outlined here will, to the best of our knowledge today, help you maintain as low a coronary risk profile as possible.

This book could not have been written without the help and support of many other individuals and institutions. We are indebted to all our colleagues whose research has resulted in the identification of cardiovascular risk factors and indicated the direction to take to avoid these risks. We are most grateful for the active advice and support of Dr. Carl Anderson of the Mayo Clinic, Mrs. Nancy Ernst of the National Heart Lung, and Blood Institute, Dr. Ivy Celender and Miss Mercedes Bates of General Mills, Inc., and the Home Economics Department of the College of Saint Elizabeth, New Jersey. We offer our heartfelt thanks to Mrs. Emelia Biskup, Mrs. Katherine Bergford, Mrs. Dianne Steiger Wellik, Miss Natalie Granito, Mrs. Suzanne Smith, Mr. William Scott, and Miss Lara Lens, all of whom contributed greatly to the finished manuscript.

In addition, we would like to thank SmithKline Corporation for its support and the United Fresh Fruit and Vegetable Association, The Tuna Research Foundation, Idaho Potato Commission, McIlhenny Company, The Florida Department of Citrus, and The Banana Bunch for giving us access to their recipe files.

Finally, we would like to thank our families for their patience and support, particularly Ellen Levy and Irene Hunt for home-testing final recipes, and Bob, Paul, and Andrew Margie, who ate the losers, as well as the winners, with a minimum of complaints.

Joyce Daly Margie, M.S.
Robert I. Levy, M.D.
James C. Hunt, M.D.

Living Better
recipes for a healthy heart

1 *Risk Factors and Cardiovascular Disease*

CARDIOVASCULAR DISEASES are disorders of the heart and blood vessels. They represent a medical, social, and economic burden of staggering proportions. An estimated 40 million Americans have some form of cardiovascular disease, and each day an estimated 3,400 Americans—more than two each minute—suffer heart attacks. Another 1,600 are victims of strokes.

Cardiovascular disease kills more than 150,000 people under the age of 65 every year, and it is the number one killer in people over 40. It accounts for about 52% of all deaths in this country; the actual number, in 1979, was nearly one million. Cancer, the number two killer, is responsible for approximately 370,000 deaths annually. Cardiovascular disorders are the major single cause of permanent disability, as reflected in Social Security disability statistics. The economic burden is enormous, exceeding $50 billion per year, which is one-fifth of the cost of all illness in the United States.

The identification of risk factors is a development of great importance to the prevention and early diagnosis of cardiovascular disease. The aim of the risk-factor approach is to try to prevent or delay the devastating effects of progressive cardiovascular disease by reducing or eliminating those risk factors that are modifiable.

WHAT ARE CARDIOVASCULAR RISK FACTORS?

Risk factors are the personal habits and inherited or acquired traits that define an individual's cardiovascular disease profile. They can be categorized as *definite, probable,* and *possible.* Most researchers in the field have associated a *definite* or *probable* cardiovascular risk with advancing age, male sex, high blood pressure, cigarette smoking, hypercholesterolemia (elevated blood cholesterol), obesity, glucose intolerance (diabetes), a sedentary lifestyle, diets rich in saturated fat and cholesterol, a family history of heart attack, stroke, or premature, sudden death (before age 65), and the use of oral contraceptives. *Possible* risk factors include stress, personality type, elevated uric acid levels (hyperuricemia), and excessive alcohol intake. The balance of trace minerals and metals in drinking water and the nature and type of fiber and carbohydrates in the diet have also been mentioned as possible risk factors.

Some risk factors can be modified, some cannot. Usually they do not appear as isolated factors; in most cases, a personal history contains multiple risk factors. It is important to keep in mind that each additional risk factor greatly increases your chance of developing cardiovascular disease.

The validity of risk factors as indicators of cardiovascular disease has been borne out in numerous epidemiological studies (long-term studies of populations) involving tens of thousands of people during the last three decades. The Framingham Heart Study, perhaps the best known, has been in progress for twenty-eight years, but major contributions have been made by many others, including the National Cooperative Pooling Project, the Tecumseh Study, the Western Collaborative Group Study, the Seven Countries Study, the Evans County Study, the Puerto Rico Study, the Ni-Hon-San Study of Japanese men, and the Goteborg Study. Most of these are *prospective* studies, in which risk factors are assessed and patients are observed over a period of time.

The prospective studies attempt to obtain representative samples of populations defined by location or occupation. (The Framingham, Tecumseh, and Evans County studies are among the few that include women.) Each participant is examined for a variety of characteristics, including weight, blood pressure, blood chemistry, smoking habits, and electrocardiographic evidence of cardiovascular disease. Some of the studies investigate other variables, such as diet, exercise, behavioral characteristics, and social factors. Participants are followed up for several years through examinations and other surveillance procedures to document the occurrence of cardiovascular disease and deaths. In these studies, the predictive value of risk factors in assessing cardiovascular prognoses in individual subjects has been firmly established.

What has not been so firmly established is the premise that altering each of the risk factors will actually decrease cardiovascular event rates. The Framingham study and the others are not *intervention* studies, and as such they do not answer the question, Does altering risk

factors alter risks? However, other studies, notably the Multiple Risk Factor Intervention Trials and the Lipid Research Clinics Primary Prevention Trial, have been set up specifically to demonstrate the effects of altering risk factors. These studies are still in progress, and because patients continue to be followed up, statements about the results of risk factor modification must be qualified.

Nevertheless, specific characteristics and personal habits strongly related to the chance of developing cardiovascular disease have been identified. Unfortunately, some of these risk factors cannot be modified or altered. If your mother or father or a sibling died of heart problems or a heart attack before the age of 65, you begin at risk. A male is more likely to have a heart attack than a female, especially before age 65, but the incidence of coronary events increases for everyone with advancing age. Your family may also be predisposed to high blood pressure, hypercholesterolemia, or diabetes, but you can work to control some of the inherent risk through diet and medical management.

Different combinations of risk factors predispose patients to different disorders of the cardiovascular system. The major risk factors for heart attack are high blood pressure, high cholesterol, and cigarette smoking. In peripheral vascular disease (diseases of blood vessels of the arms and legs), cholesterol plays a role, but the most powerful predictor is the number of cigarettes one smokes. In cerebrovascular disease, such as stroke, the risk factors change roles once again, with high blood pressure being the overwhelmingly dominant factor. In addition, each risk factor is more than cumulative in its effect. The presence of a single factor may double the risk of sustaining a heart attack, and the presence of two risk factors may increase it three to four times. With three factors, the risk increases by eightfold or more, and it continues to escalate with additional risk factors.

By far the greatest number of deaths from cardiovascular disease is caused by atherosclerosis and hypertension. Increasing attention is being focused on these two processes, and although some of the information necessary to prevent their lethal complications is still lacking, better techniques are being developed to diagnose and treat them early. The ultimate answer appears to be prevention. It is better—both physically and financially—to prevent than to repair.

A general understanding of cardiovascular disease and its consequences will enable you to adapt your lifestyle and make a personal commitment to the goal of achieving optimal cardiovascular health. (A Glossary of cardiovascular terms is provided in the back of the book.)

ARTERIOSCLEROSIS/ ATHEROSCLEROSIS

Arteriosclerosis, or hardening of the arteries, is the most common of the serious, chronic diseases affecting people of the Western industrialized countries. It is a slow, progressive process that may begin early in life, but it seldom produces symptoms until it is well advanced, and it may go undetected until middle age or even later. Then, all too often, this previously "secret" process may suddenly manifest itself as a heart attack, stroke, or other life-threatening illness. However, these complications are not inevitable. Studies show that controlling risk factors may prevent, slow down, or possibly even reverse the progress of arteriosclerosis.

The type of arteriosclerosis that most often produces serious consequences is *atherosclerosis*. In this process, the inner lining of the arteries becomes thickened by soft deposits of fatty and cellular material called *atheroma* or

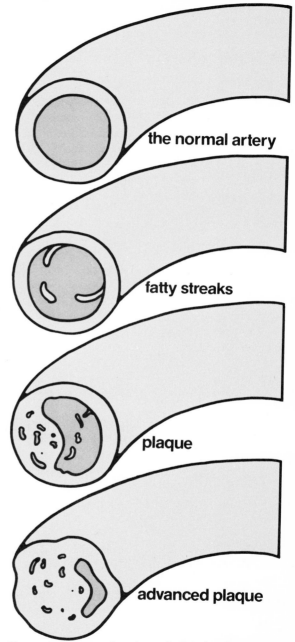

Figure 1. Progressive stages in the development of atherosclerosis. *Source:* U.S. Dept. of Health, Education, and Welfare. Publ. No. (NIH) 78–131.

atheromatous plaque (see Figure 1), which narrows the arteries and can impede or cut off blood flow. Usually, atheromatous plaque begins on the inner wall of the artery as deposits of lipids (fats, most often cholesterol) and other material from the blood. The fatty plaque narrows and roughens the normally smooth inner lining of the artery. Continued passage of blood over the plaque roughens it further as blood platelets and other components of the blood coagulation (clotting) system adhere to the site.

By encroaching on the vessel wall and making the artery less flexible, plaque encourages the further accumulation of material. Irritated areas of the plaque may become ulcerated pockets of clotted blood and cellular debris. Scar tissue may form in and around the plaque, adding to its bulk and further reducing the blood flow through the artery.

All arteries are vulnerable to atherosclerosis, but the most usual sites, and the most seriously affected, are the larger arteries serving the heart, brain, legs, and kidneys. The rate at which plaque develops may vary from one artery to the next in the same individual, and it varies widely among individuals.

Plaque build-up interferes with the body's circulatory mechanics in a number of ways. It may obstruct the artery to such an extent that little or no blood can pass. Weakening of the wall of an artery by a large plaque can lead to an *aneurysm* (a ballooning-out of the weakened vessel wall) or to a rupture of the vessel, with bleeding (hemorrhage) into the surrounding tissue. Sometimes part of a clot may break away from one plaque area and obstruct the vessel farther downstream or plug a smaller vessel elsewhere in the circulatory system. Such migrating clots are called *emboli*.

THE UNHEALTHY HEART: ISCHEMIC HEART DISEASE

To help understand what is happening in heart disease, think of the heart as a pump with two chambers for input (atria) and two chambers for output (ventricles). Blood enters the right side of the heart through the right atrium. From there it enters the right ventricle, where it is pumped under relatively low pressure into the lungs to be oxygenated. From the lungs, the oxygenated blood enters the atrium on the left side of the heart and then into the left ventricle,

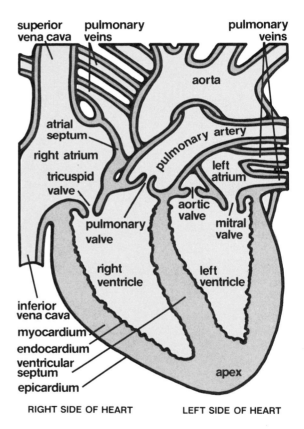

RIGHT SIDE OF HEART   LEFT SIDE OF HEART

Figure 2. The heart, cross section. Blood enters through the right atrium and is pumped to the lungs through the pulmonary artery. Oxygenated blood then enters the left atrium and ventricle and is pumped through the aortic valve to circulate to the rest of the body. *Source:* U.S. Dept. of Health, Education, and Welfare. Publ. No. (NIH) 78–131.

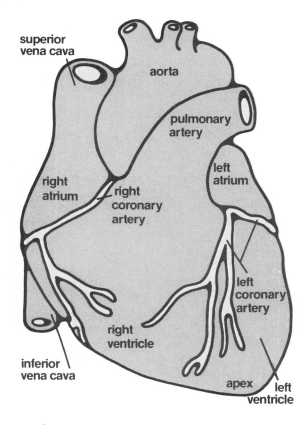

Figure 3. The heart, external view. *Source:* U.S. Dept. of Health, Education, and Welfare. Publ. No. (NIH) 78–131.

to be powered under relatively high pressure to the rest of the body, where it will supply oxygen and nutrients to all the tissues (See Figures 2 and 3).

One of the most important parts of the heart is the muscle, or *myocardium*, because it actually contracts and pumps the blood to the rest of the body. Unfortunately, the myocardium cannot obtain oxygen and nutrients directly from the blood within the chambers of the heart. Instead, it is supplied by two blood vessels that originate outside the heart, the right and left coronary arteries, which arise from the base of the aorta.

If atheromatous plaque in the coronary arteries deprives portions of heart muscle of essential blood flow, the result is *ischemic heart disease*, the blanket term for conditions resulting from an inadequate supply of blood to the heart muscle. It is a common kind of cardiovascular disease, and the names of its various clinical manifestations are well known to the public: angina, heart attack, sudden cardiac death, or congestive heart failure.

Angina Pectoris

Angina pectoris, characterized by periodic episodes of chest pain, especially during exertion, results from an inadequate supply of oxygen and other nutrients to the heart muscle because of reduced coronary blood flow. It is described as a dull ache, tightness, or sometimes crushing pain of relatively short duration under the breastbone. Ordinarily, the pain goes away in a minute or two if the victim rests, and nitroglycerin or other antianginal drugs almost always bring quick relief.

In the United States, approximately two million adults suffer from angina pectoris. These individuals must learn how to avoid anginal pain without drastically changing their lifestyles and to realize that the discomfort of angina does not necessarily mean that a heart attack or death is imminent. They must also learn to differentiate between anginal pain and heart attack pain and to recognize the characteristics of a real heart attack, which always warrants prompt medical attention.

Angina patients are generally advised to stop smoking and control high blood pressure, weight, and blood cholesterol. Most find relief with medications, but those who do not respond adequately to maximum medical management sometimes can be helped by a surgical technique called coronary artery bypass.

Myocardial Infarction

Myocardial infarction, or acute heart attack, usually results from the relatively abrupt blockage of one or more coronary artery branches, often by a blood clot (thrombus) on atheromatous plaque. The portion of the heart muscle normally supplied by the obstructed coronary branch may die or be rendered ineffective by the swift and usually drastic reduction in blood flow.

The seriousness of a heart attack is determined by the extent and location of the heart-muscle damage—that is, on the size of the blocked vessel and on the blood supply remaining in that area of the myocardium. If the stricken area is supplied by more than one vessel, the affected portion of the heart muscle may be able to tolerate a partial blockage.

Doctors describe a heart attack by various terms. They may refer to it in terms of the obstruction (coronary occlusion, coronary thrombosis, or simply coronary) or in terms of the heart-muscle damage (myocardial infarction, infarct, or M.I.). In common usage, the term *heart attack* is sometimes incorrectly used by the public to describe irregular heartbeats or attacks of angina pectoris.

If muscle tissue dies, the heart loses some of its effectiveness as a pump, since there is less muscle to contract and force blood out, and the surrounding areas may be too injured and inflamed to function well. This can lead to acute heart failure and shock, as well as to fatal disturbances in heartbeat rhythm.

Symptoms of acute myocardial infarction include severe chest pain, nearly always centered under the breastbone but often radiating to the left arm or other sites, such as the back or the point of the jaw. This pain is seldom relieved by nitroglycerin or other antianginal drugs. Some describe it as vicelike or constricting, as if a rope were being pulled tightly around the chest. Others compare it to a heavy weight crushing or pressing on the chest.

The acute attack may also be accompanied by anxiety, profuse sweating, nausea and vomiting, or loss of consciousness.

The onset of symptoms may be swift and dramatic, or symptoms may develop gradually, increasing in intensity over a period of hours. *These symptoms should never be ignored, especially by men and women in their middle or late years.*

Sudden Cardiac Death/Cardiac Arrest

Unfortunately, sudden cardiac death can be the first sign of problems with the heart and the vessels that supply it. About one-quarter of the patients who die from heart attacks have had no earlier warning and appear to be in reasonably good health.

Sudden cardiac death is thought to be caused by an *arrhythmia* (variation from normal heartbeat rhythm), which has been triggered by a transient deprivation of blood to an area of heart muscle. The arrhythmia can reduce normal heart-muscle contraction to ineffectual twitching (fibrillation) or even stop the heartbeat completely. Death ensues within minutes of onset if normal rhythm is not restored.

So swiftly do most victims succumb that only supreme good luck and exceptionally swift application of emergency resuscitation procedures promise any hope for survival. At the first sign of a suspected heart attack, the victim should be rushed to a hospital for immediate medical attention.

Ideally, cardiopulmonary resuscitation (CPR) should be started on the spot by someone thoroughly trained in its use. CPR can maintain the patient's breathing and circulation until treatment is available, even if there is no effective heartbeat. A combination of mouth-to-mouth resuscitation and closed-chest heart massage, CPR has been successfully used for some time in hospitals. CPR training courses are now recommended for the general public, and more and more people are learning the technique. Local chapters of the American Heart Association or the American National Red Cross can provide information on training centers.

Congestive Heart Failure

Congestive heart failure is a chronic condition that develops over a period of years in a heart faced with increasing circulatory burdens caused by some abnormal cardiovascular condition, such as sustained or untreated high blood pressure, a congenital or rheumatic valve defect, rheumatic inflammation, or infection. It can also be caused by the permanent heart-muscle damage resulting from one or more heart attacks.

Characteristic symptoms include fatigue after moderate exertion, or even at rest; shortness of breath in a prone position, which is relieved by getting up or by sleeping on several pillows; and swelling of the tissues, especially of the lower limbs, as a result of fluid accumulation (edema). Extensive accumulation of fluid in the lungs (pulmonary edema) can be a life-threatening complication of left-sided heart failure.

Today, many cases of congestive heart failure are arrested, before they become full-blown, by early treatment of the underlying cause. There are pharmacological controls for high blood pressure and cardiac infections, and surgical procedures exist to correct congenital heart defects and valve damage from rheumatic fever. It is hoped that the future will bring new methods for diminishing permanent heart-muscle damage after heart attacks and reducing the incidence of congestive heart

failure among recovered heart attack patients.

If congestive heart failure develops, the physician can still help the patient lead a near-normal life by prescribing any of a variety of drugs that affect the function of the heart. He or she may also advise dietary sodium restriction and a diuretic drug for alleviating fluid accumulation.

STROKE

In the brain, atherosclerosis usually manifests itself as a stroke (cerebrovascular accident). More than half of all strokes are caused by a sudden blockage of one or more blood vessels in the brain. The block can be caused by atheromatous plaque, a clot formed upon plaque (thrombus), or migrating clots of blood or fatty material (emboli) from elsewhere in the circulatory system. Strokes may also result from the rupture (hemorrhage) of cerebral blood vessels weakened by atherosclerosis and untreated high blood pressure (see Figure 4).

The portion of the brain normally serviced by the obstructed or ruptured blood vessel may be damaged or destroyed. Symptoms such as loss of sensation or paralysis in a limb, slurred speech, or loss of consciousness appear in the parts of the body controlled by the affected part of the brain. They may be permanent or temporary. Temporary symptoms may be brief, lasting for only minutes or hours if no irreversible damage has taken place, or they may be followed by a long, progressive recovery over days, weeks, or months.

Nearly 900,000 Americans are estimated to be partially or completely disabled as a result of stroke. Although the treatment of stroke has improved during recent years, a major stroke can be as lethal as an acute heart attack, and it is far more likely to produce permanent disability.

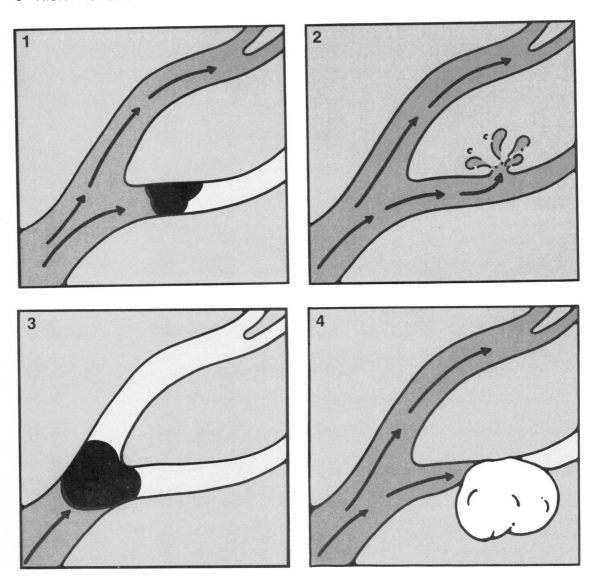

Figure 4. Strokes caused by (1) plaque clot, (2) cerebral blood vessel rupture, (3) blood clot, and (4) aneurysm. *Source:* U.S. Dept. of Health, Education, and Welfare. Publ. No. (NIH) 78–131.

Damage to the Extremities

In the extremities of the body—the hands, arms, legs, and feet—cardiovascular disease may appear, in its mildest form, as poor circulation, with the attendant feelings of cold and tingling. The two major complications that affect the blood vessels of the extremities, particularly the legs, are intermittent claudication and gangrene.

Intermittent claudication refers to transient episodes of pain and muscular weakness during exertion, usually in the calf of the leg. It results from an inadequate blood supply, and it can sometimes be controlled by drugs that dilate the blood vessels. If the response to drugs is inadequate, surgery can be performed to open or bypass the narrowed arterial segment.

Gangrene is extensive tissue death and destruction in an extremity, caused by extreme degrees of blood deprivation, and it is usually complicated by infection and tissue putrefaction. Gangrene can be prevented by surgical removal of the avascular portion of the limb or by implanting blood-vessel grafts to replace or bypass severely diseased segments of the larger blood vessels.

HIGH BLOOD PRESSURE AND ATHEROSCLEROSIS

Elevated blood pressure strains the entire cardiovascular system, but high blood pressure (hypertension), like atherosclerosis, has no early symptoms. It remains silent until major complications occur, in the form of stroke, heart attack, congestive heart failure, or kidney failure. Besides being directly responsible for 15,000 deaths each year, high blood pressure accelerates atherosclerosis, which makes it a major secondary factor in all heart attacks and strokes.

Hypertension is a mysterious disease. Its cause is unknown more than 90% of the time. It is more common in black than in white Americans, and the incidence increases with age. In general, 120/80 is considered normal blood pressure in an adult. In the United States, 25 million people have "borderline" hypertension (pressure above 140/90 but less than 160/95) and should follow weight loss and dietary sodium control programs. Another 35 million people have blood pressure of 160/95 or higher consistently and are in need of additional medical treatment.

Blood pressure is, literally, the force the flowing blood exerts against the artery walls. Primarily the circulatory system is affected, especially the blood vessels supplying the vital organs, the kidneys, brain, and heart. The earliest changes are in the small arteries and arterioles. In order to protect the organs from the elevated pressure, the arterioles constrict, and as a result they suffer the full effects of the increased pressure. The lining of the arterioles thickens, and the vessels narrow. The higher the blood pressure, the greater the damage to the blood vessels. If the pressure is extremely high, the lining of the blood vessel and the underlying elastic fibers and muscles tear and fragment. This is followed by cell destruction (necrosis) and scar tissue formation.

High blood pressure of long duration also causes changes in the large and medium-sized arteries. The vessel walls become thick and hardened, and deposits of cholesterol and other lipids (fats) accumulate and obstruct the flow of blood. In this way, the mechanisms of hypertension lead into the process of atherosclerosis, which then continues to progress slowly, even after the blood pressure has returned to normal.

Because damage to the arteries and arterioles of the body's vital organs is common in the hypertensive process, they are referred to as *target organs*. Unfortunately, by the time inadequate circulation to these organs produces symptoms, the process is often irreversible. For this reason, physicians are anxious to detect high blood pressure early and to begin an effective treatment program for lowering it. Untreated high blood pressure leads to congestive heart failure, kidney failure, heart attack, and stroke.

The major complications of high blood pressure are not inevitable. It is never too late to start a prompt and effective treatment program, even if an individual has suffered a major complication. Whatever the degree of elevation of blood pressure, and despite the presence or absence of damage to the target organs, an effective antihypertensive program can result in a greatly improved life expectancy, diminished symptoms, and fewer complications. It is thought that if treatment of hypertension is begun early—*before* the development of symptomatic atherosclerotic changes—the atherosclerotic process can be prevented or at least deferred.

CONGENITAL AND RHEUMATIC HEART DISEASE

Major advances have been made in the last thirty years in the management of the two other major forms of cardiovascular disease, congenital and rheumatic heart disease, which together claim 2,000 victims a year. Hypothermia (lowering the body temperature), the heart-lung machine, and other life-support techniques have made it possible for surgeons to operate on the heart in a stilled condition and repair even the most complex congenital defects in newborns. The incidence of rheumatic fever has been reduced by the use of antibiotics to treat streptococcal infection. The heart-lung machine and artificial heart valves have made effective surgical repair of rheumatic heart disease damage almost routine.

2 Controlling Risk Factors

THE CATALOGUE of risk factors is long and varied. Some risk factors are inherited, some are acquired, some are environmental, and some have overlapping causalities—a genetic predisposition strengthened by bad habits acquired in childhood, for example. The occurrence and effects of risk factors interweave, just as their causes do. It is rare to find a single, isolated risk factor. Typically, several can be identified in a patient's history, physical exam, and laboratory evaluation, and each added risk factor has a multiplier effect on cardiovascular health. Cigarette smoking, for example, more than triples the cardiovascular risk of an individual with mild hypercholesterolemia.

The wisdom of controlling the modifiable risk factors is apparent. Although intervention studies, which evaluate the effectiveness of risk factor alteration, are still in progress, a good deal of evidence suggests that the recent dramatic decline in cardiovascular mortality, improved cardiovascular health, and increased longevity observed in the United States is at least temporally related to changes in risk factors. The U.S. age-adjusted cardiovascular mortality rate fell by more than 25% from 1968 to 1978, and the sharp decline has coincided with striking changes in American lifestyle and habits. Between 1963 and 1975, there was a 22.4% decrease in tobacco consumption. Since 1966, the number of male smokers has decreased by more than 25%, female smokers by 10%, and smoking physicians of both sexes by more than 33%.

American dietary habits have also been changing. Between 1963 and 1977, consumption of animal fats and oils declined by 48.5%, consumption of fluid whole milk and cream by 22.5%, consumption of butter by 36.2%, and egg consumption by 14.5%. In the past ten years, the plasma cholesterol level of the average American has decreased by 4 to 8%. Simultaneously, there has been an upsurge of interest in physical fitness programs and regular exercise. Since the initiation of the National High Blood Pressure Education Program in 1972, millions of Americans with high blood pressure have been identified and their blood pressure returned to normal through treatment.

Taken together, these figures show that, as a nation, we are becoming increasingly aware of the factors involved in cardiovascular health, and that we are increasingly willing to make the hard choices and personal decisions necessary to try to prevent cardiovascular disease.

RISK: CIGARETTE SMOKING

Tobacco smoking has long been considered a health hazard, mainly because of its effect on the lungs. But numerous investigations have demonstrated that cigarette smoking is also a major risk factor for heart attack, peripheral vascular disease, and sudden cardiovascular death. In epidemiological studies of smoking effects, cigarette smokers consistently have been found to be at an increased risk for cardiovascular disease. Many studies show that the risk of cardiovascular disease is directly related to the number of cigarettes smoked per day. The more one smokes, the more likely he or she is to sustain a heart attack. A person who smokes two packs of cigarettes a day is more at risk than one who smokes one pack a day, and that person is more at risk than the occasional smoker. But all are more predisposed to a heart attack than a nonsmoker.

Furthermore, and of major importance for prevention, those who quit smoking are at lower risk than those who continue to smoke. The excess risk of cardiovascular disease in ex-smokers seems to decline dramatically within a year of discontinuation of the habit, but it remains slightly higher than the risk for non-smokers for about ten years.

A variety of mechanisms have been suggested to help explain the adverse effects of cigarette smoking on the heart and blood vessels, but none has been proven conclusively. It is theorized that nicotine increases myocardial oxygen demand and may constrict coronary blood vessels, while carboxyhemoglobin (hemoglobin carrying carbon monoxide) interferes with oxygen supply. In addition, platelet adhesiveness increases, and the threshold for ventricular fibrillation is lowered. Each of these hypothetical mechanisms could account for the reversibility of the effects.

Smoking should be the easiest risk factor to change, yet it is often the most difficult. There are many ways to quit smoking, but not one of them is effective for everyone, and the failure rate is high. A firm mental commitment and family support are required for the effort. Contrary to popular belief, weight gain is not inevitable, if the smoker defines the times when he is likely to smoke and either avoids those situations or substitutes another activity. It has been estimated that up to 150,000 fewer cardiovascular deaths would occur each year if Americans were to give up smoking entirely.

The *Selected Sources of Information* at the back of this book contains publications and names and addresses of organizations that offer help to those who want to stop smoking.

RISK: HIGH BLOOD PRESSURE

The connection between high blood pressure and the risk of cardiovascular disease is direct: The chances of developing cardiovascular disease escalate right along with the blood pressure readings. High blood pressure plays a dual role in promoting cardiovascular disease. Not only does the increased pressure make the heart work harder, but high blood pressure accelerates the process of atherosclerosis. Although blood pressure tends to rise with age, the common notion that elderly people tolerate hypertension better than younger ones has little basis. The relationship between blood pressure level and cardiovascular disease risk in women is as strong as it is in men. Like smoking, blood pressure is a graded risk: If, in a middle-aged male, a normal blood pressure of 120/80 goes up slightly to 140/90, the risk of a heart attack increases two and one-half times.

Approximately 20% of the adult population in the United States has high blood pressure. In addition to being itself a risk factor for coronary heart disease, high blood pressure has its own specific set of risk factors. They have been identified as race, age, family history, obesity, excessive salt intake, excessive alcohol intake, kidney disease, and the use of oral contraceptives. Our present state of knowledge can contribute little to the primary prevention of hypertension. Therefore, we have to rely on secondary prevention to stop its progression and prevent such consequences as heart attack, stroke, and kidney failure.

Most hypertension today can be controlled, but it cannot be cured. The key forms of secondary prevention are early detection and sustained, effective treatment. Every adult should have his or her blood pressure checked regularly, and it should be checked frequently whenever the measurement is above 140/90. If the pressure is sustained at this level or higher, most physicians advise treatment.

Blood pressure is not hard to control. The biggest problem is getting the patient to continue treatment and take prescribed medication even when he or she is feeling well. Many effective drugs are available, and physicians may prescribe them in a "stepped care" program, usually starting with diuretics to eliminate excess fluid and sodium and gradually adding other, more potent medications if necessary.

Nonpharmacological intervention, in the form of diet and exercise programs, also helps control blood pressure, sometimes to the point of reducing or eliminating the need for drugs. Control of weight and restriction of salt intake are the most effective measures.

RISK: ELEVATED BLOOD CHOLESTEROL

Almost every man, woman, and child is aware that a high blood cholesterol level is associated with an increased risk of heart disease. Evidence of the connection between cholesterol level and atherosclerosis is extensive and unequivocal. It is witnessed in animal studies and epidemiological data alike. Without a doubt, an otherwise healthy population runs a risk of coronary heart disease directly in proportion to its cholesterol levels.

Some say that any level of cholesterol is too high. The average American male's cholesterol level, 210 to 230 mg%, is probably too high. Japanese cholesterol levels are almost 100 mg% lower than ours, and their ischemic heart disease death rate is one-tenth the American

figure. As with blood pressure, the risk of cardiovascular disease rises in proportion to the cholesterol level.

Diet modification is the cornerstone of cholesterol control. In general, diet modifications should be *considered* for anyone with a cholesterol level above 210 mg%. They should *be prescribed* at levels about 250 mg% and *strictly adhered* to at cholesterol levels above 300 mg%. The risk of coronary heart disease can be predicted quite accurately from the cholesterol level in people under the age of 65. While we have not proven conclusively in man that lowering cholesterol levels will prevent or delay cardiovascular disease, there is no question that diet is often the major cause of elevated cholesterol. We see evidence for this from studies of immigrants who come to America from countries where the mean cholesterol level is low: Soon they develop the high levels characteristic of North America. Important new studies show that monkeys develop atherosclerosis when fed a typical American diet, and, more importantly, in the same group of high-risk, atherosclerotic monkeys, the progression of the disease can be stopped and even made to regress on low-cholesterol diets.

This and other evidence has led to the formulation of the *lipid hypothesis,* which states that by lowering blood cholesterol one can prevent, or at least delay, atherosclerosis and its complications. This presumption is now being tested in humans in major, long-term clinical trials.

RISK: HYPERLIPOROTEINEMIA

Cholesterol is one of several kinds of fat found in the blood. In order to travel in the bloodstream in a soluble form, the various fats must combine with protein to form compound molecules, called *lipoproteins.* The protein imparts solubility to the otherwise insoluble fat.

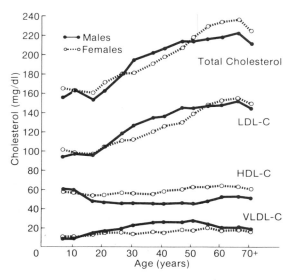

Figure 5. Average U.S. levels by age for the major lipoproteins (HDL, LDL, and VLDL) and cholesterol. *Source:* NHLBI Lipid Research Programs.

The four major lipoprotein families are the *chylomicrons*, the very low density lipoproteins (VLDL), the low-density lipoproteins (LDL), and the high-density lipoproteins (HDL). They differ from each other in size, in fat content, and in many other physical-chemical properties, which makes each one affect the body's metabolism quite differently. All lipoproteins contain cholesterol, but LDL is about 50% cholesterol by weight and carries 60 to 80% of the cholesterol in the blood. Clearly it is the most dangerous. An increase in any or all of the lipoproteins can produce hypercholesterolemia (elevated blood cholesterol), but high levels of LDL are most directly associated with coronary heart disease.

In the course of investigating the lipoproteins, researchers have made an exciting—and promising—discovery about high-density lipoproteins (HDL). While they normally carry only about 20 to 25% of the cholesterol in the blood, high levels of HDL are associated with a *de-*

creased risk of cardiovascular disease. And mounting epidemiological evidence supports the tempting hypothesis that high concentrations of HDL may be a protective factor, a deterrent to cardiovascular disease, although the cause of this effect is unknown. High HDL levels appear to go hand in hand with exercise and moderate alcohol ingestion (2 to 3 ounces per day), and low levels are found together with obesity, smoking, poor diabetes control, and the use of oral contraceptives containing progestin. Figure 5 details the average U.S. levels by age for HDL, LDL, VLDL, and total cholesterol.

Another discovery to emerge from lipoprotein research is that gross increases in blood-fat levels (hypercholesterolemia and/or hypertriglyceridemia) do not represent a single disorder. Rather, they represent a heterogeneous group of disorders—some inherited, some acquired—that differ in clinical manifestations, prognosis, and responsiveness to treatment.

RISK: DIABETES

Although diabetes mellitus (abnormal glucose tolerance) has long been recognized as a precursor of cardiovascular disease—and this association has been confirmed in prospective epidemiological studies—it is not yet clear that controlling hyperglycemia (high blood sugar) has a significant effect on the complications of atherosclerosis. Men with glucose intolerance have about a 50% greater chance of developing cardiovascular disease than men with no evidence of glucose intolerance. In women, the risk is more than doubled. Both insulin-dependent and noninsulin-dependent adult diabetics appear to be at increased risk for cardiovascular disease. Therefore, it is imperative for the diabetic to control all other risk factors by maintaining a normal weight, following a prescribed diet faithfully, taking medication, exercising regularly, and avoiding cigarettes.

RISK: OBESITY

Obesity is a major health problem that affects 30 to 50% of the American adult population. Its notable characteristic as a risk factor is its effect on other risk factors—on blood glucose, cholesterol, blood pressure, and activity levels. However, although obesity operates through its effects on these other characteristics, its role as a risk variable should not be underestimated. Like smoking, it would seem to be an easy risk factor to eliminate, but again, like smoking, the rate of backsliding among the reformed is high. Regardless of the weight-reducing method used, most people fail to lose weight or maintain weight loss for any length of time, and most of the formerly obese regain lost weight within one to six years.

The difficulties of achieving weight reduction have helped popularize a number of recent diet trends that are based on the premise that weight can be lost by changing the composition of the diet without reducing the quantity of food consumed. The high-protein, high-fat, and low-carbohydrate diets are among the most popular, but evidence shows that some of these diets have serious side effects and can be dangerous. Moreover, the weight is usually regained as soon as the diet is terminated.

Medical authorities agree that a good reducing diet should:

- Provide adequate nutrition.
- Create a negative caloric balance.
- Adapt as closely as possible to the tastes of the individual dieter.
- Be easy to obtain and reasonably inexpensive.
- Protect the dieter from hunger, satisfy the need for food, and result in a minimum of fatigue.
- Help create new eating habits that can contribute to the maintenance of a lower body weight once it is achieved.

The most widely accepted techniques for the management of obesity include diet, exercise, behavior modification, surgical intervention, pharmacological intervention, and psychotherapy. Of these, behavior modification appears to hold the most promise, because it deals directly with the cause of obesity (namely, eating behavior) and focuses on changing eating habits permanently so that weight loss may be maintained on a long-term basis.

The basic principle in weight reduction is creating a negative caloric balance, that is, expending more energy than is being ingested. This can be achieved by reducing caloric intake or increasing caloric expenditure (exercise), or by a combination of both. Numerous studies evaluating the effects of diet alone versus diet and exercise show that significantly more weight is lost by the group that both restricts caloric intake and engages in regular exercise. But this program, too, must effect permanent behavioral change to be successful.

RISK: SEDENTARY LIFESTYLE

Whatever motivates all the joggers and cyclists and tennis players, whether vanity, fashion, or a sense of well-being, they are eliminating a classic cardiovascular risk factor: a sedentary way of life. Again and again, studies have shown that individuals who are less active, especially in adult years, are more likely to sustain a heart attack than active individuals.

Regular daily exercise is recommended, but heavy, stressful, sporadic activity, such as shoveling out after snowstorms, is often not recommended for those over 40. An exercise program that will be optimal for most people cannot yet be formulated with scientific precision. But most individuals with sedentary occupations will probably benefit from some type of regular, moderate exercise.

Anyone over 40 who has not engaged in

regular exercise for a number of years should undergo a medical examination before starting an exercise program. The examination will probably include evaluation of the heart and lungs, with a resting electrocardiogram and assessment of the coronary risk factors. Some physicians also recommend a treadmill exercise test (stress test). Those with evidence of possible cardiovascular disease will probably be encouraged to engage in a carefully graded exercise program and be warned against increasing activity too rapidly.

A gradual increase in the level of physical activity over a period of weeks and even months is desirable for anyone who has been sedentary. Walking is good exercise for starters. Choosing proper equipment for a new activity will help to prevent muscle, bone, and joint problems. A reliable manual can furnish tips on gear, warm-up exercises, and training methods, which should help novice sportspeople avoid many of the acute aches and pains that come from overdoing it too early. And for safety on roads, joggers and cyclists should wear garments with reflective numbers, letters, or stripes to afford them maximum visibility at dawn and dusk.

OTHER RISK FACTORS

Modern American eating and drinking habits, with their high intake of sugar and fat and their low proportions of fiber and fresh foods, have been incriminated as possible risk factors in the development of cardiovascular disease, hyperlipidemia, obesity, and diabetes. Chemically softened water, the trace mineral content of water, and excessive alcohol intake have also been implicated. However, while evidence suggests associations, definite causal relationships in these areas have not been proven.

Studies show that diets high in sodium can produce hypertension in genetically predisposed animals. Epidemiological studies suggest an association between the role of sodium and the development of hypertension in man, but other factors, such as potassium intake, body weight, and physical activity, make it difficult to clarify this association. Although, in humans, it is not known whether limiting salt intake will prevent hypertension, sodium restriction is recommended as a prudent measure for anyone with a family history of hypertension. Large amounts of sodium can aggravate high blood pressure, and controlling sodium intake will frequently help lower the blood pressure, sometimes to within normal limits. Often, lowered sodium intake will make it possible to reduce the dosage of the drugs required to control blood pressure. How and why a reduced sodium intake makes this happen is unclear. Indeed, some people derive greater benefits from cutting back on sodium than others.

Gouty arthritis has been associated with an increased risk of cardiovascular disease, and a weak association exists between cardiovascular disease and elevated uric acid levels in the absence of clinical gout. Elevated uric acid levels (hyperuricemia) tend to be associated with higher blood pressure levels, elevated serum cholesterol and triglyceride levels, and obesity. Hyperuricemia, therefore, may merely reflect interrelated metabolic processes.

Mental and emotional stress and the so-called type-A personality—the time-oriented, overachieving, hard-driving workaholic—have also been related to cardiovascular risk. The evidence is far from conclusive, but they may play a role as additive risk factors in a person who already exhibits multiple risk factors.

3 Reducing Nutritional Risk Factors

NUTRITIONAL FACTORS—fats, calories, and sodium—play a crucial role in the development of cardiovascular disease, and they can play an equal role in the prevention and treatment of the underlying risk factors.

NUTRITIONAL GUIDELINES

In terms of diet, many Americans have been guilty of conspicuous consumption for several decades: a well-marbled steak, baked potato smothered in butter and sour cream, salad swimming in blue-cheese dressing, and a rich dessert have been held up as the ideal spread. In recent years, the "fast-food" meal of a hamburger, fries, and a shake has become a major part of the American diet. At present, the American diet consists of 38 to 43% fat, much of it saturated and of animal origin, a cholesterol intake of 400 to 600 mg per day, and a sodium intake of 100 to 400 mEq per day.

The Senate Select Committee on Nutrition, chaired by Senator George McGovern, took a look at American eating habits and recommended that *all* Americans lower their dietary intakes of salt and calories—in particular, of simple sugars, fat (to less than 30% of total calories), and cholesterol (to less than 300 mg per day). It further recommended substituting polyunsaturated fats for saturated fat and replacing refined sugar with complex carbohydrates, such as potatoes, whole-wheat breads, fresh fruits, and vegetables. The Dietary Goals as defined by the Senate Select Committee are outlined in Table 1.

Table 2 outlines the series of broad dietary guidelines for Americans recently issued by the U.S. Surgeon General.

Conservatively viewed, studies suggest an association between diet and ischemic heart disease, but they do not prove a cause-and-effect relationship. For example, animal studies do not corroborate a correlation between dietary sucrose or carbohydrates and atherosclerosis, but recent studies in man do suggest that risk *decreases* with increased consumption of starch and other complex carbohydrates when weight gain is avoided. This finding bears out earlier descriptions of population groups with a low incidence of heart disease, who derive 65 to 85% of their total energy from carbohydrates—from whole grains, potatoes, and fresh produce instead of simple sugars. High-fiber diets are in vogue, but current studies on the effects of fiber on fat metabolism show that different kinds of fiber have different effects, and further work is needed. However, many nutritionists concur with the Senate committee's recommendation that excess fats and simple sugars be replaced by complex carbohydrates.

Three basic guidelines should be followed in eating for heart health, and these guidelines become *rules* if you are at increased risk: (1) avoid weight gain and obesity, (2) reduce saturated fat and cholesterol intake, and (3) reduce salt intake.

Table 1.
U.S. Dietary Goals

To avoid overweight, consume only as much energy (calories) as is expended; if overweight, decrease energy intake and increase energy expenditure.

Increase the consumption of complex carbohydrates and "naturally occurring" sugars from about 28 percent of energy intake to about 48 percent of energy intake.

Reduce the consumption of refined and processed sugars by about 45 percent to account for about 10 percent of total energy intake.

Reduce overall fat consumption from approximately 40 percent to about 30 percent of energy intake.

Reduce saturated fat consumption to account for about 10 percent of total energy intake; and balance that with polyunsaturated and monounsaturated fats, which should account for about 10 percent of energy intake each.

Reduce cholesterol consumption to about 300 mg. a day.

Limit the intake of sodium by reducing the intake of salt to about 5 grams a day.

*The Goals Suggest the Following Changes in
Food Selection and Preparation:*

Increase consumption of fruits and vegetables and whole grains.

Decrease consumption of refined and other processed sugars and foods high in such sugars.

Decrease consumption of foods high in total fat and partially replace saturated fats, whether obtained from animal or vegetable sources, with polyunsaturated fats.

Decrease consumption of animal fat, and choose meats, poultry and fish that will reduce saturated fat intake.

Except for young children, substitute low-fat and non-fat milk for whole milk, and low-fat dairy products for high-fat dairy products.

Decrease consumption of butterfat, eggs and other high cholesterol sources. Some consideration should be given to easing the cholesterol goal for premenopausal women, young children and the elderly in order to obtain the nutritional benefits of eggs in the diet.

Decrease consumption of salt and foods high in salt content.

Source: Dietary Goals for the United States, Second Edition, December 1977.

Table 2.
Dietary Guidelines for Americans

1. Eat a variety of foods
2. Maintain ideal weight
3. Avoid too much fat, saturated fat and cholesterol
4. Eat foods with adequate starch and fiber
5. Avoid too much sugar
6. Avoid too much sodium
7. If you drink alcohol, do so in moderation

Source: "Nutrition and Your Health: Dietary Guidelines for Americans." U.S. Dept. of Agriculture and U.S Dept. of Health, Education, and Welfare, 1980.

AVOID WEIGHT GAIN AND OBESITY

Avoiding weight gain is a lifelong task that requires acknowledging that calories do count and that caloric input must be balanced by energy output. Maintenance of ideal weight should be the starting point of any prudent diet.

In the human body, maximum muscle development occurs between 20 and 25 years of age, and after that there is a gradual decrease in the amount of muscle. The average person will lose five to fifteen pounds of muscle in the years from young adult life until age 50 or 60, with a resulting shift in the proportions of muscle and fat in the body. In addition, the weight of bone decreases as people become older. So, ideally, most people (if they are to retain the same proportion of fat and muscle throughout life) should weigh less at age 50 than they did in their 20s. Most height-weight tables are reasonably good guides to ideal weight for people in their 20s, but they usually permit excessive weight for older people (see Table 3).

Dr. John Farquhar of Stanford University recommends these easy ways to calculate ideal weight for an average middle-aged American:

1. Recall what you weighed as a slim young adult. That is still your best weight.

Table 3.
Average Weights for Men and Women

Average weights for MEN 25 and over
(Weight in pounds, in indoor clothing)

Height (Shoes on 1" heels)	Small Frame	Medium Frame	Large Frame
5'2"	112–120	118–129	126–141
5'3"	115–123	121–133	129–144
5'4"	118–126	124–136	132–148
5'5"	121–129	127–139	135–152
5'6"	124–133	130–143	138–156
5'7"	128–137	134–147	142–161
5'8"	132–141	138–152	147–166
5'9"	136–145	142–156	151–170
5'10"	140–150	146–160	155–174
5'11"	144–154	150–165	159–179
6'0"	148–158	154–170	164–184
6'1"	152–162	158–175	168–189
6'2"	156–167	162–180	173–194
6'3"	160–171	167–185	178–199
6'4"	164–175	172–190	182–204

Average weights for WOMEN 25 and over
(For women between 18 and 25, subtract 1 pound for each year under 25)

Height (Shoes on 2" heels)	Small Frame	Medium Frame	Large Frame
4'10"	92– 98	96–107	104–119
4'11"	94–101	98–110	106–122
5'0"	96–104	101–113	109–125
5'1"	99–107	104–116	112–128
5'2"	102–110	107–119	115–131
5'3"	105–113	110–122	118–134
5'4"	108–116	113–126	121–138
5'5"	111–119	116–130	125–142
5'6"	114–123	120–135	129–146
5'7"	118–127	124–139	133–150
5'8"	122–131	128–143	137–154
5'9"	126–135	132–147	141–158
5'10"	130–140	136–151	145–163
5'11"	134–144	140–155	149–168
6'0"	138–148	144–159	153–173

Source: Metropolitan Life Insurance statistics.

2. Men: Calculate 110 pounds for the first five feet in height and add five pounds for each inch over that.
   Women: Calculate 100 pounds for the first five feet in height and add five pounds for every inch over that.
3. Try the pinch test: If the roll of fat at the belt line is more than the thickness of your forefinger, you are overweight.

Remember, each person is distinct, with a different physiological makeup and bone structure, so these figures are only guides.

The best way to reach your ideal weight and stay there is to develop eating habits that you can keep for life. Many "miracle" diets that promise quick weight loss are nutritionally unbalanced; they are not designed to be followed for life, and weight returns when you return to your normal diet. Too often, overweight is viewed as a problem that can be solved by a few weeks or months of agonized deprivation—and then forgotten. This is unrealistic.

The sensible approach to weight loss is to follow a nutritionally balanced, low-calorie diet with increased proportions of vegetables, fruits, and cereals and decreased proportions of fat and sugar, particularly those found in such high-calorie, high-fat desserts as pies, cakes, and ice cream. The shift from your current diet to a more sensible one should be gradual and incremental. Think of these dietary changes as a change to a healthier lifestyle, as part of a total plan aimed at reducing your risk of developing heart disease.

The goal of diet modification is what has been termed the *prudent diet*. It is a well-balanced diet that recommends a reduction in the intake of animal fat, high-cholesterol foods, and concentrated sugar sources and advocates substituting vegetable oils for animal fats, fish, poultry, and lean meat for the majority of beef and lamb, and vegetables and fruits for sweets.

It is useful in weight control and in reducing certain cardiovascular risk factors. Table 4 lists the approximate number of calories needed to maintain ideal body weight or to lose excess weight.

There are other useful tools for losing weight and keeping it off. Social scientists have developed a *behavior modification* approach to weight loss, which helps people deal with weight problems by breaking bad eating habits. Behavior modification is based on the belief that in order to lose weight and keep it off you must change habits that encourage eating and develop new ones aimed at weight control. These guidelines include:

1. Chew food slowly.
2. Never shop for food on an empty stomach.
3. Always make out a shopping list in advance. Don't add to it as you shop.
4. Learn to leave a small portion of food on your plate.
5. Do not leave open bowls of food on the table.
6. Sit down to eat.
7. Restrict eating to one or two places, such as the kitchen and dining room tables.
8. Never eat while engaging in another activity, such as watching television.
9. Become aware of your own individual eating patterns so that you can identify problems and make appropriate changes. Keep a diary of when and where you eat and under what circumstances (i.e., frustration, anger, boredom).
10. Phase out high-calorie snacks and keep a supply of low-calorie snacks readily available.
11. Enlist the help of your family in assisting you to change your eating habits.

Table 4.
Approximate Caloric Intake to Lose Weight

Calorie allowances for MEN

If you weigh (lbs)	Your daily calorie intake to maintain that weight is	Your daily calorie intake to lose 1 lb per week is	Your daily calorie intake to lose 2 lbs per week is
130	2,300	1,800	1,300
140	2,400	1,950	1,450
150	2,500	2,100	1,600
160	2,700	2,200	1,700
170	2,800	2,300	1,800
180	2,900	2,450	1,950
190	3,100	2,600	2,100
200	3,200	2,700	2,200
210	3,300	2,800	2,300
220	3,400	2,950	2,450

Calorie allowances for WOMEN

If you weigh (lbs)	Your daily calorie intake to maintain that weight is	Your daily calorie intake to lose 1 lb per week is	Your daily calorie intake to lose 2 lbs per week is
110	1,700	1,200	700
120	1,800	1,300	800
130	1,900	1,400	900
140	2,000	1,550	1,050
150	2,100	1,650	1,150
160	2,300	1,750	1,250
170	2,400	1,900	1,400
180	2,500	2,000	1,500
190	2,600	2,100	1,600
200	2,700	2,200	1,700

Note: Based on 1 pound = 3,500 calories, a one-pound weight loss per week represents a deficit of 500 calories per day or 3,500 calories per week; a two-pound weight loss represents a deficit of 1,000 calories per day or 7,000 calories per week.

12. Do not skip meals.
13. Develop a reward system for weight loss.
14. Develop a plan and continually evaluate and update it.
15. Make only one change at a time.
16. Think positively.
17. Make a personal commitment.

The books and pamphlets listed in *Selected Sources of Information* (page 276) explain the behavior modification approach in more detail.

EXERCISE REGULARLY

Exercise is very important in balancing your calorie intake. Remember, your body needs only a certain number of calories to maintain itself. Extra calories must be burned, or they will be stored as fat in the body. Table 5 outlines the number of calories expended by an average-weight individual engaged in various forms of exercise.

The key to dealing with overweight, of course, is to eat less and do more so that more energy is expended than ingested. But exercise provides many benefits in addition to burning calories. It conditions the muscles and helps the heart to handle a greater work load. Interestingly enough, moderate to vigorous exercise actually decreases appetite and so helps control weight gain.

It is vital that an exercise program be a *regular* part of your lifestyle. If you walk one mile a day, you will lose about ten pounds a year, *if* your food intake remains the same. Exercise does not have to be a torture program of push-ups and deep knee bends. Rather, it should be an activity you enjoy and can gradually and easily incorporate into your lifestyle. Exercise is one of the important contributions to a healthy heart. However, before starting a vigorous program of exercise, anyone over 40 should consult a physician.

Keep in mind that overweight is not a condition that happens overnight; it creeps upon us gradually. Most people do not deliberately set out to gain weight, but, unknowingly, they eat a few extra calories each day, and a daily excess of 200 calories can cause a gain of 16 to 18 pounds over the course of a year. Conversely, a deficit of 200 calories a day will lead to a loss of 16 to 18 pounds a year. Each pound of fat represents approximately 3,500 to 4,000 calories. The greater the deficit—created either by fewer calories eaten or more calories burned by increased exercise—the greater the weight loss.

The last element of the prescription for overweight is patience. With these guidelines for diet and exercise, your weight loss may not be rapid, but it will be steady. Eating habits and exercise habits that you can live with will keep your weight down for life.

REDUCE SATURATED FAT AND CHOLESTEROL

So far, dietary fats have been discussed as risk factors, the instigators of atherosclerosis. But they also make a positive contribution to human health. Fats help to form cell membranes, assist in absorption, transport fat-soluble vitamins (A, D, E, K), and provide essential fatty acids. Cholesterol is essential in the manufacture of cell membranes and steroid hormones. Unfortunately, we eat a great deal of it, and the body needs to take in very little, since almost all body cells are capable of synthesizing their own.

Fats should be the first nutrient you cut down on in your diet, since gram for gram fats are richest in calories. One gram of fat yields twice

Table 5.
Calories Expended in Various Activities

Activity	Calories Per Hour	Calories Per ½ Hour
Moderate Activity	**200–350**	**100–175**
Bicycling (5½ mph)	210	105
Walking (2½ mph)	210	105
Gardening	220	110
Canoeing (2½ mph)	230	115
Golf	250	125
Lawn mowing (power mower)	250	125
Lawn mowing (hand mower)	270	135
Bowling	270	135
Fencing	300	150
Rowboating (2½ mph)	300	150
Swimming (¼ mph)	300	150
Walking (3¾ mph)	300	150
Badminton	350	175
Horseback riding (trotting)	350	175
Square dancing	350	175
Volleyball	350	175
Roller skating	350	175
Vigorous Activity	**over 350**	**over 175**
Table tennis	360	180
Ice skating (10 mph)	400	200
Tennis	420	210
Water skiing	480	240
Hill climbing (100 ft. per hr)	490	245
Skiing (10 mph)	600	300
Squash and handball	600	300
Cycling (13 mph)	660	330
Scull rowing (race)	840	420
Running (10 mph)	900	450

Source: Adapted from the President's Council on Physical
Fitness and Sports, Washington, D.C.

Table 6.
Major Nutrients, Their Functions and Food Sources

Nutrient	Function in the Body	Food Sources
Protein	Basic building block of all tissues. Builds and repairs all body tissues. Supplies energy. Helps form antibodies, which fight infection.	Meat, fish, poultry, eggs, milk, cheese, dried peas and beans, soybeans, nuts, cereals breads.
Carbohydrate	Supplies energy for heat and mechanical work.	Sugars, fruits, vegetables, cereals, breads, rice, pasta.
Fat	Supplies energy to do physical work. Major storage form of excess energy in the body. Aids in absorption of vitamins A, D, E, and K and calcium.	Margarine, vegetable oils, butter, salad dressings, fatty meats, whole milk products, egg yolks, nuts, cheese, bacon, shortening, lard.
Vitamin A	Promotes normal vision in dim light. Promotes healthy skin and tissue lining. Helps maintain resistance to infection.	Liver, eggs, dark green and yellow vegetables, butter, margarine, peaches, cantaloupe, apricots, whole milk products, low-fat milk with vitamin A added, fish liver oils.
Thiamin or Vitamin B_1	Promotes normal digestion, growth, and appetite. Helps keep the nervous system healthy. Helps change food into energy.	Pork; liver; heart; kidney; dried peas and beans; nuts; wheat germ; whole-grain, restored, enriched, and fortified cereals and breads.
Riboflavin or Vitamin B_2	Necessary for the release of energy from food. Helps keep eyes, mouth, and skin healthy. Promotes vitality and growth.	Beef, pork, lamb, liver, milk and milk products, yogurt, eggs, green leafy vegetables, cheese, peanuts, enriched and fortified cereals and breads.
Niacin	Helps keep skin, mouth, and nervous system healthy. Helps convert food into energy. Aids in digestion.	Lean meat; fish; poultry; liver; kidney; peanuts; peanut butter; mushrooms; dried peas and beans; whole-grain, restored, enriched, and fortified cereals and breads.
Vitamin B_6	Aids in digestion of protein.	Meat, fish, chicken, liver, egg yolks, peanuts, peanut butter, bananas, potatoes, corn, whole-grain and fortified cereals and breads.
Vitamin B_{12}	Necessary for proper functioning of all cells.	Meat, fish, liver, kidney, eggs, milk, cheese.
Folic acid (folacin)	Necessary for the formation of blood cells.	Liver, dried beans, peanuts, walnuts, filberts, dark green vegetables.
Vitamin C or ascorbic acid	Important for healthy tissues: gums, blood vessels, bones, and teeth. Helps promote healing, stamina, and energy.	Citrus fruits and juices, strawberries, cantaloupe, broccoli, cabbage, tomatoes, tomato juice, green peppers, potatoes, leafy greens, watermelon, brussel sprouts.
Vitamin D	Aids in absorption of calcium and phosphorus, which build and maintain bones and teeth.	Fish liver oils, fortified milk, liver, egg yolks, herring, mackerel, canned salmon, sardines, sunshine.

Major Nutrients—Continued

Nutrient	Function in the Body	Food Sources
Vitamin E	Important for the stability of substances in body tissues.	Liver, eggs, whole-grain cereals and breads, whole milk, margarine, salad oil, salad dressing, green leafy vegetables.
Calcium	Needed to build bones and teeth. Helps nerves, muscles, and heart function properly. Helps blood clotting.	Milk and milk products, salmon, sardines, green leafy vegetables.
Iron	Helps build red blood cells.	Meat; liver; egg yolks; tuna; oysters; green leafy vegetables; dried fruits; whole-grain, restored, enriched, and fortified cereals and breads.
Phosphorus	Needed to build bones and teeth.	Meat, fish, poultry, eggs, dried beans, peanuts, whole-grain cereals and breads, milk and milk products.
Magnesium	Needed for proper functioning of body cells.	Dried beans, nuts, dark green vegetables, whole-grain cereals and breads.
Iodine	Needed to help regulate many body functions.	Iodized salt, seafood.

as many calories (9 calories per gram) as an equal amount of protein or carbohydrate (4 calories per gram). The Senate Select Committee on Nutrition recommends that Americans consume no more than 30% of their total calories as fat, and it further recommends that fat be distributed as 10 to 20% polyunsaturated (half of which can be monounsaturated) and 10% saturated fat. This means that the type, as well as the quantity, of the fat in the diet must be evaluated.

Fats are classified in three categories, saturated, monounsaturated, and polyunsaturated, depending on how many double bonds between carbon atoms are in the molecule. One with no available double bonds is said to be saturated (with hydrogen atoms); one with fewer than four available double bonds is monounsaturated; and one with four or more available bonds is polyunsaturated. Perhaps the best, most visible illustration of the saturation factor is peanut butter: When peanuts are ground, the oil, which is naturally monounsaturated, separates from the meat of the nuts and rises to the top of the jar. However, if the peanut oils are hydrogenated (combined with extra hydrogen), the mixture does not separate, because the peanut oil becomes more saturated and assumes a more solid form.

The degree of saturation has a different effect on blood cholesterol levels. Monounsaturated fats have little effect and are considered neutral. Saturated fats tend to raise cholesterol, and polyunsaturated fats reduce it. More-

Table 7.
The Basic Four Food Groups

	Foods in This Group Include	Major Nutrients Supplied	Recommended Servings	One Serving Equals
Meats	Beef, pork, veal, lamb, fish, poultry, eggs, organ meats, cheeses, dry beans, lentils, peas, and nuts	Protein, fat, niacin, iron, thiamine, vitamin B_{12}, vitamin E, phosphorus, copper	Adults, children, and teenagers—2; pregnant and nursing women—3	2 ounces cooked lean meat, fish, or poultry; 2 eggs; 1 cup cooked dry beans, peas, or lentils; ½ cup nuts or 4 tablespoons peanut butter; 2 ounces hard cheese; ½ cup cottage cheese; 2 cups milk may be substituted for one serving of meat
Dairy	Milk, yogurt, natural and processed cheeses, ice cream, ice milk, and food products made with milk	Protein, fat, calcium, riboflavin, vitamins A and D, magnesium, zinc	Children—3; teenagers—4; adults—2; pregnant and nursing women—4	1 cup milk or yogurt; 1 ounce cheese; ½ cup cottage cheese; ½ cup ice cream; 1 cup milk-based product (pudding, soup, or beverage)
Fruits and Vegetables	All fruits and vegetables (fresh, canned, frozen, dried, and juices)	Carbohydrate, water, vitamins A and C, iron, magnesium	Everyone—4 (including 1 citrus fruit daily and 1 deep green or yellow vegetable every other day)	1 cup cut-up raw fruit or vegetable; 1 medium apple, banana, orange, tomato, or potato; ½ melon or grapefruit; ½ cup cooked vegetable or fruit; ½ cup fruit or vegetable juice
Grains	Whole-grain or enriched white flour, pasta, rice, and cereal products	Carbohydrate, fat, protein, thiamine, niacin, vitamin E, calcium, iron, phosphorus, magnesium, zinc, copper	Everyone—4	1 slice bread; 1 ounce dry cereal; 1 roll or muffin; 1 pancake or waffle; ½ cup rice, pasta, or cooked cereal

CALORIC EXTRAS: The following foods have little nutritional value besides calories. Therefore no specific amount is recommended, and they should be added to your diet according to your caloric allowance: Butter, margarine, shortening, oils, dressings, condiments, sugars, candies, syrups, jams, unenriched refined grain products, sweetened desserts and pastries, soft drinks, and pre-sweetened fruit drinks.

over, saturated fats are twice as effective in raising the blood cholesterol levels as polyunsaturates are in lowering them.

As a general rule, moderate reduction of all fats in the diet, especially saturated fat, coupled with a decrease in dietary cholesterol intake, can lower an individual's blood cholesterol (and LDL level) by 5 to 15%.

REDUCE SALT INTAKE

Sodium is a naturally occurring mineral, and it is found in a great variety of foods. Probably the single greatest source of sodium in any diet is sodium chloride, or common table salt, which is approximately 40% sodium. It should be limited in the diet for a number of reasons. High levels of sodium can cause hypertension in some people who have a predisposition toward that disease, and it can also aggravate existing high blood pressure. Control of sodium intake will frequently lower the blood pressure, some-

times to within normal limits, and often makes it possible to reduce the dosage of certain drugs required to control blood pressure. Both the Senate Select Committee and the Surgeon General recommend a reduction in salt intake for everyone.

EAT A BALANCED DIET

Nutritionists have told us for some time that it is important to eat a nutritionally balanced diet, a diet that provides all the nutrients, including vitamins and minerals, that our bodies need (see Table 6). One system devised to help assure adequate intake of the nutrients essential for health, referred to as the Basic Four Food Groups (see Table 7): meat and meat substitutes, dairy products, bread and cereals, and fruits and vegetables. The risk factor approach to nutrition carries through the same general principles of eating for a healthy heart.

4 Eating for a Healthy Heart

EVERYONE can play a more responsible role in helping to determine his or her cardiovascular fate by making some simple dietary changes. No one is too old or too young to start on a heart-healthy program. Good eating habits formed early in life will help avoid the harder task of breaking poor eating habits later in life. So, make a decision today to follow a well-balanced diet that controls the nutrients known to promote atherosclerosis. If you think of both your health and your family's before you shop, prepare food, or sit down to eat, you will be developing a new healthier lifestyle.

The following general guidelines and directions are aimed at lowering blood cholesterol levels. Patients with diagnosed hyperlipoproteinemia should refer to page 267 for directions to follow under a physician's or dietitian's instructions.

CUT DOWN ON CHOLESTEROL

Some foods are so high in cholesterol that it is wise to cut down on them drastically: egg yolks, organ meats, shrimp, butter, and cream. Although eggs are nutritious in many ways, egg yolks are usually the greatest source of cholesterol in the diet. Luckily, most of the protein is in the egg white, which contains no cholesterol.

Eat only two or three egg yolks a week, either as whole eggs or in cooking. Whenever possible, substitute two egg whites for one

Note: This chapter is based in part on material developed by the media program of the Stanford Heart Disease Prevention Program, directed by J.W. Farquhur, M.D., and Janet Alexander, under NHLBI Grant HL-14174.

whole egg or use commercial egg substitutes. These are made from egg whites, oils, and flavorings, and they simulate whole eggs but have no cholesterol.

Put shrimp and organ meat—liver, kidneys, sweetbreads, heart, tongue, chitterlings, and brains—on the "seldom eaten" list, since they are high in cholesterol.

Butter, cream, and other dairy fats are also high in cholesterol and saturated fat and should be avoided.

CUT DOWN ON SATURATED FATS

Cutting down on cholesterol is an important step in the right direction, but it is not enough. The body is very efficient at making its own cholesterol. Saturated fats also increase the blood cholesterol level. This type of fat is found primarily in foods of animal origin—meat and dairy products—but fortunately you can get all the necessary nutrients from these foods and still avoid most of the saturated fat.

In Meat and Protein Dishes

The lean portion of meat, not the fat portion, provides most of the protein, minerals, and vitamins that are essential parts of the diet. It is not difficult to see the fat in red meat, so it should not be difficult to avoid it. Indeed, in most cases, you pay more for the extra fat when you buy meat. Prime beef, the most expensive grade, has the most fat, and Choice has more fat than the Good grade, which is the least expensive.

To maximize protein and minimize fat, eat red meat only once a day, choose lean cuts of all meats, trim off visible fat before cooking, and cook so that the fat drips off and can be discarded. The ideal ways to cook meat in order to avoid excess fat are to roast, barbecue, bake, grill, broil, or panbroil. If you boil or stew meat, skim the fat from the surface before serving, and forgo gravy or sauces made from the meat drippings.

It is more difficult to avoid the fat in ground meat than in whole meat. Hamburger is highest in fat, about 30%. Ground chuck is about 20 to 25% fat, and ground round about 15 to 20%. Prepared meatloaf mixes may be very high in fat. It actually pays—both financially and nutritionally—to buy lean or extra lean ground beef or lamb. Although they may be more expensive per pound, the meat shrinks less, so you get more meat and less fat for your money.

Substitute cold cooked turkey, chicken, or lean beef for sausage or luncheon meats, and try some of the new low-cholesterol, low-fat products. Chicken, game hens, and turkey are good sources of protein that are lower in fat, and they can be substituted for beef and lamb. If you discard the skin and the layer of fat under the skin, you can prepare them as often as you like without worrying about serving too much fat. The meat of domestic goose and duck is very fatty and should be put on the "occasional" list. Many fish are excellent sources of low-fat protein, but drain fish that has been canned in oil. Try to avoid partially prepared breaded fish and meat products, because the batter may contain egg yolks and saturated fats.

Some vegetables are very good sources of protein and contain no saturated fat or cholesterol. They are ideal sutstitutes for main meat dishes. Lentils and dried peas and beans are all good protein foods, as are nuts—walnuts, pecans, almonds, and peanuts—and some types of peanut butter. When you shop for peanut butter, be sure the terms *hydrogenated* or *partially hardened* do not appear near the beginning of the ingredient list. Peanut butter is a good source of protein, whether it is homogenized or not, but if it has been hydrogenated, some of the vegetable oil in it has been converted from polyunsaturated into saturated fat(s).

In Dairy Foods

The fat in whole milk and whole-milk products is saturated fat. The term *low-fat milk* can mean different things to different people. Whole milk contains approximately 3.5% fat, so 2% milk is really not much lower in fat content. To avoid the saturated fat and still get all the protein, vitamins, and minerals (particularly calcium) that make dairy products essential for growth and health, use skim milk and skim-milk products. Buttermilk is often nonfat. Use cultured buttermilk, and check the label for fat content.

When you buy evaporated or dried milk, look for those labeled *nonfat.* Both condensed and concentrated milk are forms of whole milk and consequently are high in fat. In addition, sugar, hence calories, is added to condensed milk.

There is no such thing as nonfat cream, but perhaps there will be someday. Sour cream and half-and-half are high in saturated fat and also contain a fair amount of cholesterol. Unfortunately, many cream substitutes, such as whipped topping and most nondairy coffee creamers, are made with saturated fats, usually coconut or palm oil, so read the labels before buying them.

Start substituting low-fat plain yogurt in recipes calling for sour cream, and make your own imitation sour cream and whipped topping (see Recipe Index). Butter is even higher than cream in saturated fat and cholesterol. So switch to margarine, but choose a margarine that lists as its first ingredient a liquid polyunsaturated vegetable oil that has not been hardened or hydrogenated.

Obviously ice cream and frozen custard are high in fat. Ice milk has a lower fat content, but it is still a form of whole milk. Use fruit ices, one of the new low-fat frozen yogurt desserts, or make your own frozen dessert (see Recipe Index).

Most cheeses are a highly concentrated form of whole milk, with a fat content of 35 to 40%. Cheeses such as uncreamed cottage cheese, farmer cheese, and part-skim-milk mozarella or ricotta have a lower fat content. Some low-fat cheeses are also available. Read the labels for fat and sodium contents.

In Vegetable Oils

In their natural state, most common vegetable oils—except coconut, palm, and macadamia nut oil—are not only free of saturated fat but are polyunsaturated. The oils that are highest in polyunsaturates are safflower, walnut, and corn oils. Olive oil is monounsaturated and is considered neutral; it does not help "balance" your saturated fat intake.

Analyze the fat content on the labels of margarine, shortening, or prepared foods carefully. Watch out for coconut oil and palm oil: They are naturally saturated oils that processors often put into products such as baked goods, whipped toppings, nondairy creamers, and packaged convenience foods. Avoid products that list *hydrogenated* or *partially hardened* vegetable oils as one of the first items on the label. Through hydrogenation, liquid fat is changed into a more solid form, to make it harder and easier to package, and hydrogen-ated vegetable oils, like the animal fats, are saturated fat.

Look for products that list poly- or monounsaturated liquid vegetable oil first. Ingredients are listed by weight in descending order. If a margarine or shortening lists partially hardened oil, hydrogenated vegetable oil, partially hardened vegetable oil, or coconut oil as its first ingredient, it should be considered a saturated fat.

CUT DOWN ON SALT

Learning to avoid sodium is an acquired skill, because it is found not only in salt but also as a preservative in many different forms in canned, frozen, commercially preserved, and convenience foods. There are large quantities of sodium in baking powder, baking soda, monosodium glutamate, meat sauces, flavoring, condiments, kosher foods, some toothpaste, and chemically softened water. So reading labels for sodium content is not always sufficient protection because it is not always listed under its own name. Do read labels for additives containing sodium. Try to avoid products that list salt, sodium, or a sodium-containing additive as the first or second item in the ingredients. As your sodium intake decreases, so will your taste for salt, and you will begin to enjoy the natural taste of food. Start by tasting your food *before* you salt it. Next, start to decrease the amount of salt used in cooking. See Chapter 8, "Using Herbs and Spices" to learn how to season your food in a way that will enhance its natural flavor. The sodium content of recipes in this book is shown in the *Nutritive Values of Recipes* table at the back of this book. In the recipe section, recipes containing more than 300 milligrams of sodium per serving are indicated by an X'd salt shaker (see Figure 6).

Figure 6. Symbols used in this book to indicate recipes containing more than 300 mg of sodium per serving (left) and recipes relatively high in calories (right).

For more low-sodium recipes and tips on diets, patients with high blood pressure should also consult *Living with High Blood Pressure: The Hypertension Diet Cookbook*, by Joyce D. Margie and James C. Hunt, M.D. (HLS Press, 1978).

WATCH YOUR CALORIES

Although sugar contains no cholesterol or saturated fat, excessive amounts of sugar contribute to overweight and elevate blood fats. In fact, sugar's only real nutritional contribution is to supply calories. So by cutting down on the amount of sugar you eat, you are not depriving your body of anything useful to health. The main sources of sugar in the diet are common granulated sugar, candy, syrup, presweetened cereal, honey, preserves, highly sweetened desserts and pastries, and liquid sugar in the form of soft drinks.

Alcohol, like sugar, can elevate blood fats in some people. In addition, because it contains 7 calories per gram, it can be a significant source of calories (see Table 8). Fortunately for our taste buds, wine in cooking is not harmful, since heating removes most of the alcohol and calories but leaves the pleasant taste of the wine.

Too much of almost any food contributes excess calories, so watch portion size. Most desserts are high not only in calories but often in fat and cholesterol. Because most of us enjoy desserts and baked goods, we have developed recipes for these foods that will enable you to cut the fat, cholesterol, and some of the calories. Recipes particularly high in calories are indicated by the symbol shown in Figure 6. The portion size for most recipes is smaller than normally called for and probably somewhat smaller than you might like, but controlling portion size will permit you to enjoy favorite foods and still stay within your calorie allowance.

SOME OTHER CONSIDERATIONS

Americans have been eating a highly refined diet for some years, and many authorities recommend that we eat more fiber. Try using whole-grain products in place of refined white flour, and eat more raw vegetables and fruit. It is not necessary to make a radical switch. Begin, as we have done in many of the recipes in this book, by replacing part of the white flour in a recipe with whole wheat, occasionally adding wheat germ to foods, and emphasizing fresh fruits and vegetables.

Replace excess fat and simple carbohydrates like candy and soft drinks with more of the *complex carbohydrates*: whole-grain breads and cereals, potatoes, fresh fruits, and vegetables. In the past few years, the word *carbohydrate* has developed a bad connotation; it has become synonymous with a high calorie intake, with soft white dinner rolls, sugar, soft drinks—and weight gain. Consequently, weight watchers have been avoiding carbohydrates in general, although many complex carbohydrates are actually low in caloric density (calories per ounce).

Table 8.
Calorie Content of Alcoholic Beverages

	Glassware Size	Calories	Alcohol (gm)	Carbohydrate (gm)
Spirits				
80 proof: gin, rum, vodka, whiskey, brandy	jigger	105	15	—
Mixed Drinks	cocktail			
Bloody Mary		80	10	3
Manhattan		183	25	2
Martini		215	27	1
Daiquiri		213	28	6
Old Fashioned		270	32	12
Brandy Alexander		237	20	10
Grasshopper		264	18	20
Cordials				
Liqueurs	cordial	66	6	7
Brandy, cognac	brandy	73	10	—
Wines				
Table:10% alcohol				
red and white, dry vermouth,	wine	90	10	4
champagne	champagne	84	11	3
Sweet: 15% alcohol				
wine, sweet vermouth,	wine	140	15	8
port, sherry	sherry	84	9	5
Beer	12 oz.			
Regular (1 can)		150	13	14
Lite (1 can)		96	12	4
Carbonated Mixes	½ cup			
Uncola		36	—	9
Cola		48	—	12
Soda		—	—	—

Note: Amounts are those of traditional glassware sizes: cordial, ²/₃ ounce; brandy, 1 ounce; jigger, 45 cc; sherry, 2 ounces; cocktail, 3 ounces; wine, 4 ounces; champagne, 5 ounces.

Source: NIH Food Values: Nutritive Content of American Foods, Food Values of Portions Commonly Used.

The recipes in this book were selected or developed to help you make the transition from a diet high in saturated fats, cholesterol, calories, and sodium. Wherever possible, calories have been trimmed by decreasing the sugar content or by adjusting portion size. Saturated fats have been replaced with unsaturated fats, and unless otherwise specified, polyunsaturated oils are used throughout. Egg whites or egg substitutes replace whole eggs, and skim milk is substituted for whole milk. Lean cuts of meat are specified, instead of the well-marbled, high-fat types. The salt in recipes is decreased or omitted, and herbs and spices are used in its place to enhance flavor. Fresh fruits and vegetables and whole-grain products are recommended throughout to help increase fiber.

HOW TO MODIFY YOUR OWN RECIPES

Using the guidelines outlined in this chapter, you can modify most of your favorite recipes to make them heart healthy. The following examples illustrate how easily this can be done. Items that can be changed are marked with an asterisk (∗). The substituted items appear in italics.

STARLIGHT CAKE

Original	*Healthier Version*
2 cups all-purpose flour	2 cups all-purpose flour
1½ cups sugar	1½ cups sugar
∗3½ teaspoons baking powder	1 tablespoon plus 2 teaspoons low-sodium baking powder
∗1 teaspoon salt	½ teaspoon salt
∗½ cup shortening (half butter or margarine, softened, if desired)	½ cup unsalted margarine, softened
∗1 cup milk	1 cup skim milk
1 teaspoon vanilla	1 teaspoon vanilla
∗3 eggs (½ to ⅔ cup)	¾ cup egg substitute

Heat oven to 350°. Grease and flour baking pan, 13 x 9 x 2 inches, or 2 round layer pans, 8 or 9 x 1½ inches. Measure all ingredients into large mixer bowl. Blend ½ minute on low speed, scraping bowl constantly. Beat 3 minutes at high speed, scraping bowl occasionally. Pour into pan(s).

Bake oblong 40 to 45 minutes, layers 30 to 35 minutes, or until wooden pick inserted in center comes out clean. Cool.

STUFFED GREEN PEPPERS

Original	*Healthier Version*
6 large green peppers	6 large green peppers
∗5 cups boiling salted water	5 cups boiling water
∗1 pound ground beef	1 pound extra lean ground beef
	2 tablespoons wheat germ
2 tablespoons chopped onion	3 tablespoons chopped onion
∗1 teaspoon salt	
∗⅛ teaspoon garlic salt	1 teaspoon garlic powder
1 cup cooked rice	1 cup cooked rice
∗1 can (15 ounces) tomato sauce	2 cups fresh tomato sauce
	½ teaspoon freshly ground pepper

Heat oven to 350°. Cut thin slice from stem end of each pepper. Remove all seeds and membrane. Wash inside and outside. Cook peppers in the boiling salted water 5 minutes; drain.

Cook and stir ground beef and onion in medium skillet until onion is tender. Drain off fat. Stir in remaining ingredients, reserving 1 cup of the tomato sauce; heat through.

Lightly stuff each pepper with ½ cup meat mixture. Stand peppers upright in ungreased baking dish, 8x8x2 inches. Pour remaining tomato sauce over peppers. Cover; bake 45 minutes. Uncover and bake 15 minutes longer.

MEATBALLS

Original	Healthier Version
* 1½ pounds ground beef	1½ pounds *extra lean* ground beef
1 medium onion, chopped (about ½ cup)	1 medium onion, chopped (about ½ cup)
* ¾ cup dry bread crumbs	¾ cup dry *whole-wheat* bread crumbs
1 tablespoon snipped parsley	1 tablespoon snipped parsley
* 1½ teaspoons salt	*¾ teaspoon salt*
⅛ teaspoon pepper	*½ teaspoon pepper, freshly ground*
* 1 teaspoon Worcestershire sauce	*1 teaspoon dry mustard*
* 1 egg	*⅓ cup egg substitute*
* ½ cup milk	½ cup *skim* milk
* ¼ cup salad oil	¼ cup *polyunsaturated vegetable* oil

Mix all ingredients except salad oil. Shape by rounded tablespoonsful into balls. In large skillet, cook meatballs in oil about 20 minutes. *Drain well on paper towels.*

CHICKEN AND RICE CASSEROLE

Original	Healthier Version
* ¼ cup chicken fat or butter	¼ cup *unsalted margarine*
⅓ cup flour	⅓ cup flour
	¼ cup chopped onion
* 1½ teaspoons salt	*¾ teaspoon salt*
* ⅛ teaspoon pepper	*½ teaspoon freshly ground* pepper
1 cup chicken broth	1 cup chicken broth
* 1½ cups milk	1½ cups *skim* milk
1½ cups cooked white or wild rice	1½ cups cooked white or wild rice
2 cups cut-up cooked chicken	2 cups cut-up cooked chicken
* 1 can (3 ounces) sliced mushrooms, drained	*3 ounces fresh mushrooms, sliced*
⅓ cup chopped green pepper	⅓ cup chopped green pepper
* 2 tablespoons chopped pimento	2 tablespoons chopped *red pepper*
¼ cup slivered almonds	¼ cup slivered almonds
Snipped parsley	Snipped parsley

Heat oven to 350°. Melt *margarine* in large saucepan over low heat. *Cook and stir onion until soft.* Blend in flour, salt, and pepper. Cook over low heat, stirring until mixture is smooth and bubbly. Remove from heat. Stir in broth and milk. Heat to boiling, stirring constantly. Boil and stir 1 minute. Stir in remaining ingredients.

Pour into ungreased baking dish, 10x6x1½ inches, or 1½ quart casserole. Bake uncovered 40 to 45 minutes. Sprinkle with snipped parsley.

A FEW REMINDERS

Cooking for a healthy heart does not have to be difficult. There are many foods that can be eaten in moderation: chicken and turkey, fin fish, lean cuts of meat, most breads, pasta, and grains, and fresh fruits and vegetables. In the beginning, you may need to consult a list, but in a few weeks you will find yourself automatically avoiding certain foods and selecting others. If you are the cook, your family probably will not notice the difference, and everyone, from the youngest to the oldest, will have a much better chance of controlling the risk factors for heart disease.

Remember to:

- Think slim! Calories do count.
- Cut down on high cholesterol foods, such as egg yolks, organ meat, and shrimp.
- Avoid high-fat cuts of meat, and switch to low-fat or nonfat milk and milk products.
- Substitute a soft margarine (one that lists liquid oil as its first ingredient) for butter; substitute vegetable oils for suet or lard.
- Use fruit ice or frozen low-fat yogurt instead of ice cream.
- Cut down on excessive quantities of sodium and avoid the salt shaker whenever possible.
- Add some fiber to your diet.
- Substitute complex carbohydrates for excess fat and sugar.
- Take a behavior-modification approach to eating. Make small, gradual changes that you can easily incorporate into your lifestyle.

We cannot say that these dietary modifications will prevent you from ever having a heart attack, but they should reduce your cardiovascular risk, and they will provide a basis for a sensible, healthful diet. And there is no question that good nutrition will help you establish the kind of lifestyle that can carry you through a long, full life.

5 Using the Food Groups to Plan Your Meals

TO FACILITATE your meal planning while assuring a balanced nutritional intake, we have broken down the Basic Four Food Groups into seven categories. The division of the four groups into seven permits you to calculate your cholesterol, fat, and caloric intake more accurately.

THE BASIC FOOD GROUPS

Basic Four Food Groups	Seven Food Groups
Meat	Lean meat and meat substitutes
Dairy	Low-fat dairy products
Grain	Breads, cereals, and starchy vegetables
Fruits and vegetables	Vegetables
	Fruits
Extras	Fats
	Caloric Supplements

In the charts that appear within each food group, serving sizes have been calculated so that, unless otherwise specified, all the foods listed in that group contain *approximately* the same number of calories and similar amounts of vitamins and minerals. (The amount of cholesterol and fat is also included.) Therefore, the foods included in each group, except the caloric supplements, are basically interchangeable. For example:

> *Meat:* 1 serving equals 3 ounces fish *or* 3 ounces of beef.

Breads: 1 serving equals 1 slice of bread *or* 1 small potato.
Vegetables: 1 serving equals ½ cup green beans *or* 1 cup of lettuce.
Fruit: 1 serving equals ½ cup orange juice *or* ½ medium grapefruit.
Fats: 1 serving equals 1 teaspoon polyunsaturated margarine *or* 1 teaspoon polyunsaturated cooking oil.

With this system, it is easy to create interesting, varied menus that incorporate all the necessary nutrients. It also makes the size of the serving as important as the kind of food you choose when you are calculating your nutrient intake. Be sure to check the serving size listed next to each item in a food group and at the bottom of every recipe.

No one category can supply all the nutrients needed for a well-balanced diet. As illustrated in Table 6, page 24, foods contribute different nutrients to an efficiently functioning body, and it takes a variety of foods working together to supply the nutritional needs for good health. A balanced diet will contain vegetables and fruit, breads and cereals, some dairy products, and poultry, fish, meat, or an equivalent protein source.

If you do not find some of your favorite foods listed here, it is because they contain excessive saturated fat, cholesterol, calories, or sodium. So, in some instances, you have to make minor adjustments by omitting them. To counterbalance these small sacrifices, remember that you are adopting a lifestyle to lessen the risk of developing cardiovascular disease, and that it may help you to live a longer, more enjoyable life. If you wish to use a food or recipe that is not listed, consult *How to Calculate the Nutritive Value of Other Recipes* (page 266) for its nutrient content or one of the publications listed at the back of this book.

All of this does not mean that you have to give up all the good things in life or live a life devoid of good foods and good cheer. Although some changes may be necessary, they can be relatively painless. The advice and recipes given in this book are intended to help you gradually make some of the necessary changes in your lifestyle. Your dedication to heart health should not be hit or miss, but should involve a commitment to a long, full life.

LEAN MEAT AND MEAT SUBSTITUTES

Meat, poultry, fish, and eggs are important sources of protein, iron, vitamin B_{12}, and other B-complex vitamins. Lean beef, crab, liver, peanut butter, oysters, and the dark meat of turkey are primary sources of zinc. Be certain to select the leanest cuts of meat, and trim off all visible fat, and remove the skin from poultry. Measure meat after it has been cooked. A three-ounce serving of cooked meat is equal to approximately four ounces of raw meat. If meat is prepared with fat, omit the equivalent number of fat servings.

Note: **Each serving is equivalent to 3 ounces (90 gm) of meat and contains approximately 200 calories.**

Food	Serving	Cholesterol (mg)	Fat (gm)
Beans, dried, cooked	¾ cup	0	0.5
Beef, lean	3 ounces	82	5.5
Egg substitutes (approximately 60 calories)	3 tablespoons	check labels	
Egg white (50 calories)	2	0	0
Fish			
Any fresh or frozen fin fish	3 ounces	60	3.6
Canned, water-packed	3 ounces	57	0.7
Clams, fresh	3 ounces	56	2.2
Crab, fresh, cooked	3 ounces	90	2.2
Lobster, fresh, cooked	3 ounces	76	1.4
Oysters, fresh	3 ounces	40	2.0
Scallops, fresh	3 ounces	47	1.2
Lamb, lean	3 ounces	90	6.3
Lentils, dried, cooked	¾ cup	0	0.3
Peanut butter (omit 1 fat serving)	2 tablespoons	0	15.1
Peas, dried, cooked	¾ cup	0	0.3
Pork, lean	3 ounces	79	9.0

LEAN MEAT AND MEAT SUBSTITUTES–Continued

Food	Serving	Cholesterol (mg)	Fat (gm)
Poultry: capon, chicken, guinea hen, pheasant, rock cornish hen, turkey	3 ounces	86	5.6
Veal, lean	3 ounces	89	6.0
Serve no more than twice a week			
Eggs, fresh, whole (75 calories)	1 egg	252	5.7
Frankfurters	2 ounces	37	16.3
Lunch meats	3 ounces	55	16.6
Sausage	2 ounces	53	27.0
Serve no more than once a month			
Heart	3 ounces	247	5.1
Kidney	3 ounces	723	10.8
Liver	3 ounces	394	3.4
Shrimp	3 ounces (½ cup or 8–10 small cooked shrimp)	130	1.0
Sweetbreads	3 ounces	419	20.8

Avoid: If you are controlling sodium intake, avoid canned, salt-cured, kosher, and commercially prepared meats such as frankfurters and lunch meats.

LOW-FAT DAIRY PRODUCTS

Milk is the leading source of calcium and a good source of phosphorus, protein, vitamins A and D, and some of the B-complex vitamins, including folic acid and vitamin B_{12}. Magnesium is also found in milk. Choose nonfat milk products and avoid cream. Use a nondairy creamer made without coconut oil, palm oil, or an unspecified vegetable oil. Except for special occasions, use low-fat cheeses.

> *Note:* **Each serving is equivalent to 1 cup of skim milk and contains approximately 7 mg cholesterol and 70 calories.**

Food	Serving	Fat (gm)
Buttermilk, cultured, fresh, skim milk, or less than 1% fat content	1 cup	2.4
Cheese		
low-fat (made with skim milk)	1 ounce	1.8
cottage cheese, uncreamed	¼ cup	0.1

LOW-FAT DAIRY PRODUCTS—Continued

Food	Serving	Fat (gm)
Cheese–continued		
cream cheese, low-calorie imitation	1 teaspoon	0.6
Farmer, skim milk	1 ounce	1.2
Mozzarella (part skim)	1 ounce	5.0
Parmesan	1 ounce (30 mg cholesterol)	9.6
Pot cheese	1 ounce	1.2
Ricotta (part skim)	1 ounce	2.5
1% milk	¾ cup	1.8
2% milk	½ cup	2.4
Skim milk	1 cup	0.2
Skim milk, evaporated, dry	2 tablespoons	0.2
Skim milk, nonfat dry	2 tablespoons	0.1
Yogurt, low-fat, plain	½ cup	2.0

Avoid: Cream, whole-milk products, cheese, ice cream, "cream" soups, and nondairy creamers made with coconut or palm oil.

BREAD, CEREALS, AND STARCHY VEGETABLES

Whole-grain or enriched breads and cereals are good sources of iron and some of the B vitamins, as are dried beans and peas and the other vegetables on this list. In addition, they are excellent sources of fiber. Magnesium is found in cooked dried beans and whole grain cereals, and dried beans, peas, and lentils are sources of zinc. When making breads, cakes, or pancakes, use soft margarine or polyunsaturated vegetable oils as shortening and an egg substitute or egg whites instead of whole eggs.

> *Note:* **Each serving is equivalent to 1 slice of bread and contains approximately 0.1 mg cholesterol, 0.5 gm fat, and 70 calories.**

Food	Serving
Angel food cake	1 slice
Bread crumbs, dry	¼ cup
Bread	
corn	1½ inch square
French	1 slice
Italian	1 slice
raisin	1 slice
white	1 slice
whole wheat	1 slice

BREAD, CEREALS, AND STARCHY VEGETABLES–Continued

Food	Serving
Buns, hamburger	1 small bun or ½ large bun
Corn	
grits, cooked	½ cup
meal, dry	2 tablespoons
Cereal	
bran flakes	½ cup
cooked, unsweetened	½ cup
corn flakes	½ cup
oats, puffed	¾ cup
rice, puffed	¾ cup
wheat flakes	½ cup
wheat, puffed	¾ cup
Crackers	
graham	2
soda	2
Flour	2½ tablespoons
Grains: rice, oats, barley	
raw	½ cup
cooked	⅓ cup
Muffins	
plain	1 small
English	½ muffin
Pasta and noodles	
dry	⅓ cup
cooked	½ cup
Popcorn, plain	1 cup
Roll, plain	1 large
Tortilla	1
Vegetables	
beans, dried, cooked	¼ cup
corn	⅓ cup
corn on the cob	1 small
grits, cooked	½ cup
lima	⅓ cup
lentils, dried, cooked	¼ cup
mixed vegetables	½ cup
parsnips, cooked	½ cup
peas, green	½ cup
peas, dried, cooked	¼ cup

BREAD, CEREALS, AND STARCHY VEGETABLES–Continued

Food	Serving
Vegetables–continued	
potatoes	
baked	1 small
pared, boiled	½ cup
french fried	5 strips
(omit 1 fat serving)	
pumpkin, canned	¾ cup
squash, winter, baked	½ cup
sweet potatoes, baked	¼ cup
canned	⅓ cup
Wheat germ	2 tablespoons

Avoid: Pastries made with butter and saturated fats. If you are counting calories, avoid sugar-coated cereals, snack foods, and desserts. If you want to reduce sodium intake, avoid salted crackers and all dry, ready-to-eat cereals except shredded wheat and puffed wheat, rice, and oats.

VEGETABLES

Dark green and deep yellow vegetables are leading sources of vitamin A. Vegetables containing vitamin C include asparagus, broccoli, brussels sprouts, cauliflower, cabbage, green peppers, greens, and tomatoes. Green leafy vegetables contain folic acid, and broccoli, cabbage, carrots, spinach, and tomatoes are good sources of vitamin B_6. Brussels sprouts, greens, tomatoes, and broccoli contain potassium. Spinach is a source of zinc, and magnesium is found in green beans, broccoli, and tomatoes. Vegetables are also good sources of fiber. Serve vegetables cooked or raw. If fat is added in preparation, omit the equivalent number of fat exchanges.

> **Note: Each serving is equivalent to ½ cup beans and contains approximately 0 mg cholesterol, 0.1 gm fat, and 20 calories. Starchy vegetables are contained in the Bread group.**

Food	Serving	Food	Serving
Artichokes, fresh or		Brussels sprouts	½ cup
water-packed	½ cup	Cabbage	½ cup
Asparagus	½ cup	Cabbage, Chinese	1 cup
Beans, snap	½ cup	Carrots	½ cup
Bean sprouts	½ cup	Cauliflower	½ cup
Beets	½ cup	Celery	½ cup
Broccoli	½ cup	Chard	½ cup

VEGETABLES–Continued

Food	Serving	Food	Serving
Chicory, raw	1 cup	Okra	½ cup
Cucumbers	1 cup	Onion	½ cup
Eggplant	½ cup	Parsley	½ cup
Endive, raw	1 cup	Rhubarb	1 cup
Escarole	1 cup	Romaine	1 cup
Green peppers	½ cup	Rutabaga	½ cup
Greens		Spinach	½ cup
beet	½ cup	Summer squash	¾ cup
collard	½ cup	Tomato juice	½ cup
dandelion	½ cup	Tomatoes	½ cup
mustard	½ cup	Turnips	½ cup
turnip	½ cup	Vegetable juice cocktail	1 cup
Kohlrabi, raw	½ cup	Watercress	1 cup
Lettuce	1 cup	Zucchini	1 cup
Mushrooms	½ cup		

Avoid: Vegetables in butter or cream sauce or deep-fat fried, and canned vegetables if you want to lower sodium intake.

FRUITS

Fruits are valuable for vitamins, minerals, and fiber. Oranges, tangerines, grapefruit, strawberries, cantaloupe, and honeydew melons are good sources of vitamin C. Apricots and peaches contain vitamin A. Mangoes and papayas contain both vitamin A and vitamin C. Bananas, nectarines, oranges, plums, and dried fruits are sources of potassium. Cantaloupe, oranges, and strawberries contain folic acid. Magnesium and vitamin B_6 are found in bananas.

Unless otherwise specified, the calories indicated for this group are for fresh and water-packed canned or frozen fruit. If you use sweetened fruit, add the appropriate number of calories.

> *Note:* **Each serving is equivalent to ½ cup orange juice and contains approximately 0 mg cholesterol, 0.2 gm fat, and 50 calories.**

Food	Serving	Food	Serving
Apple	1 small	Berries	
Apple juice	⅓ cup	blackberries	½ cup
Applesauce, unsweetened	½ cup	blueberries, fresh	½ cup
Apricots, dried	4 halves	raspberries, fresh	½ cup
Apricots, raw	2 medium	strawberries, fresh	¾ cup
Banana	½ small	Cherries, fresh	10

FRUITS—Continued

Food	Serving	Food	Serving
Cranberries	½ cup	Orange	1 small
Dates	2	Orange juice	½ cup
Figs		Papaya	½ medium
dried	2 small	Peach	1 medium
fresh	1 large	Pear	1 small
Grapefruit	½ medium	Persimmon	½ medium
Grapefruit juice	½ cup	Pineapple	½ cup
Grape juice	¼ cup	Pineapple juice	⅓ cup
Grapes, fresh	12	Plums	1 medium
Mango	½ small	Prune juice	¼ cup
Melon		Prunes	2 medium
cantaloupe	¼ small	Raisins	2 tablespoons
honeydew	⅛ medium	Rhubarb, raw	1½ cups
watermelon	1 cup	Tangerine	1 medium
Nectarine	1 medium		

Avoid: Fruit canned or frozen in syrup if you are counting calories.

FATS

Since most fats are high in calories, cholesterol, and saturated fat, foods on this list should be measured carefully to control weight and fat intake. Select margarine that lists a polyunsaturated vegetable oil as the first ingredient.

> *Note:* **Each serving is equivalent to 1 teaspoon vegetable oil and contains approximately 45 calories.**

Food	Serving	Cholesterol (mg)	Fat (gm)
Almonds	8 whole	0	4
Avocado (4 inches in diameter)	⅛	0	4
Bacon, Canadian	½ ounce	12	2.4
Margarine	1 teaspoon	0	4
Mayonnaise			
regular	1 teaspoon	10	11
low fat	1 teaspoon	3	4
imitation	1 teaspoon	2	2
Nuts, other	3 small	0	4
Oil: corn, cottonseed, safflower, soy, soybean, sunflower	1 teaspoon	0	5

FATS—Continued

Food	Serving	Cholesterol (mg)	Fat (gm)
Oil, olive	1 teaspoon	0	5
Oil, peanut	1 teaspoon	0	5
Peanuts			
Spanish	10 whole	0	3
Virginia	5 whole	0	3
Pecans	2 large whole	0	4
Salad dressing, mayonnaise type	2 teaspoons	3	2
Walnuts	3 small	0	6

Avoid: Butter; coconut, palm, and macadamia nut oils; fully hydrogenated vegetable fats; unspecified vegetable oils; lard; nondairy products such as whipped toppings and creamers which are made with saturated oils; and coconut and macadamia nuts.

CALORIC SUPPLEMENTS (including Beverages)

The foods and beverages below contain only trace amounts of cholesterol and fat. Calculate each of these items into your daily intake if you are controlling your caloric intake.

Food	Serving	Calories
Alcohol		
80 proof	1½ ounces	105
86 proof	1½ ounces	115
90 proof	1½ ounces	120
94 proof	1½ ounces	125
100 proof	1½ ounces	130
Beer, 3.6	12 ounces	150
Cola	1 cup	95
Fruit ice	½ cup	75
Fruit-flavored sodas	1 cup	110
Gelatin, unflavored	1 envelope	25
Ginger ale	1 cup	75
Hard candy	1 piece	20
Honey	1 teaspoon	20
Jam	1 tablespoon	40
Jello, flavored	½ cup	80
Jelly	1 tablespoon	40
Kool-aid	1 cup	90
Molasses, cane, medium	2 tablespoons	80
Popsicle	1 twin bar	95

CALORIC SUPPLEMENTS–Continued

Food	Serving	Calories
Root beer	1 cup	100
Sugar	1 teaspoon	20
Syrup		
cane	2 tablespoons	90
corn	2 tablespoons	100
maple	2 tablespoons	90
Wine		
dessert	6 ounces	245
table	6 ounces	150

Miscellaneous Foods

The following foods have negligible amounts of calories. However, if you want to control your sodium intake, avoid the foods marked with an asterisk (∗), which are high in sodium.

Beverages: Coffee and tea
Soups: Boullion∗ and clear broths∗
Condiments: Salt∗, pepper, spices, herbs, flavoring extracts, catsup∗, horseradish, mustard∗, pickles∗, meat sauces∗, vinegar, and lemon juice.

Avoid: Any food of unknown composition, as well as chocolate, potato chips, and shaped snacks.

SAMPLE MENUS, 1,000 CALORIES

These sample menus were compiled to show the typical selection of recipes and foods from the seven food groups. Planned for a daily calorie allowance of 1,000 and 1,500 calories (see next section), they provide a balanced, varied, and appetizing meal plan that should not be difficult to follow. Recipes for menu items beginning with capital letters are given in this book (see recipe index).

MENU I

Breakfast
½ grapefruit
½ cup cornflakes
¼ cup skim milk
1 slice whole-wheat toast
1 teaspoon margarine
coffee

Lunch
Sandwich
    2 slices rye bread
    lettuce, tomato
    2 ounces sliced turkey
    ½ teaspoon mayonnaise
1 apple
tea

Dinner
1 serving Chicken and Beef Kebabs
½ cup rice
1 serving Dilled Zucchini
½ cup tossed green salad
1 teaspoon Oil and Vinegar Dressing
1 slice Angel Food Cake
coffee or tea

MENU II

Breakfast
½ cup orange juice
1 serving Mushroom Omelet
1 slice whole-wheat toast
1 teaspoon margarine
coffee

Lunch
1 serving Chicken Salad Plate
1 whole-wheat roll
1 serving Fruit Whip
Iced tea, lemon

Dinner
1 serving Savoy Beef Stew
1 serving Citrus Slaw
1 cup chilled melon balls
coffee or tea

MENU III

Breakfast
1 slice honeydew melon
1 serving Scrambled Egg (egg substitute)
1 slice whole-wheat toast
1 teaspoon margarine
coffee

Lunch
2 ounces lean broiled hamburger
1 hamburger bun
¾ cup sliced tomato and lettuce salad
2 teaspoons Oil and Vinegar Dressing
Iced tea, lemon

Dinner
1 serving Fish Fillets
½ cup green beans
1 serving Creamy Garden Relish
1 serving Apple Snow
coffee or Sanka

SAMPLE MENUS, 1,500 CALORIES

MENU I

Breakfast
½ banana
½ cup cream of wheat
1 cup skim milk
1 teaspoon sugar
2 Doughnut Balls
coffee

Lunch
Sandwich
  2 slices whole-wheat bread
  1 serving Egg Salad
  lettuce
1 serving All American Apple Pie
Iced tea

Dinner
1 serving Rosemary Chicken
1 serving Ratatouille
1 serving Broccoli Vinaigrette
1 serving Cafe Diable Mold
coffee or tea

MENU II

Breakfast
1 cup orange juice
1 serving Omelet
2 slices rye toast
2 teaspoons margarine
2 teaspoons jelly
coffee

Lunch
1 serving Downhome Vegetable Soup
1 serving Hamburger Deluxe
1 serving Green and Red Cabbage Slaw
1 Brownie
Iced or hot tea

Dinner

1 serving Poached Bass
½ cup asparagus
1 serving Grilled Melon
1 lettuce wedge
1 tablespoon French Dressing
coffee or tea

MENU III

Breakfast

1 wedge fresh pineapple
2 slices rye toast with
　　2 ounces low-fat mozzarella cheese
　　melted on top
coffee

Lunch

1 cup vegetable broth
1 serving Citrus Slimmer Salad
2 plain muffins
½ cup skim milk
1 serving Peach Parfait
Iced or hot tea, lemon

Dinner

1 serving Lentil Soup
1 serving Eggplant and Tomato Casserole
1 cup spinach salad
2 teaspoons Oil and Vinegar Dressing
1 serving Banana-Yogurt Cake
coffee or tea

6 Eating Away from Home

THERE is no reason why you cannot eat out, even though you are controlling your food intake or altering your diet. Armed with an awareness of the nutrient content of foods, you can choose foods from almost any menu. If you are counting calories, you may not always be able to eat the whole portion, but be brave, leave some on your plate, and ask for a doggie bag. If it is a special occasion, go easy at breakfast and lunch and save a little extra for dinner. You should not make this a regular practice, but you can follow it for weddings, holidays, anniversaries, birthdays, and other special occasions.

EATING IN RESTAURANTS

If you ask, most restaurants will prepare simple food at your request, such as chicken or fresh fish without a sauce. Order fresh vegetables, but specify that they be cooked without additional fat. Ask for margarine and skim milk. Choose clear soups, avoid fried foods and mixed casserole dishes, and trim fat and skin from poultry and meat. Avoid prepared gravy, sauces, and salad dressings: Instead, ask for oil and vinegar or lemon juice for your salad dressing. Select a baked potato, if it has not been prepared with fat. Have fresh fruit, fresh fruit cocktail, or broth for an appetizer, and fruit ice, angel food cake, or fresh fruit for dessert. Remember to plan ahead so that you save some calories during the day for an extra something that catches your eye. But watch portion sizes on desserts.

Here are some ideas to help you when you are going out to eat or traveling. Remember to keep the portion size in mind.

Breakfast
Fresh fruit or juice
- Melon
- Orange juice
- Grapefruit half
- Sliced banana
- Fruit cup
- Prunes
- Prune juice
- Cranberry juice
- Apricot nectar

Cereal or Bread
- Unsweetened cereal
- Unbuttered toast
- Margarine

Milk
- Skim milk or low-fat yogurt

Egg
- Remember: Only 2 fresh eggs a week. Request an egg substitute, if possible, and ask that your egg be cooked in vegetable oil if you want it fried or scrambled.

Lunch or Supper
Appetizer
- Juice
- Fruit Cocktail
- Grapefruit half or sections
- Melon
- Broth, bouillon, or jellied consommé

Main Dish
- Roast beef

Sliced chicken or turkey sandwich
Small steak
Hamburger, broiled
Yogurt
Fruit salad
Chef's salad with chicken, turkey, beef
(no cheese)
Salad or Vegetable
Lettuce and tomato
Tossed green
Sliced tomato
Hearts of lettuce
Oil and vinegar dressing or lemon juice
Cooked vegetable without butter or
cream sauce
Dessert
Fresh fruit
Fruit compote
Fruit ice
Angel food cake

Dinner

Appetizer
Juice
Fresh fruit cup
Melon
Grapefruit half or sections
Broth, bouillon, or jellied consommé
Entree
Turkey
Veal
Steak
Center-cut roast
Lamb
Fresh fish

Watch the portion size, and specify that meat be cooked without extra fat. Avoid casseroles, fried foods, and foods cooked in sauces, and trim the fat from meat and the skin from poultry.

Potato or Pasta
Order baked potato; most others are cooked with extra fat. Check portion size on pasta, and avoid cream or cheese sauces.
Salad or Vegetable
Lettuce and tomato
Tossed green
Sliced tomato
Hearts of lettuce
Fruit salad
Oil and vinegar dressing or lemon juice
Cooked vegetable without butter or cream sauce
Bread
French
Italian
Avoid egg breads
Dessert
Stewed fruit
Fruit ice
Fresh fruit
Fruit cup
Baked apple
Fruit compote
Angel food cake
Beverage
Coffee, tea, Sanka, fruit juice

In this diet-conscious age, restaurants are accustomed to requests for special dietary items, so do not be reluctant to ask for them. Even some fast-food restaurants will prepare french fries and hamburgers without extra fat or salt. You probably are not the first to make such a request, so do not be shy about asking for broiled items, foods without sauces, or smaller portions. After all, it is the nouvelle cuisine. Most restaurants will be happy to accommodate you, and if you frequent a particular restaurant, most likely they will be glad to stock such things as margarine, salad dressings, or fruit ice for you.

In many Chinese and Japanese restaurants, you can order your food prepared without monosodium glutamate, although it is a primary seasoning in Oriental cooking. Avoid shrimp and egg dishes. Italian restaurants pose no problem: veal, fish, chicken, and pasta dishes abound. Just avoid cream sauces and watch portion sizes. French restaurants are known for their sauces, but simpler types of foods are available. Order foods without sauces, and stay away from high-calorie pastries.

EATING AT THE HOME OF A FRIEND

Being invited to dinner at the home of a friend need not pose a problem if you tell your hostess in advance that you are watching your diet. This will save embarrassment for you and for her because she can plan the menu accord-ingly. It will also alleviate the problem of being urged to eat "just a little more," and she will understand if you ask for small portions or pass up dessert. Think ahead: Eat less during the day and save some calories for dinner.

There is no reason to feel ill at ease about being on a controlled dietary regime. In fact, most people will be happy to help you.

EATING ON AIRPLANES

Most airlines offer a variety of meals to meet special medical, religious, or other dietary spec-ifications. All they ask is that you notify their reservations personnel at least twenty-four hours in advance of your flight so that proper preparation can be made. Low-fat, low-cholesterol, or calorie-controlled meals are routinely offered. Just remind the flight atten-dant or the gate agent upon check-in that you have ordered a special meal.

7 Nutrition Labeling: What It Means to You

TODAY, most of us no longer get our food directly from the farm. Nor are we content to eat the plain mealtime fare that was consumed by our forebears. Modern advances in food technology, storage techniques, and rapid transportation have enabled us to choose from a vast variety of both fresh and packaged foods. However, as prepared foods and recipes become increasingly complex, it becomes harder to know how to fit them into the basic four groups. And it becomes more and more difficult to assess the nutrient content of the food we consume.

To help identify nutrients in the foods we buy, the Food and Drug Administration has formulated a new labeling program. It requires a nutrition label on all foods that have nutrients added or that make a special nutritional claim. The regulations are optional for most foods now, but many companies are voluntarily labeling their products in an effort to help consumers. Nutrition labeling is an important tool that can help you ensure nutritious meals for you and your family by enabling you to select or reject and to control your intake of specific nutrients, such as cholesterol, fat, calories, or sodium.

When you shop, buy brands with a label whenever possible so that you can examine the nutrient composition of the foods you serve. The label assures that the manufacturer has certified the levels of nutrients listed. As you become more familiar with the terminology, and as more brands are labeled, nutrition labeling will become indispensable in your menu planning.

Nutritional information as it appears on most labels is illustrated in Figure 7. The upper portion of the label states the serving size and the number of calories per serving and lists, in grams, the amount of protein, carbohydrate, and fat, the three major nutrients in food. The lower portion of the label gives the percentage per serving of the United States Recommended Daily Allowances (U.S. RDA) for protein and the seven key vitamins and minerals: vitamin A, vitamin C, thiamin, riboflavin, niacin, calcium, and iron. Values have also been established for twelve other vitamins and minerals, and these may be included on the nutrition label if they are present in significant amounts. They are folic acid, phosphorus, iodine, magnesium, zinc, copper, biotin, pantothenic acid, and vitamins D, E, B_6, and B_{12}.

Keep track of your daily intake of each nutrient and add up the percentages you consume throughout the day. When the daily total approaches 100, you are getting an ample supply of that nutrient. Table 9 gives the U.S. RDA for specific nutrients.

WHAT ARE THE U.S. RDAs?

The U.S. RDAs have been established by the Food and Drug Administration to replace the outdated MDR (Minimum Daily Requirement), which used to appear on some labels. The U.S. RDA values are guidelines for the quantities of protein, vitamins, and minerals needed each

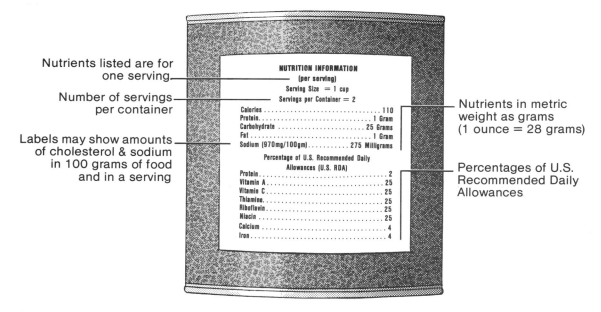

Nutrients listed are for one serving

Number of servings per container

Labels may show amounts of cholesterol & sodium in 100 grams of food and in a serving

Nutrients in metric weight as grams (1 ounce = 28 grams)

Percentages of U.S. Recommended Daily Allowances

NUTRITION INFORMATION
(per serving)
Serving Size = 1 cup
Servings per Container = 2

Calories 110
Protein............................... 1 Gram
Carbohydrate .... 25 Grams
Fat .... 1 Gram
Sodium (970mg/100gm).......... 275 Milligrams

Percentage of U.S. Recommended Daily
Allowances (U.S. RDA)
Protein................................... 2
Vitamin A............................... 25
Vitamin C............................... 25
Thiamine................................ 25
Riboflavin.............................. 25
Niacin 25
Calcium 4
Iron 4

Figure 7. Nutrition labels list amounts of nutrients and U.S. RDAs per serving.

day for growth, development, and health, based on body needs for most healthy adults. Set at general levels, they provide a considerable margin of safety, above actual body needs for most people.

Obviously, recommended daily allowances are not the same for every individual. The requirements for teenagers and pregnant or lactating women are higher than those for the general population. Certain other factors, such as age, activity levels, and physical health, can also influence nutrient needs.

Nutrition labels list U.S. RDA *by percentage* per serving. For example, if the label reads "Vitamin A . . . 10," one serving contains 10% of the U.S. RDA for vitamin A.

The U.S. RDAs on the label indicate what that product contributes to your diet. Because of space availability, not all essential nutrients are listed. The standard format requires only the U.S. RDA listing for protein, five vitamins,

and two minerals. However, approximately twenty to thirty micronutrients are needed to support good health. The seven chosen by the FDA to be included on the label are considered "indicator" nutrients, and they are the ones we know most about. In most instances, if you are getting 100% of these seven indicator nutrients, you are probably getting a sufficient amount of the other micronutrients.

LEARN TO READ LABELS

Starting at the top of the label, the first item shown is the individual serving size. This figure is very important because all the other information on the label is based on it. The serving size for the same food can differ from product to product, and it may vary greatly from what *you* consider a correct size. So look at this measurement carefully.

Listed next is the number of servings in the container, followed by the number of calo-

Table 9.
U.S. Recommended Daily Allowances
(U.S. RDA)

For adults and children over 4 years old

Nutrients	Amounts
Protein	45 or 65 grams*
Vitamin A	5,000 International Units
Vitamin C (ascorbic acid)	60 milligrams
Thiamine (vitamin B_1)	1.5 milligrams
Riboflavin (vitamin B_2)	1.7 milligrams
Niacin	20 milligrams
Calcium	1.0 gram
Iron	18 milligrams
Vitamin D	400 International Units
Vitamin E	30 International Units
Vitamin B_6	2.0 milligrams
Folic acid (folacin)	0.4 milligram
Vitamin B_{12}	6 micrograms
Phosphorus	1.0 gram
Iodine	150 micrograms
Magnesium	400 milligrams
Zinc	15 milligrams
Copper	2 milligrams
Biotin	0.3 milligram
Pantothenic acid	10 milligrams

* 45 grams if protein quality is equal to or greater than milk protein; 65 grams if protein quality is less than milk protein.

ries per serving and then the grams per serving of protein, carbohydrate, and fat. This information can help you see where your calories are coming from. Multiply the grams indicated per serving by the number of calories per gram of protein, fat, and carbohydrate to find out the number of calories contributed by each nutrient.

For example, using the information in Figure 7:

Nutrients	Grams per serving		Calories per gram		Total calories
Protein	1	×	4	=	4
Carbohydrate	25	×	4	=	100
Fat	1	×	9	=	9

This section of the label can also give op-

tional information about the type and amount of fat and the amount of cholesterol and sodium (see Figure 8). The FDA regulations allow only two kinds of fat to be listed: polyunsaturated and saturated. To calculate the amount of monounsaturated fat, add the polyunsaturated and saturated fat figures and subtract this sum from the figure given for the amount of total fat. The amounts of cholesterol and sodium are given in milligrams per serving and milligrams per 100 grams.

The lower portion of the label gives the percentage of the U.S. RDA for protein, five vitamins, and two minerals. It is important to note

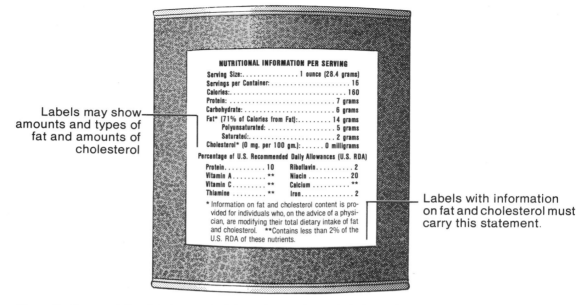

Labels may show amounts and types of fat and amounts of cholesterol

NUTRITIONAL INFORMATION PER SERVING

Serving Size:.............. 1 ounce (28.4 grams)
Servings per Container:..................... 16
Calories:.............................. 160
Protein:........................... 7 grams
Carbohydrate:...................... 6 grams
Fat* (71% of Calories from Fat):........ 14 grams
   Polyunsaturated:.................. 5 grams
   Saturated:...................... 2 grams
Cholesterol* (0 mg. per 100 gm.):...... 0 milligrams

Percentage of U.S. Recommended Daily Allowances (U.S. RDA)

Protein...........10	Riboflavin..........2
Vitamin A..........**	Niacin...........20
Vitamin C..........**	Calcium..........**
Thiamine.........**	Iron..............2

* Information on fat and cholesterol content is provided for individuals who, on the advice of a physician, are modifying their total dietary intake of fat and cholesterol. **Contains less than 2% of the U.S. RDA of these nutrients.

Labels with information on fat and cholesterol must carry this statement.

Figure 8. Some nutrition labels contain information on fat and cholesterol.

the differences in the protein information: The top part of the label notes the actual *amount* of protein per serving, in *grams,* whereas the bottom notes the *quality* of the protein, expressed as the *percentage* of the U.S. RDA. This is the percentage of protein that can be used by the body efficiently to meet its needs.

Information on the other vitamins and minerals that have U.S. RDA values may also appear on the lower portion of the label, if the manufacturers voluntarily choose to include it.

THE INGREDIENT LIST

Another important part of a label is the ingredient list, which is simply a statement of what is in a particular product. The FDA requires that most ingredients be listed by their common name. The ingredients are listed in descending order by weight. This means that the ingredient that makes up the largest part of the product will be listed first, and so on down to the ingredient that makes up the smallest part.

In addition to food items, the ingredient list includes additives such as flavorings or colorings, which are often unfamiliar to the consumer. Table 10 lists the types of additives you might find on a label and gives the purposes and examples of each. Table 11 lists the function of some additives that are used in many convenience foods.

In two cases, you may not find an ingredient list. The first is when the whole product is just one ingredient. The second involves a *standard of identity.* The FDA has defined standards of identity for some common, familiar foods, such as macaroni, noodle products, cheeses, or canned fruits, and a listing of ingredients is not required for them. But in both these special cases, the manufacturer must state any ingredients he has added to the basic product.

The label can be an effective starting point to help you learn about the food you eat. Used correctly, it can help you to achieve a balanced nutritional intake. And it can provide you with information about calories and fat content of foods. See *Selected Sources of Information* for booklets you can obtain for more information on nutrition labeling.

Recently, some supermarkets have initiated color-coded labeling systems to assist their shoppers who need to follow controlled diets. Red, yellow, and green are used to indicate low-sodium, low-calorie, and low-fat products. Stores using this system have instructions to help you find the appropriate products.

Table 10.
Types of Food Additives

Type	Purpose	Examples	Foods in which Additives are Used
Nutrient supplements	To improve the nutritive value.	Potassium iodide, ascorbic acid, niacin, riboflavin, iron, vitamins A and D.	Iodized salt, fortified cereal, milk, margarine, enriched flour, breads, macaroni, noodle products.
Preservatives and antioxidants	To prevent mold growth, darkening of color; to keep fats from becoming rancid.	Calcium propionate.	Bread.
		Sulfur dioxide or sodium sulfite.	Dried fruits, vegetables, wine.
		BHT (butylated hydroxytoluene), BHA (butylated hydroxyanisole).	Lard and shortening, dessert mixes, beverages, dehydrated potatoes, baked goods, sausage.
Emulsifiers, stabilizers, and thinners	To keep water and oil portions of foods mixed; to improve and maintain a certain texture.	Monoglycerides and diglycerides, lecithin, polysorbate 60, sorbitan monosterate, propylene glycol monoesters.	Canned spaghetti, coffee whiteners, baked goods, shortenings, ice cream, peanut butter, margarine, toppings, cereals, candy.
		Modified food starches, methylcellulose, guar gum, gelatin, sodium alginate, pectin.	Marshmallows, cream cheese, pudding, ice cream, baked goods, soft drinks, toppings, jelly, candy.
Acidulants, buffers, alkalis, and neutralizers	To control acidity and alkalinity; to contribute flavor; to leaven baked goods.	Sodium bicarbonate, cream of tartar (potassium bitartrate), monocalcium phosphate, vinegar, acetic acid.	Baking powder, catsup, baked goods, gelatin desserts.
		Disodium hydrogen phosphate, lactic acid, potassium hydroxide.	Processed cheese, cocoa processed with alkali.

Table 11.
Food Additives and Their Functions

Additive	Functions
BHT (butylated hydroxytoluene) and BHA (butylated hydroxyanisole)	Prevents rancidity in products such as frosting mixes, casserole mixes, snacks, and cereals.
Calcium chloride	Helps ensure better texture and imparts greater tolerance to recipe variations in angel food cake mixes.
Calcium phosphate	Added to salt to prevent it from lumping; mineral supplement.
Cellulose gum	Prevents "weeping" and gives body to products such as frosting mixes.
Citric acid	Adjusts acidity and adds a citrus flavor to products such as cakes and frosting mixes; leavens angel food cake mixes; prevents rancidity in foods such as casserole mixes and snacks.
Cream of tartar	Stiffens egg whites in products such as frosting mixes.
Disodium guanylate and disodium inosinate	Intensify and enhance flavors in foods such as casserole mixes and soups.
Gelatin	Gives body to foods such as frosting mixes and marshmallows.
Guar gum	Aids in moisture retention to provide moist eating quality.
Gum arabic	Aids in uniform distribution of flavor in products such as cake mixes and frosting mixes.
Iron	Mineral supplement in foods such as cereals.
Lactic acid	Accentuates cheese flavors in products such as cheese casserole mixes.
Mono- and diglycerides	Aid in making a uniform mixture of oil and water, which gives good texture to products such as cake mixes; keeps dehydrated mashed potatoes from becoming sticky; prevents cereals from clumping together during processing.
Monosodium glutamate (MSG)	Intensifies and enhances the flavor in foods such as casserole mixes and soups.
Niacinamide (niacin)	Vitamin B supplement in products such as flour and cereals.
Polysorbate 60	Contributes light, creamy texture to products such as frosting mixes.
Potassium sorbate	Inhibits mold growth in ready-to-use products such as frostings.
Propyl gallate	Prevents rancidity in foods.
Propyl glycol monesters	Helps incorporate air during beating and aids in making a uniform mixture of oil and water to give good texture to products such as cake mixes.
Pyridoxine (vitamin B_6)	Vitamin B supplement in foods such as cereals.
Riboflavin (vitamin B_2)	Vitamin B supplement in products such as flour and cereal.
Soda (baking)	Leavens and gives flavor to products such as snacks.
Sodium ascorbate	Vitamin C supplement in foods such as cereals.
Sodium caseinate	Protein supplement; aids in processing ingredients for dry mixes, such as casseroles.
Sodium lauryl sulfate	Makes egg whites easier to whip in products such as angel food cake mixes.
Sodium phosphate	Aids in processing dried cheese for casserole mixes; preserves color in snacks; prevents curdling of milk in foods such as puddings.

Food Additives and Their Functions –Continued

Additive	Functions
Sodium sulfite	Prevents browning of dried vegetables and fruits in products such as snacks, casserole mixes, and cake mixes.
Soy lecithin	Makes a smoother texture in products such as frosting and cake mixes; improves the appearance of a baked cake.
Thiamin mononitrate (vitamin B_1)	Vitamin B supplement in foods such as flour and cereal.
Vitamin A palmitate	Vitamin A supplement in products such as margarine and cereals.
Cyanocobalamin (vitamin B_{12})	Vitamin B supplement in foods such as cereals.
Calciferol (vitamin D)	Vitamin D supplement in milk and other products.
Alpha tocopherol (vitamin E)	Vitamin E supplement in cereals and other products.

8 Using Herbs and Spices

THE SKILLFUL USE of herbs and spices will increase the mealtime pleasure of your whole family and add a new taste dimension to even long-familiar recipes and menus.

Unsalted foods are more tasty if they are flavored with herbs and spices, which you can learn to use as easily as salt and pepper.

The spice and herb chart on page 60 suggests which combinations of herbs go best with particular foods. In cooking with herbs, remember that they should accentuate, not overpower, the flavor of your food. Use them discreetly. If you follow the rules listed below, you should be successful. It is a good rule of thumb to plan just one strongly seasoned dish per meal.

1. Use no more than ¼ teaspoon of dried herbs or ¾ teaspoon of fresh herbs for a dish that serves four. Start with that amount, then increase it to suit your taste.
2. Add herbs during the last hour of cooking to soups and stews that must be cooked a long time.
3. Add herbs before cooking hamburgers, meat loaf, and stuffing.
4. Sprinkle herbs on roasts before cooking, or top with herb-flavored margarine after cooking.
5. Steaks and chops can either be sprinkled with herbs while the meat is cooking or brushed with oil and sprinkled with herbs one hour before cooking.
6. Add herbs to vegetables, sauces, or gravies while they are cooking. If you wish, moisten the herbs first with a small amount of oil and let them stand half an hour, before adding them.
7. Add herbs several hours before serving cold foods, such as tomato juice, salad dressing, and cottage cheese. These foods can be stored in the refrigerator for three or four hours or overnight to enhance their flavor.
8. To bring out the essence of the herbs in your food, put the dried herbs in a tea strainer and dip the strainer into piping hot water for 20 seconds. After draining, add the moistened herbs to your food. (Heat and moisture bring out the fragrance and flavor of dried herbs.)
9. If you do not want bits of herbs in the food, tie the herbs in a small piece of cheesecloth and remove the bag before serving.
10. Combine herbs with margarine to flavor steaks, roasts, or vegetables after cooking.
11. If your diet allows it, marinate meats in a wine and herb mixture before cooking.
12. Crush dried herbs in the palm of your hand before adding them to your food. This hastens the flavor release.
13. When substituting fresh herbs for dried herbs, use three or four times the amount specified.

14. Do not combine too many herbs and spices in one dish, even though many would complement it.

The correct combination of herbs and spices for any food is the one that tastes best to you. Remember that seasoning foods is not a science but an expressive art—and you are the artist. When experimenting with a new herb, crush some of it and let it warm in your hand; then sniff it and taste it. If it is delicate, you can be bold and adventurous. If it is very strong and pungent, be cautious.

DRYING YOUR OWN HERBS

Herbs are easy to grow, whether in a vegetable or flower garden or in pots in an indoor window garden. With little effort, most home-grown herbs can be preserved.

Drying is the most popular method of preserving herbs, and while the flavor changes somewhat in the process, herbs home-dried and properly stored are always superior to their commercial counterparts. Most herbs can be frozen, which preserves their freshness and character even more. Some can be combined with other flavorings—in bouquets garnis or tarragon vinegar, for example—to perk up winter cooking.

To dry herbs, pick them early in the day after the dew has evaporated, when the air is dry. Shake them and check to make sure they are free of garden pests. Do not wash them unless it is absolutely necessary, because any bruising will result in a loss of flavor. If you have to wash them to remove clinging soil or insecticides, dry them thoroughly and carefully.

Tie the herbs in small bunches of 4 to 6 stalks or mix varieties for a bouquet garni (parsley, thyme, and bay leaves are a good combination). Hang the bunches in an airy place to dry or put them in a single layer on a window screen in any shaded, well-ventilated place. This method, like oven-drying, tends to turn the herbs brown, but the damage is only cosmetic. The drying process can take as little as six hours or as long as eighteen hours. The herbs must be totally dry before storing, or they will rot.

Drying herbs in the oven is a less satisfactory method, because it diminishes the flavor and drains the color. If you must prepare them that way, heat the oven to 200° and turn it off. Place herbs on oven racks or on a baking sheet and let the oven cool. Check the herbs for dryness when the oven has cooled and repeat the procedure until they are completely dry. Three or four dryings are usually required.

To test for dryness, put a sprig or two in an airtight container in a warm, bright place for two or three hours. If there is any condensation, the herbs have not dried sufficiently.

Herb leaves can be stripped from the stem or left on it for storage. Do not, however, pulverize the leaves until you are ready to use them. Store them in an airtight container and keep it in a cool, dark place—never over or near the range.

To freeze fresh herbs, rinse, shake, and discard any bruised, damaged leaves. Place in a large saucepan with enough water to cover. Heat to boiling, count to 10, and immediately drain herbs and plunge in iced water. Count to 30, drain and dry thoroughly and carefully with paper towels. Seal in plastic wrap and freeze.

Basil can be preserved by either freezing or drying, but it also lends itself well to another method of freezing, which is especially speedy and convenient. Wipe the basil leaves clean with a damp paper towel, being careful not to bruise them. Brush both sides of the leaves with olive oil and place them in a single row on a length of waxed paper. Fold the paper over the leaves and repeat, finishing with a fold of paper. Make a tight packet, wrap in plastic wrap, and freeze. To use, peel off the number of leaves needed, rewrap the packet, and return the rest to the freezer. Wipe the leaves with a paper towel and add them to the recipe.

Basil can also be refrigerated. Use a large clean, wide-mouthed jar with a screw cap. Pick over the leaves, wipe them, and pack them tightly in the jar. Pour in enough vegetable oil to cover. Seal with plastic wrap, then screw the cap on tightly and refrigerate. Basil leaves and oil can be added until the jar is filled, but make sure that the top leaves are always completely under the oil.

To make a flavorful oil, pour out one cup of oil from a one-pint bottle of vegetable oil and reserve it. To the bottle, add 4 to 5 sprigs of tarragon or 6 to 7 sprigs of thyme that have been rinsed and dried. Pour in reserved oil to cover herbs completely. Recap and let stand at least 24 hours. For tarragon vinegar, substitute white wine vinegar for the oil.

Table 12.
Dictionary of Herbs and Spices

Approximately ⅓ teaspoon ground herbs or 1 teaspoon dried herbs is equal in strength to 1 tablespoon fresh herbs.

Herb or Spice	Form	Flavor	Uses
ALLSPICE	Whole or ground	Blend of cinnamon, nutmeg, and cloves	Spices meat, fish, seafood dishes, soups, juices, fruits, spicy sauces, spinach, turnips, peas, red and yellow vegetables
ANISE	Whole or ground	Aromatic, sweet licorice flavor	Sweet rolls, breads, fruit pies and fillings, sparingly in fruit, stews, shellfish dishes, carrots, beets, cottage cheese
BASIL, sweet	Fresh, whole or ground	Aromatic, mild mint-licorice flavor	Meat, fish, seafood dishes, eggs, soups, stews, sauces, salads, tomato dishes, most vegetables, fruit compotes
BAY	Dried whole leaves, ground	Aromatic, woodsy, pleasantly bitter	Meat, game, poultry, stews, fish, shellfish, chowders, soups, pickled meats and vegetables, gravies, marinades
BURNET	Fresh, dried leaves	Delicate cucumber flavor	Soups, salads, dressings, most vegetables, beverages, as a garnish
CARAWAY	Whole or gound, seed	Leaves and root delicately flavored, seeds sharp and pungent	Beans, beets, cabbage soup, breads, cookies, dips, variety meats, casseroles, dressings, cottage cheese, cheese spreads, sauerbraten

Dictionary of Herbs and Spices—Continued

Herb or Spice	Form	Flavor	Uses
CARDAMOM	Whole or ground, seed	Mild pleasant ginger flavor	Pastries, pies, cookies, jellies, fruit dishes, sweet potatoes, pumpkin
CAYENNE	Ground	Blend of hottest chili peppers	Sparingly in sauces, meat or seafood dishes, casseroles, soups, curries, stews, Mexican recipes, vegetables, cottage and cream cheeses
CHERVIL	Fresh, whole	Delicate parsley flavor	Soups, salads, stews, meats, fish, garnishes, eggs, sauces, dressings, vegetables, cottage cheese
CHILI POWDER	Powder	Blend of chilies and spices	Sparingly in Mexican dishes, meats, stews, soups, cocktail sauces, eggs, seafoods, relishes, dressings
CHIVES	Fresh, frozen, dried	Delicate onion flavor	As an ingredient or garnish for any dish complemented by this flavor
CINNAMON	Whole sticks or ground	Warm spicy flavor	Pastries, desserts, puddings, fruits, spiced beverages, pork, chicken, stews, sweet potatoes, carrots, squash
CLOVES	Whole or ground	Hot, spicy, penetrating	Sparingly with pork, in soups, desserts, fruits, sauces, baked beans, candied sweet potatoes, carrots, squash
CORIANDER	Whole or ground, seed	Pleasant lemon-orange flavor	Pastries, cookies, cream or pea soups, Spanish dishes, dressings, spiced dishes, salads, cheeses, meats
CUMIN	Ground, seed	Warm, distinctive, salty-sweet, reminiscent of caraway	Meat loaf, chili, fish, soft cheeses, deviled eggs, stews, beans, cabbage, fruit pies, rice, Oriental meat cookery
CURRY	Powder	Combination of many spices, warm, fragrant, exotic, combinations vary	Meats, sauces, stews, soups, fruits, eggs, fish, shellfish, poultry, creamed and scalloped vegetables, dressings, cream or cottage cheeses
DILL	Fresh, dried (whole or ground), seed	Aromatic, somewhat like caraway, but milder and sweeter	Seafood, meat, poultry, spreads, dips, dressings, cream or cottage cheeses, potato salads, many vegetables, soups, chowders

Dictionary of Herbs and Spices—Continued

Herb or Spice	Form	Flavor	Uses
FENNEL	Fresh, dried (whole or ground), seed	Pleasant licorice flavor somewhat like anise	Breads, rolls, sweet pastries, cookies, apples, stews, pork, squash, eggs, fish, beets, cabbage
GINGER	Fresh whole root, ground, crystallized	Aromatic, sweet, spice, penetrating	Cakes, pies, cookies, chutneys, curries, beverages, fruits, meats, poultry, stews, yellow vegetables, beets, soups, dressings, cheese dishes
MACE	Whole or ground	This dried pulp of the nutmeg kernel has a strong nutmeg flavor	Chicken, creamed fish, fish sauces, cakes, cookies, spiced doughs, jellies, beverages, yellow vegetables, cheese dishes, desserts, toppings
MARJORAM	Fresh, dried (whole or ground)	Faintly like sage, slight mint after-taste, delicate	Pork, lamb, beef, game, fish, fish sauces, poultry, chowders, soups, stews, sauces, cottage or cream cheeses, omelets, soufflés, green salads, many vegetables
MINT	Fresh, dried	Fruity, aromatic, distinctive flavor	Lamb, veal, fish, soups, fruit, desserts, cottage or cream cheeses, sauces, salads, cabbage, carrots, beans, potatoes
MUSTARD	Fresh, dried (whole or ground)	Sharp, hot, very pungent	Salads, dressings, eggs, sauces, fish, spreads, soups, many vegetables
NUTMEG	Whole or ground	Spicy, sweet, pleasant	Desserts of all kinds, stews, sauces, cream dishes, soups, fruits, beverages, ground meats, many vegetables
OREGANO (wild marjoram)	Fresh, dried (whole or ground)	More pungent than marjoram, but similar, reminiscent of thyme	Italian cooking, Mexican cooking, spaghetti, tomato sauces, soups, meats, fish, poultry, eggs, omelets, spreads, dips, many vegetables, green salads, mushroom dishes
PARSLEY	Fresh, dried flakes	Sweet, mildly spicy, refreshing	As a garnish, ingredient in soups, spreads, dips, stews, butters, all meats, poultry, fish, most vegetables, omelets, eggs, herb breads, salads

Dictionary of Herbs and Spices—Continued

Herb or Spice	Form	Flavor	Uses
POPPY SEED	Tiny, whole dried seed	Nut flavor	Breads, rolls, cakes, soups, cookies, dressings, cottage or cream cheeses, noodles, many vegetables, fruits, deviled eggs, stuffings
ROSEMARY	Fresh, whole	Refreshing, piny, resinous, pungent	Sparingly in meats, game, poultry, soups, fruits, stuffings, eggs, omelets, herb breads, sauces, green salads, marinades, vegetables
SAFFRON	Whole or ground	Exotic, delicate, pleasantly bittersweet	Expensive, but a little goes far; use for color and flavor in rice dishes, potatoes, rolls, breads, fish, stew, veal, chicken, bouillabaisse, curries, scrambled eggs, cream cheese, cream soups, sauces
SAGE	Fresh, whole, or rubbed	Pungent, warm, astringent	Sparingly in pork dishes, fish, veal, lamb, stuffings, cheese dips, fish chowders, consommé, cream soups, gravies, green salads, tomatoes, carrots, lima beans, peas, onions, brussels sprouts, eggplant
SAVORY	Fresh, dried (whole or ground)	Warm, aromatic, resinous, delicate sage flavor, winter savory stronger than summer savory	Egg dishes, salads, soups, seafoods, pork, lamb, veal, poultry, tomatoes, beans, beets, cabbage, peas, lentils, summer squash, artichokes, rice, barbecue dishes, stuffings
SESAME	Whole seed	Toasted, it has a nutlike flavor	Breads, rolls, cookies, fish, lamb, eggs, fruit or vegetable salads, chicken, thick soups, vegetables, casseroles, toppings, noodles, candies
TARRAGON	Fresh, dried (whole or ground)	Licorice-anise flavor, pleasant, slightly bitter	Sparingly in egg dishes, fish, shellfish, veal, poultry, chowders, chicken, soups, butters, vinegar, sauces, marinades, beans, beets, cabbage, cauliflower, broccoli, vegetable juices, fresh sprigs in salads

Dictionary of Herbs and Spices—Continued

Herb or Spice	Form	Flavor	Uses
THYME	Fresh, dried (whole or ground)	Strong, pleasant, pungent clove flavor	Sparingly in fish, gumbo, shellfish, soups, meats, poultry, tomato juice or sauces, cheeses, eggs, sauces, fricasees, tomatoes, artichokes, beets, beans, mushrooms, potatoes, onions, carrots
TURMERIC	Whole or ground	Aromatic, warm, mild	Substitutes for saffron in salads, salad dressings, butters, creamed eggs, fish, curries, rice dishes without saffron, vegetables, used partially for its orange color
WATERCRESS	Fresh	Pleasing, peppery	Garnish or ingredient in salads, fruit or vegetable cocktails, soups, cottage cheese, spreads, egg dishes or sprinkled on vegetables or salads

FLAVORING EQUIVALENTS

If you are temporarily out of a particular seasoning ingredient or want to substitute items called for in recipes, follow this convenient guide.

ARROWROOT

1 teaspoon	1 tablespoon flour
1 tablespoon	3 tablespoons flour
2 teaspoons	1 tablespoon cornstarch
1 tablespoon	1 tablespoon flour plus 1 teaspoon cornstarch

BAY LEAF (dried)

½ teaspoon, cracked	1 whole bay leaf

BELL PEPPERS (green, dried)

1 tablespoon, rehydrated	3 tablespoons chopped fresh green pepper

BELL PEPPERS (red, dried)

1 tablespoon, rehydrated	3 tablespoons chopped fresh red pepper or 2 tablespoons chopped pimiento

CHIVES (see ONIONS, shredded green)

CORNSTARCH (see ARROWROOT)

GARLIC CHIPS

⅛ teaspoon, ground or crushed	1 medium clove garlic or ⅛ teaspoon garlic powder

GARLIC POWDER

⅛ teaspoon	1 medium clove garlic or ⅛ teaspoon ground or crushed garlic chips

GINGER (dried)

1 teaspoon whole (soak several hours, then mince or grate)	2 teaspoons chopped fresh ginger
2 teaspoons crystallized chopped or slivered	1 teaspoon chopped fresh ginger
¼ teaspoon ground	1 teaspoon chopped fresh ginger or 2 teaspoons chopped crystallized ginger

HORSERADISH (dried)

| 1 tablespoon, rehydrated in 1 tablespoon water mixed with 1 tablespoon vinegar and sugar and salt to taste | 2 tablespoons bottled horseradish |

LEMON PEEL (dried)

| 1 teaspoon | 1 teaspoon grated fresh lemon peel or grated peel of 1 medium lemon or ½ teaspoon lemon extract |

MINT (see PEPPERMINT or SPEARMINT)

MUSHROOMS (powdered)

| 1 tablespoon | 3 tablespoons whole dried mushrooms or 4 ounces fresh mushrooms |

MUSTARD (dry)

| 1 teaspoon mild | 1 tablespoon mild prepared mustard |
| 1 teaspoon hot | 1 tablespoon hot prepared mustard |

ONION POWDER

| 1 tablespoon rehydrated | 1 small onion, chopped or ¼ cup chopped onion |

ONION (instant minced)

| 1 tablespoon rehydrated | 1 very small onion, chopped or 2 tablespoons chopped fresh onion |
| 1 tablespoon, not rehydrated | 1 tablespoon instant toasted onion |

ONION (instant toasted)

| 1 tablespoon | 1 tablespoon instant minced onion |

ONION (shredded green)

| ½ teaspoon | 2 teaspoons finely chopped fresh chives or 2 teaspoons finely chopped green onion tops |

ORANGE PEEL (dried)

| 1 tablespoon | 1 tablespoon grated fresh orange peel or grated peel of 1 medium orange |
| 2 teaspoons | 1 teaspoon orange extract |

PARSLEY FLAKES

| 1 teaspoon | 3 teaspoons chopped fresh parsley |

PEPPER

| Cayenne | Nepal pepper (equal amount) |

PEPPERMINT (dried)

| 1 tablespoon | ¼ cup chopped fresh mint |

PIMIENTO (see BELL PEPPERS, red)

SPEARMINT (dried)

| 1 tablespoon | ¼ cup chopped fresh mint |

VANILLA BEAN

| 1-inch piece | 1 teaspoon vanilla |

IMPORTANT: If you are on a low-salt diet, avoid the following seasonings and condiments: Salt, and all seasonings containing salt or sodium, bottled meat sauce, catsup, and prepared mustard.

9 Appetizers and Beverages

FRESH FRUIT CUP

½ pineapple, cut into pieces (see *Note*)
2 oranges, pared and sectioned
1 tablespoon slivered crystallized ginger
½ cup orange juice
2 bananas
Fresh mint leaves

Combine pineapple pieces, orange sections, and ginger in bowl. Pour orange juice on fruits. Cover and refrigerate.

Just before serving, slice bananas into bowl and mix lightly. Divide among four sherbet glasses and garnish with fresh mint.

4 servings.

    1 serving = 120 calories
                  0 cholesterol
                  0 fat

Note: To cut pineapple, twist off top; cut pineapple in half, then into quarters. Hold pineapple quarter securely, slice fruit from rind. Cut off pineapple core and remove any "eyes." For pieces, slice quarters lengthwise, then cut crosswise.

ICED MELON MORSELS

Divide 2 cups chilled melon balls (cantaloupe, honeydew, crenshaw, watermelon, or mixture) among 4 sherbet dishes. Garnish each with slice of lime.

4 servings.

    1 serving = 25 calories
                  0 cholesterol
                  0 fat

FRUIT CORNUCOPIA

3 tablespoons sugar
½ cup water
3 tablespoons fresh lemon juice
½ teaspoon vanilla
1 cup diced cantaloupe
1 cup sliced peaches
1 cup blueberries
½ cup seedless green grapes
Fresh mint leaves

Heat sugar and water in small saucepan to boiling; boil ½ minute. Remove from heat; stir in lemon juice and vanilla. Cool.

Combine fruits in bowl. Pour sugar syrup on fruit and chill. Serve in sherbet dishes and garnish with mint leaves.

6 servings.

    1 serving = 71 calories
                  0 cholesterol
                  0 fat

STEWED FRUIT COMPOTE

1 pound mixed dried fruits
4 oranges, pared and sectioned
2 grapefruit, pared and sectioned

Cook dried fruits as directed on package. Cool and refrigerate. Mix orange and grapefruit sections and mixed dried fruits.

8 servings.

    1 serving = 213 calories
                  0 cholesterol
                  0 fat

WONDERFUL WINGS

3 pounds chicken wings (15 to 16)
½ cup lemon juice
½ cup vegetable oil
3 cloves garlic, crushed

Cut bony wing tips from chicken wings and discard. Separate chicken wings at joint. Place wing halves in shallow baking dish. Mix lemon juice, oil, and garlic and pour on wing halves. Cover and refrigerate at least 4 hours.

Remove wing halves from marinade; place on rack in broiler pan. Bake at 400° for 45 minutes.

30 pieces.
 1 piece = 41 calories
    14 mg cholesterol
    3 gm fat

Note: Wings can be frozen after baking. To serve, thaw at room temperature. Place on rack in broiler pan; broil until hot, 3 to 4 minutes.

Fifteen pounds will serve 40 guests.

CRUNCHY VEGETABLE CURLS

Scrape 2 long, thick carrots. Cut lengthwise with vegetable parer into paper-thin slices. Roll each slice around index finger to form a curl; fasten curl with wooden pick. Place in bowl of ice and water to keep curled and crisp.

At serving time, unroll each curl; place cherry tomato on end and roll curl around tomato. Fasten with wooden picks. Insert picks with curls in long, narrow cucumber and serve with a dip.

Note: Substitute cubes of cucumber, zucchini, apple, or celery for the cherry tomatoes.

STUFFED CHERRY TOMATOES

Cut off tops of cherry tomatoes and remove pulp, leaving a ¼-inch wall. Stuff each with Chicken Salad (page 91), Tuna Salad (page 92), Egg Salad (page 92), or Zucchini Spread (page 73).

BROILED STUFFED MUSHROOMS

1 pourd small mushrooms
1 green pepper, finely chopped
2 or 3 green onions (with tops), chopped
2 tablespoons margarine
¼ cup dry bread crumbs
¼ cup snipped parsley
¼ teaspoon oregano
Dash cayenne pepper
3 tablespoons shredded part skim milk
 mozzarrella cheese
2 teaspoons white wine
3 tablespoons margarine, melted
Paprika

Trim mushrooms; remove stems and reserve caps for stuffing. Chop stems. Cook and stir mushroom stems, green pepper, and onion in 2 tablespoons margarine until mushrooms are brown. Stir in bread crumbs, parsley, oregano, cayenne pepper, cheese, and wine; heat through.

Brush mushroom caps with 3 tablespoons melted margarine. Press stuffing into caps and place on broiler rack. Sprinkle with paprika. Set oven at broil and/or 550°. Broil mushroom caps 3 to 4 inches from heat until tender, 4 to 5 minutes.

60 to 70 mushrooms.
 1 mushroom = 15 calories
    trace cholesterol
    1 gm fat

ARTICHOKES

Allow 1 artichoke for each serving. Remove any discolored leaves and the small leaves at base; trim stem even with base. Cutting straight across, slice 1 inch off top; discard top. Snip off points of the remaining leaves with scissors. Rinse artichoke under cold water.

Cook artichokes in large kettle. For 4 medium artichokes, heat 6 quarts water, 1 teaspoon salt, and juice of 1 lemon to boiling. Add artichokes; heat to boiling. Reduce heat; simmer uncovered until leaves pull out easily and bottom is tender when pierced with a knife, 30 to 40 minutes. Remove artichokes carefully from water (use tongs or 2 large spoons); place upside down to drain. Remove choke (fuzzy center) from centers with a teaspoon. Serve with Lemon-Margarine Sauce (below).

> 1 serving = 53 calories
> 0 cholesterol
> 0 fat

Lemon-Margarine Sauce: Mix ½ cup unsalted margarine, melted, and 2 tablespoons lemon juice.

> *½ cup (enough for 4 artichokes).*
> 1 serving = 217 calories
> 0 cholesterol
> 24 gm fat

Note: To serve artichokes cold, cover and refrigerate several hours. Serve with your favorite dipping sauce or mayonnaise.

BOHEMIAN MUSHROOMS

1 pound mushrooms, trimmed and sliced
1 onion, finely chopped
1 tablespoon plus 1½ teaspoons margarine
1 tablespoon plus 1½ teaspoons safflower oil
¾ cup low-fat yogurt
½ teaspoon salt
½ teaspoon dried mint leaves
Freshly ground pepper

Cook and stir mushrooms and onion in margarine and oil until mushrooms are lightly cooked, about 3 minutes. Remove from heat; stir in yogurt, salt, and mint leaves. Season with pepper. Cover and refrigerate at least 2 hours. Serve as first course or as a salad substitute.

> *6 servings.*
> 1 serving = 99 calories
> 2 mg cholesterol
> 7 gm fat

CAROUSEL KEBABS

12 pineapple chunks
12 cantaloupe balls
12 honeydew melon balls
12 strawberries
6 thin melon wedges

Place a pineapple chunk, cantaloupe ball, honeydew ball, and strawberry on each of 12 wooden skewers. Insert 2 skewers in each melon wedge.

> *6 servings.*
> 1 serving = 37 calories
> 0 cholesterol
> 0 fat

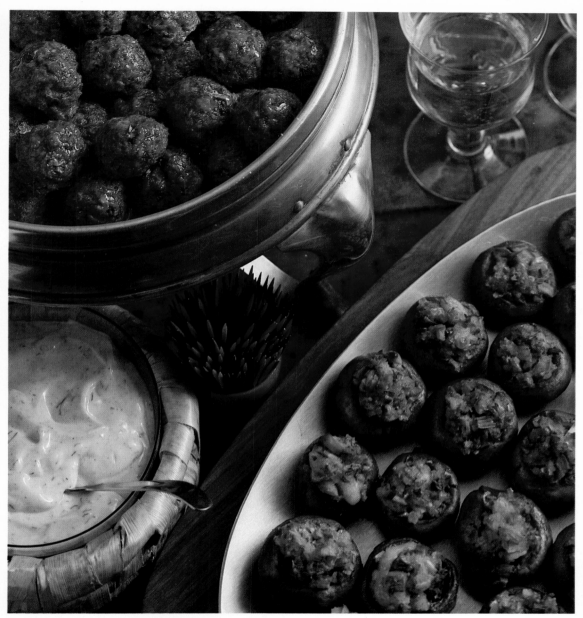
Hot Meatballs; Broiled Stuffed Mushrooms.

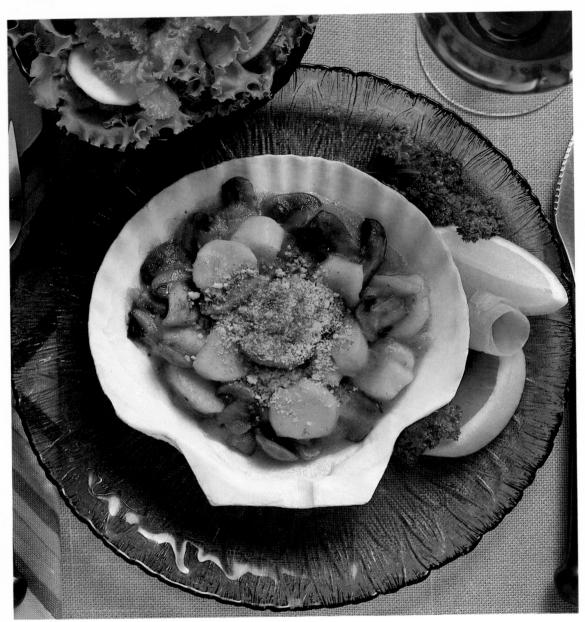

Coquilles St. Jacques.

BAKED CLAMS BRETONNE

12 cherrystone clams, opened (reserve shells)
½ pound mushrooms, finely chopped
2 shallots, minced
1 clove garlic, minced
2 tablespoons margarine
½ cup plus 2 tablespoons soft bread crumbs
1 parsley sprig, snipped
1 tablespoon tarragon leaves
2 tablespoons dry sherry
½ teaspoon Pernod or other anise-flavored aperitif
⅛ teaspoon salt
⅛ teaspoon white pepper
2 tablespoons margarine, melted

Dice clams; place in bowl and set aside. Heat oven to 350°. Cook and stir mushrooms, shallots, and garlic in 2 tablespoons margarine until mushrooms begin to brown. Pour mushroom mixture into bowl with clams. Stir in ¼ cup of the bread crumbs, the parsley, tarragon leaves, sherry, Pernod, salt, and pepper. Spoon 1 tablespoon clam mixture into each reserved shell and pack lightly. Top each with ½ teaspoon of the remaining bread crumbs and ½ teaspoon melted margarine. Place shells on baking sheet. Bake until brown, about 30 minutes.

6 servings.
1 serving = 137 calories
19 mg cholesterol
9 gm fat

Note: Filled clam shells can be frozen before baking.

BROILED SCALLOPS

2 pounds sea scallops, washed and drained
½ cup safflower oil
½ cup olive oil
1 cup dry white wine
1 clove garlic, minced
1 teaspoon tarragon leaves
½ teaspoon salt
Freshly ground pepper
½ cup snipped parsley

Place scallops in deep bowl. Mix remaining ingredients and pour over scallops. Cover and refrigerate at least 2 hours, turning scallops occasionally.

Set oven at broil and/or 550°. Arrange scallops on small skewers and place on broiler rack. Broil 2 inches from heat, turning frequently to cook scallops on all sides, about 5 minutes.

32 appetizer servings.
1 serving = 63 calories
12 mg cholesterol
5 gm fat

8 main-course servings.
1 serving = 253 calories
48 mg cholesterol
19 gm fat

SHISH KEBABS (Without Skewers)

**2 pounds boneless lamb shoulder or leg,
cut into 1-inch cubes**
½ cup lemon juice
½ cup vegetable oil
3 cloves garlic, crushed
1 pint cherry tomatoes
2 medium onions, sliced
**2 medium green peppers, cut into ½-inch
slices**
8 ounces large mushroom caps, trimmed
Freshly ground pepper

Place meat in shallow baking dish. Mix lemon juice, oil, and garlic; pour on meat. Cover and refrigerate at least 4 hours.

Remove meat from marinade; reserve marinade. Line broiler pan with aluminum foil; poke holes in foil and arrange meat and vegetables in pan. Season with pepper and sprinkle reserved marinade on vegetables.

Set oven at broil and/or 550°. Broil meat and vegetables 3 inches from heat, turning until brown on all sides.

12 appetizer servings.
1 serving = 198 calories
60 mg cholesterol
12 gm fat

6 main-dish servings.
1 serving = 397 calories
120 mg cholesterol
25 gm fat

BENGAL SAUSAGES

1 pound ground lean beef
1 pound ground lean lamb
1 small onion, minced
Juice of ½ lemon
¼ cup soft bread crumbs
½ cup egg substitute
2 tablespoons snipped parsley
¼ teaspoon garlic powder
½ teaspoon white pepper
½ teaspoon ground coriander
½ teaspoon ground cumin
Hot cooked rice
Dilled Onions (below)
Mustard Sauce (below)

Mix all ingredients except rice, Dilled Onions, and Mustard Sauce. Shape mixture to resemble link sausages, each about 3 x 1 inch.

Set oven at broil and/or 550°. Arrange sausages on rack and broil about 4 inches from heat, turning each to brown on all sides. Serve on rice and sprinkle Dilled Onions on top. Pass Mustard Sauce.

30 sausages (8 servings).
1 serving = 215 calories
95 mg cholesterol
9 gm fat

Dilled Onions: Mix ½ cup chopped onion and ½ teaspoon dill weed.

1 serving = 5 calories
0 cholesterol
0 fat

Mustard Sauce: Mix 2 teaspoons Dijon-Type Mustard (page 187) and 1 cup imitation sour cream.

1 serving = 63 calories
0 cholesterol
5 gm fat

Note: Sausages can be served as an appetizer. Omit hot cooked rice, mix Dilled Onions and Mustard Sauce, and serve as dip for sausage.

BEEF KEBABS

1 pound ground lean beef
1 slice bread, soaked in water and
squeezed
2 onions, finely chopped
2 cloves garlic, crushed
2 teaspoons chopped fresh coriander or
½ teaspoon ground coriander
¼ teaspoon cayenne pepper
2 teaspoons curry powder
½ teaspoon salt
1-inch piece ginger root, chopped
1 to 2 green chili peppers, thinly
sliced
¼ teaspoon cloves
½ teaspoon cinnamon
¼ cup vegetable oil

Mix all ingredients except oil. Shape mixture into small balls. Heat oil in large skillet. Cook meatballs until brown and thoroughly cooked. Drain. Serve as appetizers. Mixture can be shaped into larger meatballs for main dish.

50 to 60 appetizer meatballs.

1 meatball = 21 calories
7 mg cholesterol
1 gm fat

Note: Fresh ginger root is available in Chinese food stores, or substitute preserved ginger, drained.

SYRIAN MEATBALLS

1½ pounds lean ground lamb
2 cloves garlic, minced
3 tablespoons egg substitute
Freshly ground pepper
1 tablespoon dry mustard
½ cup snipped parsley
2 tablespoons olive oil
Vegetable oil
Curry-Dill Dip (page 73)

Mix meat, garlic, egg substitute, parsley, mustard, and pepper. Moisten mixture with 1 tablespoon of the olive oil. Shape mixture into 48 small balls.

Heat remaining 1 tablespoon olive oil and just enough vegetable oil in large skillet to cover bottom. Brown meatballs in skillet, shaking skillet briskly to cook meatballs evenly. Serve with Curry-Dill Dip.

8 servings.

1 serving = 203 calories
75 mg cholesterol
13 gm fat

HOT MEATBALLS

Substitute ground round steak for lean ground beef in Hamburgers (page 133) and shape mixture into 1-inch balls (about 48).

Heat just enough vegetable oil in large skillet to cover bottom; brown meatballs in hot oil but do not cook through. Turn meatballs into chafing dish; keep warm. Serve with Dijon-Type Mustard (page 187) and provide wooden picks for guests to spear meatballs.

1 meatball = 16 calories
8 mg cholesterol
1 gm fat

ALOHA DIP

1 pineapple
1 carton (8 ounces) orange low-fat yogurt
2 tablespoons brown sugar
1 pint strawberries

Cut thick slice from bottom and top of pineapple. Cut remaining pineapple into 1-inch slices; remove rind and core. Cut ¾ of rings into cubes; place in bowl. Cover and refrigerate.

Finely chop remaining rings. Mix chopped pineapple, yogurt, and brown sugar in small bowl. Cover and refrigerate to blend flavors.

Insert wooden picks in pineapple cubes. Arrange strawberries (with hulls) and pineapple cubes on serving plate. Place bowl with yogurt mixture in center. Guests spoon some of the yogurt mixture onto dessert plates, then dip pineapple and strawberries into mixture.

6 servings.

1 serving = 136 calories
2 mg cholesterol
1 gm fat

HERB CHEESE DIP

2 cups low-fat cottage cheese
¼ teaspoon dill weed
¼ teaspoon dry mustard
Freshly ground pepper
2 tablespoons snipped parsley
1½ teaspoons snipped chives
Crisp Vegetable Dippers (this page)

Place cottage cheese, dill weed, mustard, and pepper in blender. Blend on high speed until smooth. Mix in parsley and chives. Serve with Crisp Vegetable Dippers.

2 cups.

1 tablespoon = 21 calories
1 mg cholesterol
trace fat

CRISP VEGETABLE DIPPERS

Asparagus tips
Broccoli buds
Cherry tomatoes
Turnip sticks
Cabbage fingers
Cauliflower flowerets
Watercress sprigs
Green onions
Zucchini sticks
Cooked green or wax beans
Carrot sticks
Cucumber fingers
Green or red sweet pepper strips
Artichoke leaves, cooked
Button mushroom caps
Cooked eggplant spears
Chinese pea pods

CURRIED TUNA DIP

½ cup chopped onion
½ cup chopped pared apple
1 teaspoon curry powder
1 tablespoon unsalted margarine
1 cup low-fat cottage cheese
1 tablespoon skim milk
1 teaspoon lemon juice
1 can (6½ or 7 ounces) tuna in water, drained and flaked
Crisp Vegetable Dippers (above)

Cook and stir onion, apple, and curry powder in margarine until onion is tender. Turn into blender container; add cottage cheese, milk, and lemon juice. Cover and mix on high speed until smooth. Mix in tuna on low speed. Cover and refrigerate. Serve with Crisp Vegetable Dippers.

2 cups.

1 tablespoon = 18 calories
4 mg cholesterol
1 gm fat

CURRY DILL DIP

½ cup low-fat mayonnaise
½ cup low-fat yogurt
1 teaspoon lemon or lime juice
1 teaspoon grated onion
1 teaspoon curry powder
½ teaspoon dill weed
½ teaspoon dry mustard
Crisp Vegetable Dippers (page 72)

Mix all ingredients except vegetable dippers. Cover and refrigerate at least 1 hour. Serve with vegetable dippers.

1 cup.

1 tablespoon = 28 calories
1 mg cholesterol
2 gm fat

CALCUTTA VEGETABLE DIP

1 cup shredded unpared zucchini
**   (about 1 medium)**
½ cup shredded carrot (about 2 medium)
1 cup low-fat yogurt
3 tablespoons low-fat mayonnaise
1 small onion, grated
⅓ teaspoon garlic powder or ¼ teaspoon
**   salt**
1 teaspoon curry powder
Crisp Vegetable Dippers (page 72)

Place shredded zucchini in strainer and press out excess liquid. Turn into bowl; add remaining ingredients, except vegetable sticks, and toss. Cover and refrigerate at least 2 hours to blend flavors. Serve with Crisp Vegetable Dippers.

2 cups.

¼ cup = 44 calories
4 mg cholesterol
3 gm fat

ZUCCHINI SPREAD

¼ cup egg substitute
1 tablespoon low-fat yogurt
¼ teaspoon salt
Dash freshly ground pepper
½ cup diced unpared zucchini
1 green onion (with top), minced
2 teaspoons margarine
Crackers or Melba toast

Mix egg substitute, yogurt, salt, and pepper; set aside. Cook and stir zucchini and onion in margarine in small skillet over low heat until hot. Pour egg substitute mixture on vegetables; stir lightly with fork. Cook over low heat until light brown on bottom; turn and brown on other side. Serve with crackers.

¾ cup.

1 tablespoon = 12 calories
trace cholesterol
1 gm fat

Bean Sprout Spread: Omit yogurt; mix in 1 teaspoon soy sauce with egg substitute. Substitute ½ cup bean sprouts for the zucchini.

1 tablespoon = 12 calories
0 cholesterol
1 gm fat

TUNA-CHUTNEY DIP

1 package (8 ounces) imitation cream
  cheese, softened
¼ cup low-fat mayonnaise
2 tablespoons prepared mustard
¼ teaspoon cayenne pepper
2 cans (6½ or 7 ounces each) tuna in
  water, drained and flaked
¼ cup chopped chutney
Crisp crackers

Blend cheese, mayonnaise, mustard, and cayenne pepper until fluffy. Mix in tuna and chutney. Serve with crackers.

About 2½ cups.

  2 tablespoons = 56 calories
              16 mg cholesterol
              3 gm fat

MOCK SOUR CREAM

Mix 1 carton (8 ounces) low-fat cottage cheese and 1 tablespoon low-fat yogurt in blender container on high speed until smooth and creamy. Use as a base for dips.

1 cup.

  1 tablespoon = 11 calories
              1 mg cholesterol
              trace fat

SUMMER SLUSH

½ pint lime ice
¾ cup apple juice, chilled

Soften lime ice. Gradually stir in apple juice until mixture is smooth. Pour into chilled glasses. Serve with cinnamon-stick stirrers.

2 servings (about 1 cup each).

  1 serving = 180 calories
            4 mg cholesterol
            1 gm fat

HONEY-LEMON TEA

6 cups boiling water
6 orange pekoe tea bags
¼ cup plus 2 tablespoons honey
1 stick cinnamon
½ cup lemon juice

Pour boiling water on tea bags in saucepan. Cover; let steep 5 minutes. Stir and remove tea bags. Stir in remaining ingredients; heat to boiling. Reduce heat and simmer 5 minutes. Remove stick cinnamon and serve.

6 servings (about 1 cup each).

  1 serving = 82 calories
            0 cholesterol
            trace fat

HOT GRAPEFRUIT TODDY

1 can (46 ounces) unsweetened
  grapefruit juice
1 teaspoon whole cloves
One 4-inch stick cinnamon
1 tablespoon sugar

Simmer all ingredients 10 minutes, stirring occasionally. Remove from heat. Remove cloves and stick cinnamon and pour into mugs. Serve with cinnamon stick muddlers if desired.

Six 5-ounce servings.

  1 serving = 99 calories
            0 cholesterol
            0 fat

BANANA CITRUS SHAKE

Place 1 banana, cut up, and 1 cup orange juice in blender container. Blend on high speed until smooth.

2 servings.

  1 serving = 113 calories
            0 cholesterol
            0 fat

EGGNOG

¼ cup egg substitute
1 cup skim milk
1 tablespoon sugar
½ teaspoon vanilla

Mix all ingredients in tall glass.

Two 6-ounce servings.

1 serving = 91 calories
2 mg cholesterol
1 gm fat

SPICY ICED TEA

2 cups boiling water
3-inch stick cinnamon
4 whole cloves
¼ teaspoon ground ginger
2 cups boiling water
2 tablespoons Darjeeling tea
Juice of ½ lemon
1 tablespoon honey

Pour 2 cups boiling water on stick cinnamon, cloves, and ginger in saucepan. Simmer 15 minutes.

Pour 2 cups boiling water on tea in heatproof container. Cover and steep 5 to 7 minutes. Strain spiced water and the tea into large pitcher. Stir in lemon juice and honey. Cover and refrigerate. Serve over crushed ice.

4 to 6 servings.

1 serving = 19 calories
0 cholesterol
0 fat

ICED TEA LEMONADE

4 cups boiling water
2 tablespoons plus 1½ teaspoons loose tea
⅓ cup water
¼ cup sugar
⅓ cup lemon juice
Fresh mint sprigs

Pour boiling water on tea in heatproof container. Cover; let steep 5 to 7 minutes.

Heat ⅓ cup water and the sugar to boiling, stirring until sugar is dissolved. Reduce heat and simmer 3 minutes. Strain tea into large pitcher. Stir in syrup and lemon juice. Cool. Serve over crushed ice and garnish with mint sprigs.

5 servings.

1 serving = 47 calories
0 cholesterol
0 fat

TROPICAL COOLER

2 cups unsweetened grapefruit juice, chilled
1 cup unsweetened orange juice, chilled
½ cup unsweetened pineapple juice, chilled
1 bottle (12 ounces) club soda, chilled
Mint leaves

Mix fruit juices and soda. Serve in glasses with ice cubes or crushed ice and garnish with mint leaves.

6 servings (about ¾ cup each).

1 serving = 83 calories
0 cholesterol
0 fat

Note: If you do not have fresh mint, substitute thin slice of orange, lemon, or lime.

CRANBERRY TEA COOLER

1½ cups boiling water
3 orange-spice-flavored tea bags
2 tablespoons sugar
1 cup cranberry cocktail
½ cup orange juice
2 tablespoons lemon juice
¾ cup water

Pour boiling water on tea bags. Cover and brew 5 minutes. Remove tea bags; pour tea into large pitcher. Stir in sugar until dissolved. Stir in remaining ingredients. Pour over ice in tall glasses.

6 servings.

1 serving = 56 calories
0 cholesterol
0 fat

Note: For a tart flavor, add ½ teaspoon lemon juice to each serving.

NEW ENGLAND MULLED CIDER

2 quarts apple cider
Two 3-inch sticks cinnamon
12 whole cloves
Dash nutmeg
1 tablespoon brown sugar
½ cup lemon juice
2 oranges

Heat cider, stick cinnamon, cloves, nutmeg, and brown sugar, stirring until sugar is dissolved. Reduce heat and simmer 1 hour. Strain mixture and stir in lemon juice.

Cut oranges into paper-thin slices; place orange slice in each cup. Pour in hot cider mixture. If desired, cider can be cooled and served cold.

9 servings.

1 serving = 135 calories
0 cholesterol
0 fat

10 Salads and Salad Dressings

SALADS

The most popular leafy bases for salads are head and leaf lettuce and endive.

Head Lettuce

Boston: Tender, rather soft leaf, slightly buttery in texture, center of head bleaches to a soft yellow, outer leaves are green in color.

Iceberg: Crisp leaves tightly curled into a compact head, center of head is bleached to a pale greenish white, outer leaves are fresh green in color.

Leaf Lettuce

Nonheading Leafy: Leaves are somewhat feathered with crinkled edges, leaf is uniformly a fresh green in color.

Romaine or Cos: Leaves are long and narrow, leaf edge is smooth, color is uniformly green, texture is brittle and juicy.

Endive

Curly chicory: Open head that spreads widely, leaf has a feathery edge, color is deep green at leaf ends and bleaches to a creamy yellow at center of open head.

Belgian, Witloof, or French: Satin-smooth leaves tightly folded into a slender elongated head, color is creamy yellow because of bleaching underground.

Escarole or Batavian: Leaf is long, rather narrow with heavy midrib, color is fresh green, texture is crisp.

MOLDED TUNA SUPPER

2 envelopes unflavored gelatin
¾ cup water
2 tablespoons white vinegar
2 cups low-fat cottage cheese
2 cups low-fat yogurt
2 tablespoons snipped chives
¼ cup chopped green pepper
¼ cup chopped red pepper
2 cans (6½ or 7 ounces) tuna in water, drained and broken into chunks
Salad greens
Cherry tomatoes

Sprinkle gelatin on water in saucepan to soften. Stir over low heat until gelatin is dissolved. Remove from heat; stir in vinegar, cottage cheese, and yogurt. Refrigerate until thickened.

Fold in chives, red pepper, green pepper, and tuna. Turn into 8 individual molds or a 6-cup mold. Refrigerate until set. Unmold onto salad greens and garnish with cherry tomatoes.

8 servings.

1 serving = 149 calories
40 mg cholesterol
3 gm fat

CINNAMON FRUIT MOLD

1 envelope unflavored gelatin
½ cup water
1 can (15¼ ounces) pineapple chunks in unsweetened pineapple juice, drained (reserve juice)
1 can (11 ounces) mandarin oranges, drained (reserve syrup)
2 cups water
1 cinnamon stick (3 inches)
1 teaspoon whole cloves
¼ teaspoon ginger
1 medium red apple, diced

Sprinkle gelatin on ½ cup water to soften. Measure reserved pineapple juice into medium saucepan and add enough reserved orange syrup to measure 1 cup. Add 2 cups water and the spices; heat to simmering and simmer 10 minutes.

Remove cinnamon stick and cloves; pour liquid on gelatin mixture. Stir over low heat until gelatin is dissolved, about 2 minutes. Refrigerate until slightly thickened. Stir in fruit. Pour into 8 individual molds or into 5-cup ring mold. Refrigerate until firm.

8 servings.

1 serving = 78 calories
0 cholesterol
trace fat

CURRIED FRUIT SALAD

Arrange banana chunks, pineapple chunks or slices, seedless green grapes, apple slices, and melon wedges on platter. Serve with Curried Fruit Salad Dressing (page 95).

1 serving from
fruit group = 50 calories
0 cholesterol
0 fat

LAYERED FRUIT SALAD

2 envelopes unflavored gelatin
⅓ cup sugar
3 cups water
½ cup lemon juice
1 cup melon balls
1 cup blueberries
1 cup sliced peaches
1 cup halved strawberries

Mix gelatin and sugar in small saucepan. Stir in 1 cup of the water and heat to boiling, stirring until sugar is dissolved. Remove from heat; stir in remaining 2 cups water and the lemon juice. Pour 1 cup gelatin mixture into each of 4 bowls. Refrigerate 1 cup gelatin mixture until thickened.

Fold melon balls into the 1 cup thickened gelatin. Pour into 6-cup mold. Refrigerate until almost set. Refrigerate second cup gelatin mixture until thickened. Fold blueberries into second cup thickened gelatin. Pour over melon ball gelatin in mold. Refrigerate until almost set.

Repeat with remaining cups of gelatin mixture and the peaches and strawberries. Refrigerate mold until set, 3 to 4 hours.

10 servings.

1 serving = 65 calories
0 cholesterol
trace fat

SPRING SALAD

Arrange grapefruit sections and orange slices on lettuce. Top with scoop of low-fat cottage cheese and garnish with fresh strawberries.

1 serving = 157 calories
9 mg cholesterol
2 gm fat

COMBINATION VEGETABLE GELS

1 envelope unflavored gelatin
¼ cup sugar
½ cup water
¼ teaspoon Tabasco sauce
¼ cup lemon juice
1 cup water
Choice of Vegetable Combination (below)

Mix gelatin and sugar in saucepan. Stir in ½ cup water. Stir over low heat until gelatin is dissolved. Remove from heat; stir in Tabasco sauce, lemon juice, and 1 cup water. Refrigerate until mixture is slightly thickened.

Fold in vegetable combination. Pour into 3-cup mold or into 6 individual molds. Refrigerate until firm.

6 servings.

VEGETABLE COMBINATIONS

1½ cups shredded carrot
¼ cup chopped cauliflower
¼ cup diced green pepper

> 1 serving = 56 calories
> 0 cholesterol
> trace fat

2 cups canned unsalted mixed vegetables
2 tablespoons snipped dill or parsley

> 1 serving = 77 calories
> 0 cholesterol
> trace fat

1½ cups finely shredded cabbage
¼ cup sliced radish
¼ cup minced green onion

> 1 serving = 50 calories
> 0 cholesterol
> trace fat

CREAMY GARDEN SALAD

1 envelope unflavored gelatin
1 tablespoon sugar
¾ cup water
1 cup low-fat yogurt
2 tablespoons white vinegar
2 drops Tabasco sauce
1 cup shredded unpared cucumber, drained
¼ cup shredded radish
2 tablespoons minced scallions or green onion
Lettuce

Mix gelatin and sugar in small saucepan. Stir in water and heat to boiling, stirring constantly until sugar is dissolved. Remove from heat; stir in yogurt, vinegar, and Tabasco sauce. Refrigerate until thickened.

Fold in cucumber, radish, and scallions. Pour into loaf pan, 9 x 5 x 3 inches. Refrigerate until set, about 3 hours. Cut into slices and serve on lettuce.

8 servings.

> 1 serving = 32 calories
> 2 mg cholesterol
> trace fat

CITRUS SLIMMER SALAD

½ cup low-fat cottage cheese
1½ teaspoons thawed frozen orange juice concentrate
1 tablespoon chopped green pepper
1 teaspoon slivered orange peel
Lettuce
1 cup orange and grapefruit sections

Mix cottage cheese, orange juice concentrate, green pepper, and orange peel. Spoon onto lettuce. Arrange orange and grapefruit sections around cottage-cheese mixture.

> 1 serving = 210 calories
> 3 mg cholesterol
> 1 gm fat

MOLDED VEGETABLE SALAD

1 envelope unflavored gelatin
2 tablespoons sugar
⅛ teaspoon salt
½ cup water
¼ cup lemon juice
¾ cup water
12 thin unpared cucumber slices
¾ cup thinly sliced radish
¼ cup shredded cabbage
½ cup diced celery

Mix gelatin, sugar, and salt in small saucepan. Stir in ½ cup water. Stir over low heat until gelatin is dissolved. Remove from heat; stir in lemon juice and ¾ cup water. Arrange cucumber slices and several radish slices in loaf pan, 7⅛ x 3⅝ x 2¼ inches. Spoon in enough gelatin mixture to cover vegetables.

Refrigerate until almost firm. Refrigerate remaining gelatin mixture until thickened. Stir in remaining radish slices, the cabbage, and celery. Pour on gelatin mixture in loaf pan; refrigerate until firm. Cut into slices and, if desired, serve on lettuce.

4 servings.

1 serving = 46 calories
0 cholesterol
0 fat

TURKEY SALAD SURPRISE

2 cups diced cooked turkey
1 can (16 ounces) unsweetened peach halves, drained and cut up
1 cup diced celery
½ cup diced green pepper
¼ cup toasted blanched slivered almonds
1 teaspoon curry powder
1 tablespoon lemon juice
½ cup low-fat mayonnaise
Salad greens

Combine turkey, peaches, celery, green pepper, and almonds in bowl. Mix curry powder, lemon juice, and mayonnaise; pour over turkey mixture and toss. Serve on salad greens.

6 servings.

1 serving = 212 calories
41 mg cholesterol
12 gm fat

GAZPACHO GELATIN SALAD

1 envelope unflavored gelatin
1½ cups (unsalted) vegetable juice
½ cup low-fat mayonnaise
¼ cup red wine vinegar
2 tablespoons vegetable oil
¼ teaspoon hot pepper sauce
1 clove garlic, crushed
1 cup diced cucumber
½ cup diced green pepper
½ cup minced onion

Sprinkle gelatin on vegetable juice in saucepan to soften. Stir over low heat until gelatin is dissolved. Stir in mayonnaise, vinegar, oil, pepper sauce, and garlic. Chill until thickened.

Fold in cucumber, green pepper, and onion. Pour into 4-cup mold. Chill until set.

6 servings.

1 serving = 131 calories
0 cholesterol
11 gm fat

CRANBERRY-APPLE GELATIN

1 envelope unflavored gelatin
½ cup water
2 cups cranberries
1 cup water
1 cup sugar
⅛ teaspoon mace
½ cup chopped pared apple

Sprinkle gelatin on ½ cup water to soften.
Heat cranberries, 1 cup water, the sugar, and mace in large saucepan to boiling, stirring constantly. Cook until cranberries pop, 5 to 10 minutes.

Stir gelatin into hot cranberry mixture. Place pan in bowl of ice and water or refrigerate until mixture mounds slightly when dropped from a spoon. Fold in apple. Pour into 4-cup mold and refrigerate until firm.

6 servings.

1 serving = 159 calories
0 cholesterol
trace fat

LUAU COTTAGE CHEESE and PINEAPPLE

1 can (8¼ ounces) crushed pineapple in unsweetened pineapple juice, drained
½ teaspoon rum extract
2 cups low-fat cottage cheese
Eight ½-inch center slices cantaloupe, pared (2 medium)
Lettuce

Sprinkle pineapple with rum extract and let stand 5 minutes. Fold in cottage cheese. For each serving, place cantaloupe slice on lettuce and top with about ½ cup cottage cheese mixture.

8 servings.

1 serving = 111 calories
5 mg cholesterol
1 gm fat

SPICED MINTED PEARS

1 can (20 ounces) unsweetened pear halves, drained (reserve juice)
1 stick cinnamon
6 whole cloves
½ teaspoon ginger
2 tablespoons lemon juice
1 teaspoon sugar
½ teaspoon mint extract
Few drops green food color
Crisp salad greens

Heat reserved pear juice, cinnamon, cloves, ginger, lemon juice, and sugar in large skillet to simmer; simmer uncovered 3 minutes. Add pears; cover and simmer 5 minutes. Cool pears in syrup. Remove pears to bowl. Stir mint extract and food color into syrup; pour on pears. Cover and refrigerate.

To serve, remove pears from syrup, drain and place on greens.

6 servings.

1 serving = 66 calories
0 cholesterol
trace fat

Note: This recipe is also an excellent garnish for lamb or veal.

YOGURT VEGETABLE MOLD

2 envelopes unflavored gelatin
2 tablespoons sugar
1 cup water
1¾ cups low-fat yogurt
2 tablespoons vinegar
1½ cups cooked cut green beans
1½ cups sliced pared cucumber
1 medium tomato, peeled and chopped

Mix gelatin and sugar in small saucepan. Stir in water and heat to boiling, stirring constantly until sugar is dissolved. Remove from heat and cool. Stir in vinegar and yogurt. Refrigerate until thickened.

Fold in green beans, cucumber, and tomato. Pour into 5-cup mold. Refrigerate until set.

6 main-dish servings.

1 serving = 81 calories
5 mg cholesterol
1 gm fat

10 salad servings.

1 serving = 48 calories
3 mg cholesterol
trace fat

FLORIDA HEALTH SALAD

2 envelopes unflavored gelatin
3 cups unsweetened grapefruit juice
⅛ teaspoon salt
1¼ cups grapefruit sections
⅔ cup shredded carrot
⅔ cup diced celery
1 cup low-fat yogurt

Sprinkle gelatin on 1 cup of the grapefruit juice in small saucepan to soften. Stir over heat until gelatin is dissolved. Remove from heat; stir in remaining grapefruit juice and the salt. Refrigerate until thickened.

Fold in grapefruit sections, carrot, celery, and yogurt. Pour into 6-cup mold and refrigerate until set. Unmold and, if desired, garnish with grapefruit sections and carrot slices.

8 servings.

1 serving = 83 calories
2 mg cholesterol
trace fat

Note: If fresh grapefruit sections are not available, use 2 cans (16 ounces each) unsweetened grapefruit sections, drained.

JELLIED CRANBERRY RELISH MOLD

1 can (18 ounces) pineapple juice
2 envelopes unflavored gelatin
2 tablespoons sugar
½ teaspoon salt
1 can (1 pound 4½ ounces) crushed pineapple
¼ cup vinegar
Juice of 1 lemon (3 tablespoons)
½ cup chopped celery
½ cup chopped green pepper
1 cup chopped cranberries

Measure 1 cup of the pineapple juice into medium saucepan. Sprinkle gelatin on juice to soften. Stir over low heat until gelatin is dissolved, 4 to 5 minutes. Remove from heat. Stir in remaining juice, the sugar, salt, pineapple (with syrup), vinegar, and lemon juice. Refrigerate until slightly thickened. Stir in celery, green pepper and cranberries. Pour into 6-cup mold. Refrigerate until firm.

10 servings.

1 serving = 93 calories
0 cholesterol
trace fat

FROZEN GRAPEFRUIT MEDLEY

1 can (16 ounces) unsweetened grapefruit sections
1 cup watermelon cubes
1 cup honeydew melon cubes
1 cup cantaloupe cubes
1 cup cherries, halved and pitted
Lettuce

Freeze unopened can of grapefruit sections until solid, about 6 hours.

Run warm water over can. Remove one end from can and slide frozen grapefruit sections onto platter. Cut into 4 slices.

Combine the melon cubes and cherries. Place frozen grapefruit slices on lettuce and top each with melon-cherry mixture.

4 servings.

   1 serving = 113 calories
              0 cholesterol
              trace fat

TOMATO-CUCUMBER MARINADE

2 medium tomatoes, sliced
1 medium cucumber, scored and thinly sliced (about 2 cups)
¼ cup sliced green onion (with tops)
½ cup vegetable oil
¼ cup plus 2 tablespoons tarragon wine vinegar
2 teaspoons dried salad herbs
½ teaspoon garlic salt
¼ teaspoon dry mustard

Alternate layers of tomato, cucumber, and onion in deep bowl. Shake remaining ingredients in tightly covered jar. Pour on vegetables in bowl. Cover and refrigerate 5 to 6 hours to blend flavors.

6 servings.

   1 serving = 100 calories
              0 cholesterol
              9 gm fat

FOURTH-OF-JULY POTATO SALAD

¼ teaspoon mustard seed
¼ teaspoon dill seed
1 tablespoon water
1½ cups diced cooked potatoes
2 tablespoons thinly sliced celery
1 tablespoon sliced green onion
1 teaspoon lemon juice
1 hard-cooked egg, chopped
¼ cup Cooked Dressing (below)
2 red radishes

Mix mustard seed, dill seed, and water; let stand at least 1 hour. Toss seed mixture, potatoes, celery, onion, and lemon juice. Stir in egg and dressing. Cover and refrigerate.

Remove stem and root ends from radishes. Cut thin petals around radishes; place in bowl of ice and water to crispen. At serving time, garnish potato salad with radish "roses."

8 servings.

   1 serving = 46 calories
              32 mg cholesterol
              1 gm fat

1 tablespoon flour
1 tablespoon sugar
¾ tablespoon dry mustard
Dash cayenne pepper
3 tablespoons egg substitute
⅓ cup skim milk
2 tablespoons vinegar
1 teaspoon unsalted margarine

Mix flour, sugar, mustard, and cayenne pepper in small saucepan. Stir in egg substitute and milk. Heat to boiling, stirring constantly, until mixture thickens and boils. Remove from heat; stir in vinegar and margarine. Store in covered container in refrigerator.

About ½ cup.

   1 tablespoon = 24 calories
                 trace cholesterol
                 trace fat

VEGETABLE SALAD

3 medium unpared potatoes
5 beets, pared
1 onion
3 or 4 peppercorns
1 bay leaf
1 slice lemon
¼ cup low-fat mayonnaise
1 tablespoon wine vinegar
Freshly ground pepper
Red cabbage leaves

Wash potatoes. Place potatoes, beets, onion, peppercorns, bay leaf, and lemon slice in large saucepan. Add water to cover vegetables. Cover and cook until tender, 30 to 40 minutes. As each vegetable becomes tender, remove with tongs and cool. Peel potatoes and cut into cubes. Cut beets into julienne strips and chop onion; place in bowl. Mix mayonnaise and vinegar; pour on vegetables and mix gently. Season with pepper. Cover and refrigerate at least 2 hours. Serve salad in bowl lined with cabbage leaves.

6 servings.

1 serving = 104 calories
0 cholesterol
3 gm fat

Note: Because of the beets, the potatoes will pick up a red tinge.

BROCCOLI VINAIGRETTE

1½ pounds broccoli
1 small onion, sliced
¼ cup lemon juice
¼ cup wine vinegar
½ cup vegetable oil
¼ teaspoon Tabasco sauce
¼ teaspoon ginger
2 teaspoons tarragon

Trim large leaves from broccoli; remove tough ends of lower stems. Wash broccoli. If stems are thicker than 1 inch in diameter, make lengthwise gashes in each stem. Heat 1 inch water to boiling in saucepan. Add broccoli; cover and heat to boiling. Cook until crisp-tender, 12 to 15 minutes. Drain and cool under running cold water.

Place broccoli in shallow baking dish; top with onion. Beat remaining ingredients or shake in tightly covered jar; pour on vegetables in dish. Cover and refrigerate 2 to 3 hours. Drain excess oil and serve.

6 servings.

1 serving = 151 calories
0 cholesterol
12 gm fat

MINTED CUCUMBERS

2 medium cucumbers
1 carton (8 ounces) low-fat yogurt
1 teaspoon garlic powder
1 teaspoon dried mint leaves, crushed

Pare cucumbers; cut lengthwise into halves and thinly slice into bowl. (There should be about 2 cups.) Mix yogurt and garlic powder; pour on cucumber slices and toss. Sprinkle mint leaves on top.

6 servings.

1 serving = 28 calories
3 mg cholesterol
trace fat

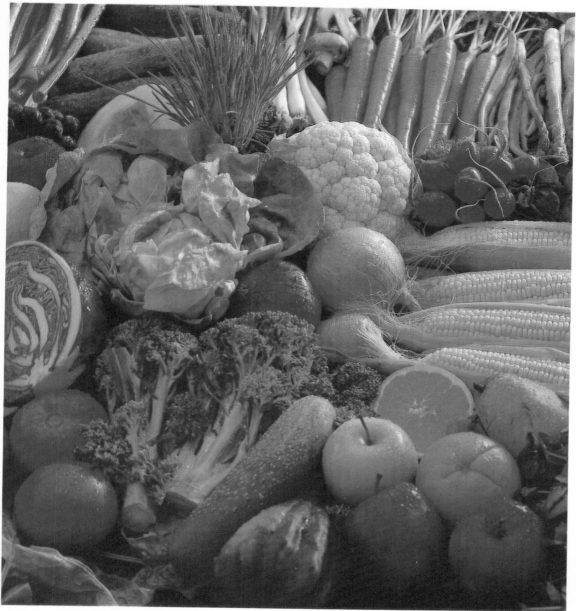

Fruits and Vegetables.

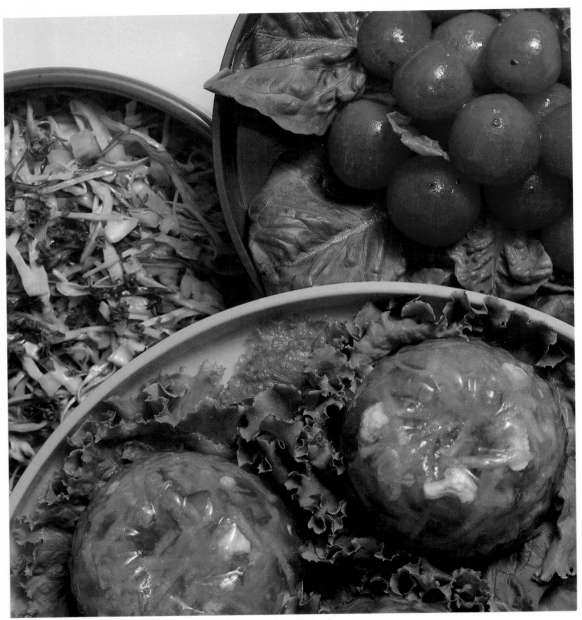

Cherry Tomatoes with Garlic; Molded Vegetable Salad;
Green and Red Cabbage Slaw.

CABBAGE and CARROT SLAW

½ cup low-fat mayonnaise
1 tablespoon sugar
2 tablespoons lemon juice
½ teaspoon pepper
6 cups shredded cabbage
2 cups shredded carrot
2 cups orange sections, cut up

Mix mayonnaise, sugar, lemon juice, and pepper in large bowl. Add cabbage, carrots, and orange sections and toss until coated. Cover and refrigerate 2 to 3 hours.

12 servings.

1 serving = 74 calories
0 cholesterol
3 gm fat

CITRUS SLAW

1 can (16 ounces) unsweetened grapefruit sections
1 medium head cabbage, shredded (about 4 cups)
1 green pepper, thinly sliced
¾ cup low-fat mayonnaise
¼ teaspoon mace
¼ teaspoon ginger
¼ teaspoon Tabasco sauce

Drain grapefruit sections; reserve juice. Combine cabbage and green pepper in salad bowl. Mix ¼ cup plus 2 tablespoons reserved grapefruit juice, the mayonnaise, mace, ginger, and Tabasco sauce. Stir in grapefruit sections; pour over cabbage mixture and toss.

Twelve ½-cup servings.

1 serving = 69 calories
0 mg cholesterol
5 gm fat

HOT CABBAGE SLAW

1 small green cabbage (about 1 pound)
¼ cup chopped onion
1 tablespoon margarine
2 tablespoons vinegar
3 tablespoons water
⅛ teaspoon salt
⅛ teaspoon freshly ground pepper
¼ teaspoon basil
1 teaspoon caraway seed
¼ teaspoon dry mustard

Remove outside leaves of cabbage and discard. Cut cabbage into wedges; remove core and cut cabbage into thin shreds.

Cook and stir onion in margarine in large skillet until tender. Stir in vinegar, water, salt, pepper, basil, caraway seed, and mustard. Stir in cabbage, cover, and cook over medium-low heat until cabbage is crisp-tender, about 10 minutes.

4 servings.

1 serving = 68 calories
0 cholesterol
3 gm fat

GREEN and RED CABBAGE SLAW

1 cup shredded green cabbage
1 cup shredded red cabbage
½ cup chopped celery
¼ cup minced onion
⅛ teaspoon pepper
2 teaspoons lemon juice
2 tablespoons low-fat mayonnaise
Snipped parsley

Measure all ingredients except parsley into salad bowl and toss. Garnish with parsley.

4 servings.

1 serving = 39 calories
0 cholesterol
2 gm fat

MARINATED MUSHROOM SALAD

½ pound mushrooms, sliced
½ cup thinly sliced onion
⅓ cup vegetable oil
1 clove garlic, minced
¼ teaspoon dry mustard
3 tablespoons snipped parsley
¼ cup wine vinegar
2 drops Tabasco sauce
1 head lettuce

Combine mushrooms and onion in salad bowl. Mix oil, garlic, mustard, parsley, vinegar, and pepper sauce; pour on mushrooms and onion and toss. Cover and refrigerate at least 4 hours.

At serving time, tear lettuce into bite-size pieces and toss with mushroom-onion mixture.

6 servings.

1 serving = 145 calories
0 cholesterol
12 gm fat

HERBED TOMATOES

1 teaspoon basil
1 teaspoon snipped chives
¼ teaspoon tarragon
Freshly ground pepper
Grated peel and juice of 1 lemon
1 teaspoon grated orange peel
1 tablespoon orange juice
3 tablespoons (unsalted) tomato juice
4 medium tomatoes, peeled and sliced

Shake all ingredients except tomatoes in tightly covered jar. Refrigerate 2 hours. At serving time, pour on tomatoes.

6 servings.

1 serving = 25 calories
0 cholesterol
trace fat

CHICK-PEA SALAD

2 cans (20 ounces each) chick peas (garbanzo beans), drained
1 green pepper, finely chopped
½ red pepper, finely chopped
1 onion, chopped
2 tablespoons snipped parsley
½ cup olive oil
½ cup vinegar
1 teaspoon dry mustard
1 teaspoon Dijon-style mustard
Freshly ground pepper
¼ teaspoon salt
¼ teaspoon crushed thyme
1 tablespoon minced shallot
1 clove garlic, crushed

Combine chick peas, green pepper, red pepper, onion, and parsley in large salad bowl.

Shake remaining ingredients in tightly covered 16-ounce jar. Pour over chick-pea mixture and toss until ingredients are well coated. Cover and refrigerate at least 2 hours. Toss and drain before serving.

8 servings.

1 serving = 226 calories
0 cholesterol
6 gm fat

WATERCRESS and ORANGE SALAD

1 bunch watercress, washed and chilled
1 head romaine lettuce, washed and chilled
1½ cups orange sections
Gourmet Dressing (page 95)

Tear greens into bite-size pieces into bowl. Add orange sections; pour dressing on salad mixture.

6 servings.

1 serving = 56 calories
0 cholesterol
trace fat

TOMATO SALAD

⅓ cup French Dressing (page 95)
1 tablespoon snipped parsley
1 teaspoon dill seed
1 teaspoon chervil
½ teaspoon rosemary
3 tomatoes, peeled and sliced
1 medium cucumber, thinly sliced
2 medium onions, thinly sliced and
   separated into rings

Mix dressing, parsley, dill seed, chervil, and rosemary in large bowl. Add tomatoes, cucumber, and onions and toss. Cover and refrigerate to blend flavors.

6 servings.
   1 serving = 106 calories
                 0 cholesterol
                 8 gm fat

ZUCCHINI SALAD

6 cups thinly sliced zucchini (3 medium)
2 tablespoons snipped parsley
3 tablespoons lemon juice
2 tablespoons vegetable oil
¼ teaspoon salt
¼ teaspoon freshly ground pepper
1 clove garlic, peeled and slit
3 cups shredded salad greens
⅓ cup thinly sliced radish

Measure zucchini, parsley, lemon juice, oil, salt, pepper, and garlic into bowl. Cover and refrigerate 1 hour.

Remove garlic. Arrange ½ cup salad greens on each of 6 plates. Top each with 1 cup zucchini mixture. Garnish with radish and, if desired, cherry tomatoes.

6 servings.
   1 serving = 71 calories
               0 cholesterol
               4 gm fat

FRESH CORN VINAIGRETTE

8 ears corn, husks and silk removed
½ cup vegetable oil
¼ cup cider vinegar
1½ teaspoons lemon juice
3 tablespoons snipped parsley
¼ teaspoon dry mustard
1 teaspoon sugar
½ teaspoon basil
¼ teaspoon cayenne pepper
2 large tomatoes, peeled and chopped
½ cup chopped green pepper
½ cup chopped scallions

Fill large kettle half full with water; heat to boiling. Add corn; cover and heat to boiling. Remove from heat and let stand 5 minutes. Drain corn and cool.

Mix oil, vinegar, lemon juice, parsley, mustard, sugar, basil, and cayenne pepper in large bowl. Cut corn from cobs. Stir corn, tomatoes, green pepper, and scallions into oil-vinegar mixture. Cover and refrigerate 2 to 3 hours. Drain and serve.

8 servings.
   1 serving = 166 calories
                 0 cholesterol
                 8 gm fat

TOMATO PREPARATION

Wash and cut into quarters or ¾-inch slices. If desired, peel tomatoes before cutting. To remove skin easily, dip tomato in boiling water ½ minute, then in cold water. Or scrape surface of tomato with blade of knife to loosen.

CHERRY TOMATOES with GARLIC

2 pints cherry tomatoes
Boiling water
¼ cup vegetable oil
2 tablespoons wine vinegar
2 cloves garlic, crushed
¼ teaspoon salt
Freshly ground pepper
6 Bibb lettuce leaves
3 tablespoons snipped parsley

Dip tomatoes into boiling water; peel off skins. Place tomatoes in shallow bowl. Mix oil, vinegar, garlic, salt, and pepper ; pour on tomatoes. Cover and refrigerate at least 1 hour.

Drain tomatoes, reserving marinade; arrange tomatoes on lettuce leaves and sprinkle with parsley. If desired, serve marinade as dressing.

6 servings.
1 serving = 46 calories
0 cholesterol
2 gm fat

CUCUMBERS in YOGURT

3 medium cucumbers
1 cup low-fat yogurt
1 tablespoon lemon juice
1 tablespoon snipped chives
⅛ teaspoon paprika

Pare cucumbers and slice thinly. Mix remaining ingredients with fork. Cover and refrigerate yogurt mixture and cucumbers separately.

Just before serving, add cucumbers to yogurt mixture and toss until all slices are coated.

6 servings.
1 serving = 29 calories
3 mg cholesterol
trace fat

SPINACH SALAD PROVENÇAL

1 clove garlic, peeled and halved
¼ cup olive or vegetable oil
¼ pound spinach
1 head curly endive, washed and chilled
10 cherry tomatoes, cut into halves
¾ teaspoon oregano leaves
¼ teaspoon freshly ground pepper
1 tablespoon wine vinegar
1 tablespoon lemon juice
¼ teaspoon dry mustard
¼ teaspoon salt

Add garlic to oil and let stand 1 hour. Wash spinach; remove stems and dry leaves. Remove garlic from oil and rub on inside of salad bowl. Tear spinach leaves and endive into bite-size pieces into bowl. Add tomato halves. Mix remaining ingredients and garlic oil; pour on salad mixture and toss.

8 servings.
1 serving = 82 calories
0 cholesterol
7 gm fat

THREE-GREEN SALAD

2 heads endive, washed
2 heads Bibb lettuce, washed and chilled
½ bunch watercress, washed and chilled
Leaf lettuce, washed and chilled
Gourmet Dressing (page 95)

Cut endive into quarters, place in large bowl, pour lukewarm water on endive and let stand 10 minutes to remove bitterness. Drain and chill.

Tear Bibb lettuce into bite-size pieces into salad bowl. Tear leaf lettuce into bite-size pieces to measure ¼ cup. Add watercress and endive. Pour dressing on greens and toss.

4 servings.
1 serving = 43 calories
0 cholesterol
trace fat

ENDIVE SALAD

2 tablespoons red wine vinegar
3 tablespoons olive oil
3 tablespoons safflower oil
2 teaspoons Dijon-type mustard
2 teaspoons lemon juice
½ teaspoon salt
Freshly ground pepper
5 to 6 heads endive
2 tablespoons snipped parsley

Shake vinegar, oils, mustard, lemon juice, salt, and pepper in tightly covered jar.

Remove core from each endive head by cutting wedge-shaped piece from root end, then slice endive diagonally for long oval pieces. Place endive in large salad bowl; add parsley and dressing and toss.

6 to 8 servings.

> 1 serving = 122 calories
> 0 cholesterol
> 10 gm fat

CAESAR SALAD

1 clove garlic, split
¼ cup olive oil
3 tablespoons wine vinegar
⅛ teaspoon dry mustard
⅛ teaspoon onion powder
⅛ teaspoon garlic powder
1 teaspoon sugar
Freshly ground pepper
1 head romaine lettuce
1 egg, beaten

Rub wooden salad bowl with cut clove of garlic. Measure oil, vinegar, and seasonings into bowl and mix thoroughly. Tear lettuce into bite-size pieces (about 8 cups) into bowl. Toss until leaves glisten. Add egg and toss until leaves are well coated.

8 servings.

> 1 serving = 96 calories
> 31 mg cholesterol
> 7 gm fat

LOBSTER SALAD

2 quarts water (8 cups)
1 bay leaf
2 packages (8 ounces each) frozen lobster tails
2 tablespoons lemon juice
1 apple, pared and diced
1 orange, pared and sectioned
½ cup halved green grapes
¼ cup plus 2 tablespoons low-fat mayonnaise
2 tablespoons skim milk
1 tablespoon Dijon-Type Mustard (page 187)
1 tablespoon minced scallion
1 teaspoon tarragon
Lettuce

Heat water and bay leaf in large saucepan to boiling. Add lobster tails and lemon juice; cook over medium heat 15 minutes, or cook lobster tails as directed on package. Drain and cool. Remove meat from shell; cut into pieces and chill.

Combine lobster and fruits in bowl. Mix mayonnaise, milk, mustard, scallion, and tarragon; pour on salad and mix. Serve in lettuce-lined bowl.

4 servings.

> 1 serving = 221 calories
> 76 mg cholesterol
> 10 gm fat

SPINACH and CAULIFLOWER SALAD

3 tablespoons wine vinegar
¼ cup plus 2 tablespoons vegetable oil
⅛ teaspoon pepper
½ teaspoon dry mustard
2 tablespoons snipped parsley
1 large clove garlic, peeled and halved
1 bag (10 ounces) spinach
½ cauliflower, separated into flowerets
½ red onion, sliced and separated into rings
½ cup sliced radish

Mix vinegar, oil, pepper, mustard, and parsley in salad bowl; add garlic and let stand ½ to 1 hour.

Wash spinach; remove stems and dry leaves. Remove garlic from bowl and discard. Tear spinach leaves into bite-size pieces into bowl. Add cauliflowerets, onion, and radish slices and toss until vegetables are well coated.

6 servings.

1 serving = 159 calories
0 cholesterol
13 gm fat

JUBILATION SALAD

2 bunches watercress
3 green onions (with tops), chopped
¼ cup slivered green pepper
1 medium navel orange, pared, sectioned, and cut up
½ cup grapefruit sections, cut up
3 tablespoons wine vinegar
1 tablespoon vegetable oil
Freshly ground pepper

Remove imperfect leaves and stems from watercress and discard. Toss watercress leaves, onion, and green pepper. Cover with damp towel and refrigerate.

Just before serving time, add remaining ingredients and toss.

4 servings.

1 serving = 64 calories
0 cholesterol
3 gm fat

CHICKEN SALAD PLATE

Chicken Salad (page 91)
2 small tomatoes
2 lettuce leaves
Freshly ground pepper

Prepare Chicken Salad. Cut off stem ends of tomatoes. With cut side down, cut each tomato into sixths, cutting through to within 1 inch of bottom. Carefully spread sections, forming a "flower." Sprinkle inside of each tomato flower with freshly ground pepper and fill with chicken salad. Serve on lettuce.

2 servings.

1 serving = 153 calories
51 mg cholesterol
6 gm fat

Variations: Substitute small red apples, pineapple wedges, or halves of green pepper, artichoke, cucumber, or cantaloupe for the tomatoes.

CHICKEN SALAD

½ green pepper, finely chopped
1 tablespoon finely chopped onion
4 ounces diced cooked chicken
1 tablespoon low-fat mayonnaise
½ teaspoon sugar
½ teaspoon dry mustard
¼ teaspoon freshly ground pepper
¼ teaspoon paprika
⅛ teaspoon salt

Combine green pepper, onion, and chicken in bowl. Mix mayonnaise and remaining ingredients; pour on chicken mixture and toss.
2 servings.

Variations: Substitute 4 ounces drained tuna, crabmeat, salmon, or cooked white fish for the chicken.

1 serving
Crabmeat
Salad Plate = 125 calories
61 mg cholesterol
4 gm fat

1 serving
Tuna
Salad Plate = 139 calories
38 mg cholesterol
3 gm fat

1 serving
Salmon
Salad Plate = 148 calories
21 mg cholesterol
7 gm fat

1 serving
Fish
Salad Plate = 135 calories
40 mg cholesterol
5 gm fat

FISH SALAD

2 pounds poached fish (page 152), cooled, or 2 cups cooked fish and shellfish
4 scallions (with tops), chopped, or 2 tablespoons minced onion
1 medium green pepper, finely chopped
¼ cup vegetable oil
2 tablespoons tarragon vinegar
½ teaspoon dry mustard
⅛ teaspoon garlic powder
½ teaspoon oregano
2 tablespoons snipped parsley
Freshly ground pepper
2 tablespoons imitation sour cream
Juice of ½ lemon
Lemon wedges (2½ lemons)

Cut fish into bite-size pieces and place in bowl. Mix remaining ingredients except sour cream, lemon juice, and lemon wedges. Pour on fish and toss. Cover and refrigerate 2 to 3 hours.

Stir in sour cream and lemon juice. Just before serving, squeeze juice from wedges of half lemon on salad. Serve with remaining wedges. If desired, serve salad on chicory and garnish with cherry tomatoes.

4 servings.

1 serving = 362 calories
84 mg cholesterol
28 gm fat

TUNA SALAD

2 cans (7 ounces each) tuna packed in
water, drained and flaked
½ cup chopped celery
¾ cup chopped onion
2 tablespoons lemon juice
½ cup low-fat mayonnaise
Freshly ground pepper
Salad greens
4 medium tomatoes, quartered
2 cucumbers, sliced
Lemon wedges

Combine tuna, celery, and onion in bowl. Mix lemon juice, mayonnaise, and pepper; pour on tuna mixture and toss.

Serve on salad greens with tomato wedges, cucumber slices, and lemon wedges.

6 servings.

1 serving = 175 calories
42 mg cholesterol
6 gm fat

EGG SALAD

1 tablespoon margarine or vegetable oil
1 cup egg substitute
¼ cup chopped onion
¼ cup chopped green pepper
½ cup chopped celery
¼ cup low-fat mayonnaise

Melt margarine in large skillet. Add egg substitute and cook over low heat until set. (Do not stir.) Turn onto large plate; cool.

Cut mixture into small pieces; turn into bowl. Stir in onion, green pepper, celery, and mayonnaise.

4 servings.

1 serving = 123 calories
0 cholesterol
9 gm fat

MAYONNAISE

1 tablespoon plus 2 teaspoons
white wine vinegar
3 tablespoons egg substitute
1 teaspoon sugar
1 teaspoon dry mustard
¼ teaspoon white pepper
Dash cayenne pepper
1 cup vegetable oil

In small mixer bowl, beat vinegar, egg substitute, sugar, mustard, pepper, and cayenne pepper until blended. Continue beating, adding oil by the teaspoonful; as mixture thickens, increase amounts of oil. Store in tightly covered container in refrigerator.

About 1½ cups.

1 tablespoon = 82 calories
0 cholesterol
9 gm fat

LOW-CALORIE SALAD DRESSING

1 teaspoon unflavored gelatin
1¼ cups tomato juice
2 tablespoons vinegar
1 clove garlic, peeled
⅛ teaspoon salt
¼ teaspoon Tabasco sauce
1 tablespoon vegetable oil

Sprinkle gelatin on ¼ cup of the tomato juice in small saucepan to soften. Stir over low heat until gelatin is dissolved, 2 to 3 minutes. Remove from heat; stir in remaining ingredients. Cover and refrigerate. Shake or stir before using.

1¼ cups.

1 tablespoon = 21 calories
0 cholesterol
trace fat

LEMON SESAME DRESSING

⅓ cup vegetable oil
Juice of 1 lemon
1 tablespoon toasted sesame seed,
  (see *Note*)
2 teaspoons sugar
½ teaspoon onion salt
  Shake all ingredients in tightly covered jar.
  About ½ cup.

    1 tablespoon = 83 calories
                    0 cholesterol
                    9 gm fat

  Note: To toast sesame seed, heat in 350°
oven 10 to 15 minutes until golden.

FRUIT SALAD DRESSING

½ cup olive oil
½ cup unsweetened pineapple juice
1 teaspoon brown sugar
1 teaspoon lemon juice
1 banana, cut up
¼ orange, cut up
  Place all ingredients in blender; blend on
high speed until smooth. Store in tightly covered jar in refrigerator. Shake before using.
  1½ cups.

    1 tablespoon = 48 calories
                    0 cholesterol
                    4 gm fat

HONEY DRESSING

½ cup honey
2 tablespoons lemon or lime juice
⅛ teaspoon Tabasco sauce
  Mix all ingredients.
  About ½ cup.

    1 tablespoon = 63 calories
                    0 cholesterol
                    0 fat

CREAMY COOKED DRESSING

1 tablespoon flour
1 tablespoon sugar
¾ teaspoon dry mustard
⅛ teaspoon salt
Dash cayenne pepper
3 tablespoons egg substitute
⅓ cup skim milk
2 tablespoons vinegar
1 teaspoon margarine
  Mix flour, sugar, mustard, salt, and cayenne
pepper in small saucepan. Stir in egg substitute and milk. Heat to boiling, stirring constantly, until mixture thickens and boils. Remove from heat; stir in vinegar and margarine.
Store in covered container in refrigerator.
  About ½ cup.

    1 tablespoon = 25 calories
                    trace cholesterol
                    1 gm fat

OIL-AND-VINEGAR DRESSING

½ cup safflower oil
¼ cup olive oil
¼ cup wine vinegar
Salt and pepper
5 cloves garlic, crushed
2 teaspoons dried tarragon
2 teaspoons dried basil
2 teaspoons dried chervil
Snipped fresh chives, if available
¼ cup snipped parsley or 5
  tablespoons parsley flakes
  Shake all ingredients in tightly covered jar.
Refrigerate at least 2 hours to blend flavors.
Shake before serving.
  1 cup.

    1 tablespoon = 96 calories
                    0 cholesterol
                    10 gm fat

CONNOISSEUR FRENCH DRESSING

½ cup vegetable oil
3 tablespoons wine vinegar
2 tablespoons lemon juice
1 tablespoon chopped onion or snipped
  chives
2 teaspoons snipped parsley
1¾ teaspoons paprika
½ teaspoon basil
⅛ teaspoon pepper
1½ cloves garlic, peeled

Shake all ingredients in tightly covered jar. Refrigerate at least 12 hours to blend flavors. Remove garlic. Shake before serving.

About ¾ cup.

1 tablespoon = 84 calories
0 cholesterol
9 gm fat

VINAIGRETTE DRESSING and VARIATIONS

¾ cup safflower oil
¼ cup wine vinegar
⅛ teaspoon salt
Dash freshly ground pepper

Shake all ingredients in tightly covered jar.

1 cup.

1 tablespoon = 89 calories
0 cholesterol
10 gm fat

VARIATION 1

⅔ cup safflower oil
⅓ cup lemon juice
⅛ teaspoon salt
Dash freshly ground pepper
1 clove garlic, minced

Shake all ingredients in tightly covered jar.

1 tablespoon = 80 calories
0 cholesterol
9 gm fat

VARIATION 2

1 cup safflower oil
⅓ cup wine vinegar
¼ teaspoon Dijon-type mustard
⅛ teaspoon salt
Dash freshly ground pepper
1 egg white
2 tablespoons snipped parsley

Shake all ingredients in tightly covered jar.

1 tablespoon = 120 calories
0 cholesterol
13 gm fat

VARIATION 3

¾ cup safflower oil
¼ cup red wine vinegar
1 tablespoon minced shallot
2 tablespoons snipped fresh herbs
  (chervil, tarragon, basil, thyme, chives)
⅛ teaspoon salt
Dash freshly ground pepper

Shake all ingredients in tightly covered jar.

1 tablespoon = 94 calories
0 cholesterol
10 gm fat

VARIATION 4

¾ cup safflower oil
¼ cup lemon juice
½ teaspoon dry mustard
3 tablespoons evaporated skim milk
⅛ teaspoon salt
Dash freshly ground pepper
1 teaspoon sweet paprika

Shake all ingredients in tightly covered jar.

1 tablespoon = 93 calories
0 cholesterol
10 gm fat

CURRIED FRUIT SALAD DRESSING

¾ cup low-fat yogurt
¼ cup low-fat mayonnaise
1 teaspoon sugar
1 teaspoon curry powder
⅛ teaspoon salt
1 teaspoon finely chopped crystallized
   ginger
½ teaspoon lemon juice

Mix all ingredients. Cover and refrigerate at least 2 hours.

1 cup.

1 tablespoon = 19 calories
                      trace cholesterol
                      1 gm fat

ZESTY FRENCH DRESSING

⅔ cup vegetable oil
⅓ cup lemon juice or vinegar
½ teaspoon Tabasco sauce
1 teaspoon paprika
1 teaspoon dry mustard
½ teaspoon sugar

Shake all ingredients in tightly covered jar. Serve with avocado, tomato, and onion salad or with salad greens.

1 cup.

1 tablespoon = 83 calories
                      0 cholesterol
                      9 gm fat

BASIC SALAD DRESSING

¼ cup vegetable oil
1 tablespoon low-fat mayonnaise
1 tablespoon wine vinegar
⅛ teaspoon salt
⅛ teaspoon pepper
Dash garlic powder

Mix all ingredients thoroughly. Cover and refrigerate until ready to use.

About ¼ cup.

1 tablespoon = 124 calories
                      0 cholesterol
                      14 gm fat

FRENCH DRESSING

1 cup vegetable oil
½ cup cider vinegar
1 tablespoon sugar
1 teaspoon paprika
1 teaspoon lemon juice
½ teaspoon dry mustard
1 clove garlic, peeled

Shake all ingredients in tightly covered jar. Refrigerate. Remove garlic and shake again before serving.

About 1½ cups.

1 tablespoon = 83 calories
                      0 cholesterol
                      9 gm fat

GOURMET DRESSING

¾ cup vegetable oil
1 tablespoon olive oil
2 tablespoons wine vinegar
1 tablespoon sugar
¼ teaspoon salt
Freshly ground pepper
¼ cup snipped parsley
1 tablespoon tarragon
1 tablespoon snipped chives
1 tablespoon snipped dill
2 shallots, chopped

Measure all ingredients into blender; blend until smooth.

1½ cups.

1 tablespoon = 71 calories
                      0 cholesterol
                      7 gm fat

Eggs, Soups, and Sandwiches

OMELET

1 tablespoon margarine
1 cup egg substitute

Stir Method: Melt margarine in 8-inch skillet or omelet pan over medium heat. Pour egg substitute into skillet. With left hand, slide skillet back and forth rapidly over heat. At the same time, stir quickly with fork to spread egg substitute continuously over bottom of skillet as it thickens. Let stand over heat a few seconds to cook.

Tilt skillet; run fork under edge of omelet, then jerk skillet sharply to loosen omelet from bottom of skillet. If filling is used, spoon on center. With fork, fold portion of omelet nearest you just to center.

Grasp skillet handle and turn omelet onto warm plate, flipping folded portion of omelet over so that far side is on bottom.

Lift Method: Melt margarine in 8-inch skillet or omelet pan over medium heat. Pour egg substitute into skillet. Do not stir. As mixture begins to set at bottom and side, gently lift cooked portion with spatula so that thin uncooked portion can flow to bottom. When almost set, cover pan and cook until top of omelet is set, 2 minutes. If desired, spoon filling on half of omelet. Fold other half onto filling. With large spatula, lift or slide omelet onto warm plate.

2 servings.

1 serving = 143 calories
0 cholesterol
10 gm fat

Ratatouille Omelet: Fill omelet with 1 cup Ratatouille (page 183).

1 serving = 254 calories
0 cholesterol
19 gm fat

Herb Omelet: Before pouring egg substitute into skillet, sprinkle 1 tablespoon each snipped chives and snipped parsley on margarine in skillet.

1 serving = 146 calories
0 cholesterol
10 gm fat

Mushroom Omelet: Before pouring egg substitute into skillet, cook and stir ¼ cup chopped mushroom and 1 tablespoon snipped parsley in margarine 1 minute.

1 serving = 122 calories
0 cholesterol
8 gm fat

Green Pepper Omelet: Before pouring egg substitute into skillet, cook and stir ¼ cup chopped green pepper and 2 tablespoons minced onion in margarine 1 minute.

> 1 serving = 150 calories
>   0 cholesterol
>   10 gm fat

Apple Omelet: Before pouring egg substitute into skillet, cook and stir 1 small apple, sliced, in margarine. Stir in 1 teaspoon sugar and ¼ teaspoon cinnamon. Remove apple mixture and set aside. Before removing omelet, spoon apple mixture on half the omelet.

> 1 serving = 177 calories
>   0 cholesterol
>   10 gm fat

Cheese Omelet: Before pouring egg substitute into skillet, sprinkle 1 tablespoon snipped chives and 1 tablespoon snipped parsley on margarine. Sprinkle ¼ cup shredded skim-milk mozzarella cheese on omelet when rolling it.

> 1 serving = 211 calories
>   16 mg cholesterol
>   14 gm fat

OMELET FRANÇAIS

3 eggs
2 tablespoons snipped parsley
1 teaspoon snipped fresh or ½ teaspoon dried tarragon leaves
½ teaspoon snipped fresh or ¼ teaspoon dried thyme leaves
⅛ teaspoon pepper
2 teaspoons chopped shallots or green onions
1 tablespoon margarine

Beat eggs with fork until whites and yolks are blended. Stir in parsley, tarragon, thyme, pepper, and shallots. Heat margarine in 8-inch skillet or omelet pan over medium-high heat. As margarine melts, tilt skillet in all directions to coat side thoroughly. When margarine just begins to brown, skillet is hot enough to use.

Quickly pour egg mixture all at once into skillet. With left hand, slide skillet back and forth rapidly over heat. At the same time, stir quickly with fork to spread eggs continuously over bottom of skillet as they thicken. Let stand over heat a few seconds to brown bottom of omelet lightly; do not overcook. (Omelet will continue to cook after folding.)

Tilt skillet; run fork under edge of omelet, then jerk skillet sharply to loosen eggs from bottom of skillet. With fork, fold portion of omelet nearest you just to center. (Allow for portion of omelet to slide up side of skillet.)

Grasp skillet handle and turn omelet onto warm plate, flipping folded portion of omelet over so that far side is on bottom. If necessary, tuck sides of omelet under.

3 servings.

> 1 serving = 123 calories
>   252 mg cholesterol
>   10 gm fat

IRISH OMELET

1 small potato, pared and cubed
1 tablespoon vegetable oil
1 egg white
2 tablespoons egg substitute
1 tablespoon snipped chives
Freshly ground pepper

In small skillet, cook and stir potato cubes in oil until tender but not brown. Remove from skillet; drain and cool to lukewarm. Beat egg white and egg substitute with fork until just blended; stir in potato cubes, chives, and pepper. Heat skillet. Pour egg mixture into skillet. Slide skillet back and forth rapidly over heat. At same time, stir quickly with fork to spread egg mixture continuously over bottom of skillet as it thickens. Let stand over heat a few seconds to brown bottom of omelet lightly; do not overcook. (Omelet will continue to cook after folding.)

Tilt skillet; run fork under edge of omelet, then jerk skillet sharply to loosen egg mixture from bottom of skillet. With fork, fold portion of omelet nearest you just to center. (Allow for portion of omelet to slide up side of skillet.)

Grasp skillet handle and turn omelet onto warm plate, flipping folded portion of omelet over so that far side is on bottom. (If necessary, tuck sides of omelet under.)

1 serving.

1 serving = 219 calories
0 cholesterol
14 gm fat

OMELET SOUFFLÉ

4 eggs, separated
2 tablespoons water
Dash pepper
1 teaspoon unsalted margarine

Beat egg whites in small mixer bowl until stiff but not dry. Beat egg yolks, water, and pepper until thick and lemon colored. Fold into egg whites.

Heat oven to 325°. Heat margarine in large skillet with ovenproof handle until just hot enough to sizzle a drop of water. Pour egg mixture into skillet; level surface gently. Reduce heat; cook slowly until puffy and light brown on bottom, about 5 minutes. (Lift omelet at edge to judge color.)

Place in oven; bake until knife inserted in center comes out clean, 12 to 15 minutes. Tip skillet and loosen omelet by slipping pancake turner or spatula under. Fold omelet in half, being careful not to break it; slip onto warm platter. Serve immediately.

4 servings.

1 serving = 88 calories
252 mg cholesterol
7 gm fat

MUSHROOM OMELET

½ pound mushrooms, trimmed and sliced
½ cup thinly sliced onion
¼ cup finely chopped green pepper
2 tablespoons vegetable oil
4 egg whites
½ cup egg substitute
Freshly ground pepper

Cook and stir mushrooms, onion and green pepper in oil until onion is tender, 3 to 4 minutes. Mix egg whites and egg substitute until just blended. Pour on vegetables in skillet. Slide skillet back and forth rapidly over heat. At the same time, stir quickly with fork to spread egg mixture continuously over bottom of skillet as it thickens. Let stand over heat a few seconds to brown bottom of omelet lightly; do not overcook. (Omelet will continue to cook after folding.)

Tilt skillet; run fork under edge of omelet, then jerk skillet sharply to loosen egg mixture from bottom of skillet. With fork, fold portion of omelet nearest you just to center. (Allow for portion of omelet to slide up side of skillet.)

Grasp skillet handle and turn omelet onto warm plate, flipping folded portion of omelet over so that far side is on bottom. If necessary, tuck sides of omelet under. Season with pepper.

4 servings.

1 serving = 122 calories
0 cholesterol
8 gm fat

JELLY OMELET

4 eggs
¼ cup skim milk
2 teaspoons margarine
1 tablespoon strawberry jam or jelly
1 teaspoon powdered sugar

Beat eggs until light and fluffy. Stir in milk. Heat margarine in large skillet until just hot enough to sizzle a drop of water. As margarine melts, tilt pan to coat bottom. Pour egg mixture into skillet. Cook over medium heat, lifting edge to allow uncooked portion to flow to bottom, until omelet is light brown on bottom.

Drop jam by small amounts on half the omelet. Tip skillet and loosen omelet by slipping pancake turner or spatula under. Fold omelet in half, being careful not to break it. Slip onto heated platter; sprinkle sugar on top.

4 servings.

1 serving = 110 calories
252 mg cholesterol
8 gm fat

ITALIAN OMELET

½ green pepper, chopped
4 mushrooms, trimmed and sliced
¼ cup chopped pimiento
2 eggs
2 tablespoons vegetable oil
Freshly ground pepper

Spray small skillet with vegetable spray. Cook and stir green pepper in skillet until tender. Add mushrooms and pimiento; cook and stir 1 to 2 minutes. Remove from heat and cool.

Heat oven to 325°. Beat eggs until fluffy. Stir in vegetable mixture. Heat oil in skillet until just hot enough to sizzle a drop of water. Pour egg mixture into skillet. Reduce heat; cook slowly until puffy and light brown on bottom, about 5 minutes. (Lift omelet at edge to judge color.)

Place in oven; bake until knife inserted in center comes out clean.

2 servings.

1 serving = 209 calories
252 mg cholesterol
18 gm fat

OMELET ROLL

1 teaspoon margarine
⅓ cup egg substitute
Freshly ground pepper

Melt margarine in 10-inch skillet; rotate pan to coat bottom with margarine. Pour egg substitute into skillet; slowly rotate pan to spread mixture into thin circle. Cook over medium heat 2 to 3 minutes. Loosen edge; roll up, using small spatula and fork. Season with pepper.

When preparing more than one, keep Omelet Roll warm on ungreased baking sheet in 275° oven.

1 roll = 81 calories
0 cholesterol
5 gm fat

Herb Omelet Roll: Just before rolling egg, sprinkle basil, chervil, thyme, or marjoram and snipped chives on top.

1 roll = 81 calories
0 cholesterol
5 gm fat

Cheese Omelet Roll: Just before rolling egg, sprinkle 2 teaspoons shredded part-skim mozzarella cheese and 1 tablespoon snipped chives on top.

1 roll = 103 calories
5 mg cholesterol
6 gm fat

Jelly Omelet Roll: Just before rolling egg, spread 1 teaspoon jelly or orange marmalade on top.

1 roll = 95 calories
0 cholesterol
5 gm fat

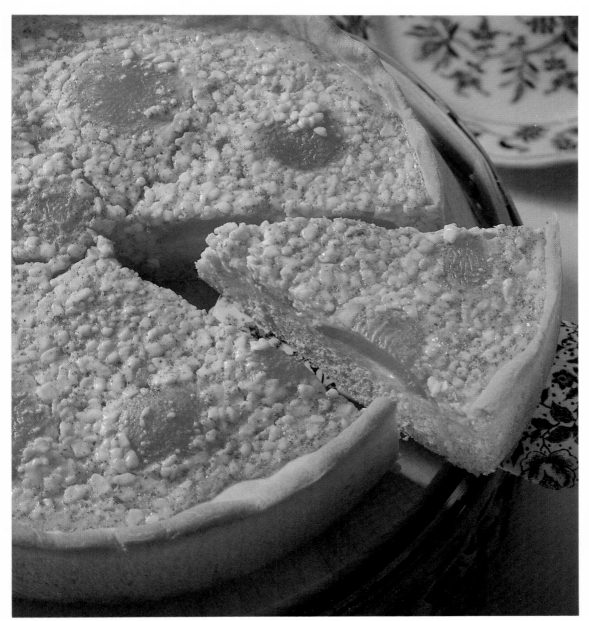

Apricot Coffee Cake.

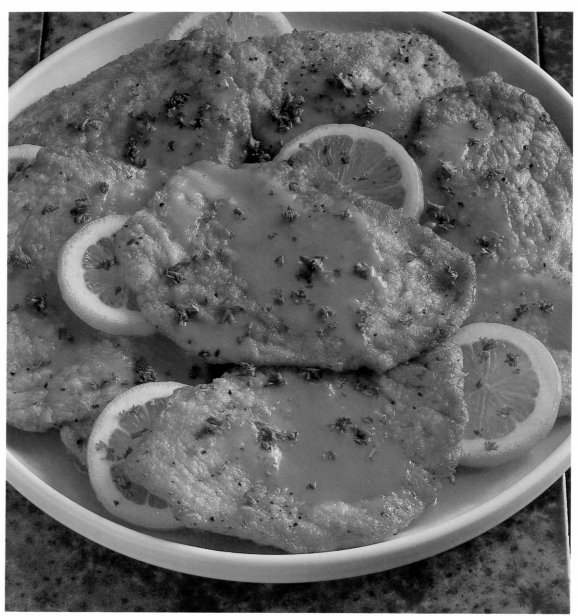

Escalopes de Veau au Citron.

OMELET ROLL with MUSHROOM FILLING

4 ounces mushrooms, trimmed and sliced
¼ cup thinly sliced onion
2 tablespoons finely chopped green
** pepper**
1 tablespoon vegetable oil
Freshly ground pepper
4 Omelet Rolls
2 teaspoons snipped parsley

Cook and stir mushrooms, onion, and green pepper in oil until onion is tender, 3 to 4 minutes. Season with pepper; remove from heat and keep warm.

Prepare 4 Omelet Rolls, cooking one at a time as directed on page 100, except just before rolling egg, place ¼ of mushroom mixture on top. Keep filled rolls warm on ungreased baking sheet in 275° oven. Just before serving, sprinkle rolls with parsley.

4 rolls.

1 roll = 131 calories
         0 cholesterol
         9 gm fat

OMELET ROLL with CREOLE SAUCE

3 Omelet Rolls
1 tablespoon margarine
1 medium onion, chopped
1 small green pepper, chopped
1 large tomato, peeled and diced
¼ teaspoon paprika
2 teaspoons oregano
Dash pepper

Prepare 3 Omelet Rolls, cooking one at a time as directed on page 100. Keep rolls warm on ungreased baking sheet in 275° oven while preparing sauce.

Melt margarine in small saucepan. Cook and stir onion in margarine until tender. Stir in remaining ingredients. Reduce heat; simmer until green pepper is tender, about 10 minutes. Serve ⅓ cup sauce on each Omelet Roll.

3 rolls.

1 roll = 155 calories
         0 cholesterol
         9 gm fat

RATATOUILLE OMELET ROLL

1 small onion, thinly sliced
2 tablespoons vegetable oil
1 medium zucchini, sliced
2 medium tomatoes, peeled and chopped
1 small clove garlic, minced
¼ teaspoon freshly ground pepper
⅛ teaspoon dry mustard
½ teaspoon lemon juice
12 Omelet Rolls
2 tablespoons snipped parsley

Cook and stir onion in oil until tender. Stir in remaining ingredients except Omelet Rolls and parsley. Reduce heat; cover and simmer 3 minutes. Remove from heat and keep warm.

Prepare 12 Omelet Rolls, cooking one at a time as directed on page 100, except just before rolling egg, place 2 tablespoons ratatouille on top. Keep filled rolls warm on ungreased baking sheet in 275° oven. Just before serving, sprinkle rolls with parsley.

12 rolls.

1 roll = 108 calories
0 cholesterol
7 gm fat

CALICO SCRAMBLED EGGS

½ cup green pepper slices
2 tablespoons chopped onion
2 tablespoons vegetable oil
½ cup chopped peeled tomato (seeds removed)
Small bay leaf
2 teaspoons basil
Dash paprika
1 cup egg substitute

Cook and stir green pepper and onion in oil until onion is tender, 3 to 4 minutes. Stir in tomato, bay leaf, basil, and paprika. Heat just to boiling, stirring constantly. Reduce heat; pour egg substitute into skillet and stir with fork until eggs are set. Remove bay leaf.

4 servings.

1 serving = 119 calories
0 cholesterol
9 gm fat

POACHED EGG

2 teaspoons vinegar
1 egg
1 slice bread, toasted
1 teaspoon margarine
Freshly ground pepper
Dash curry powder, sage, or dry mustard

Heat 1½ inches water in small skillet to boiling; reduce to simmer and add vinegar. Break egg into cup or saucer; slip into water, holding cup or saucer close to surface of water.

Cook to desired doneness, 3 to 5 minutes. Remove egg from water with slotted spoon. Place on toast and dot with margarine. Season with pepper and, if desired, with dash curry powder, sage, or dry mustard.

1 serving = 184 calories
252 mg cholesterol
11 gm fat

SCRAMBLED EGGS

4 eggs
2 tablespoons water
¼ teaspoon dry mustard
Dash freshly ground pepper
1 tablespoon margarine

Mix eggs, water, mustard, and pepper with fork, stirring thoroughly for a uniform yellow, or mixing just slightly if streaks of white and yellow are preferred.

Heat margarine in skillet over medium heat until just hot enough to sizzle a drop of water. Pour egg mixture into skillet. As mixture begins to set at bottom and side, gently lift cooked portions with spatula so that thin uncooked portion can flow to bottom. Avoid constant stirring. Cook until eggs are thickened throughout but still moist, 3 to 5 minutes.

4 servings.

        1 serving = 108 calories
                        252 mg cholesterol
                            9 gm fat

Herbed Scrambled Eggs: Substitute snipped chives, snipped parsley, tarragon leaves, or chervil leaves for the dry mustard.

        1 serving = 107 calories
                        252 mg cholesterol
                            9 gm fat

SCRAMBLED EGGS (Egg Substitute)

2 teaspoons vegetable oil or margarine
1 pint (2 cups) egg substitute

Heat oil in large skillet over medium heat. Pour egg substitute into skillet. Cook, stirring frequently with spatula until set, about 2 minutes.

4 servings.

        1 serving = 111 calories
                            0 cholesterol
                            6 gm fat

Variation 1: Before cooking, add 2 tablespoons snipped parsley, 1 teaspoon chopped chives, or ¼ teaspoon tarragon leaves, dill weed, basil, or fines herbes to egg substitute.

        1 serving = 113 calories
                            0 cholesterol
                            6 gm fat

Variation 2: Before removing from heat, sprinkle ½ cup shredded skim-milk mozzarella cheese on top.

        1 serving = 176 calories
                          16 mg cholesterol
                          11 gm fat

MULLIGATAWNY SOUP

¼ cup margarine
6 ounces cut-up, cooked, unsalted chicken
¼ cup sliced carrot (1 medium)
¾ cup sliced unpared apple (1 medium)
1 small onion (2 inches in diameter), sliced
¼ cup diced celery
½ cup water
2 tablespoons flour
1 teaspoon curry powder
¼ teaspoon salt
⅛ teaspoon mace
1 can (16 ounces) tomatoes
2 whole cloves
1 sprig parsley, snipped
1 bay leaf
1 tablespoon lemon juice
¾ cup diced green pepper (1 medium)

Melt margarine in 2-quart saucepan. Cook and stir chicken, carrot, apple, onion, and celery in margarine for 10 minutes. Reduce heat; cover and simmer until carrot is tender, about 20 minutes.

Mix water, flour, curry powder, salt and mace until smooth. Stir flour mixture, tomatoes (with liquid), and remaining ingredients except green pepper into saucepan. Heat to boiling, stirring constantly. Boil and stir 1 minute. Stir in green pepper. Reduce heat; simmer uncovered 10 minutes.

4 servings (1 cup each).

1 serving = 274 calories
39 mg cholesterol
15 gm fat

LENTIL SOUP

4 cups lentils
1 turkey carcass
2 onions, peeled, and 1 whole clove inserted in each
3 carrots, sliced
2 cups chopped onion (2 large)
1 cup sliced celery (with leaves)
3 sprigs parsley
2 bay leaves
1½ teaspoons salt
1 teaspoon thyme
1 tablespoon dry mustard
Dash Tabasco sauce
4 to 5 quarts water
½ cup snipped parsley
½ cup chopped onion
Salt and freshly ground pepper

Soak lentils covered in water 8 to 12 hours.

Drain lentils; place in large kettle with turkey carcass and next 11 ingredients. Heat to boiling. Reduce heat to simmer; cover and simmer 4 to 6 hours.

Remove carcass, all bones, and onions with cloves from broth. Stir in ½ cup snipped parsley and ½ cup chopped onion and heat to boiling. Season to taste with salt and freshly ground pepper.

12 servings.

1 serving = 115 calories
5 mg cholesterol
1 gm fat

Note: Leftover soup can be frozen.

MINESTRONE

To Make the Broth

1½ pounds beef shanks, cracked
1 veal knuckle, cracked
3 pounds marrow bones
1 tablespoon salt
1 teaspoon peppercorns
2 leeks, cut into halves
1 large onion, peeled, and 2 whole
   cloves inserted
2 stalks celery, cut up
2 carrots, sliced
1 small bunch parsley
2 pounds tomatoes, peeled and
   coarsely chopped
1 teaspoon thyme
1 bay leaf
6 quarts water

Heat ingredients in large kettle to boiling. Remove any foam that forms on top. Reduce heat and simmer at least 2 hours or until liquid is reduced about one third and meat on bones is tender.

Remove bones from broth; cut meat from bones and reserve. Strain broth; cover and refrigerate 8 hours.

To Complete the Soup

3 cloves garlic, minced
1 leek, sliced
3 tablespoons olive oil
½ cup coarsely chopped carrot
½ cup chopped celery
3 cups coarsely chopped cabbage
2 cups dried red kidney beans
½ cup dried great northern beans
½ cup lentils
1 small zucchini, thinly sliced
1 medium potato, pared and diced
1 carrot, sliced
1 cup uncooked macaroni
½ cup fresh peas
Salt and pepper

Remove fat from broth. Cook and stir garlic

and leek in oil until leek is tender. Stir in chopped carrot, chopped celery, cabbage, beans, lentils, reserved meat, and broth. Heat to boiling; reduce heat and simmer, partially covered, until beans and lentils are tender. Stir in zucchini, sliced carrot, sliced celery, and the macaroni, cook until macaroni is tender. Stir in peas, heat through and season with salt and pepper.

8 servings.

   1 serving = 244 calories
                 10 mg cholesterol
                 7 gm fat

DOWNHOME VEGETABLE SOUP

3-pound beef knuckle bone
1 large onion, chopped
3 quarts water (12 cups)
6 beef bouillon cubes
2 cups cut fresh green beans
1 large potato, pared and diced
2 cups coarsely chopped cabbage
1 pound tomatoes, peeled and coarsely
   chopped
3 small carrots, sliced
¼ teaspoon lemon juice
Bouquet garni (1 bay leaf, 1 sprig thyme,
   2 sprigs parsley, 1 sprig rosemary)

If necessary, trim fat from bone. Heat bone, onion, water, and bouillon cubes in 4-quart dutch oven or covered large kettle to boiling. Reduce heat; cover and simmer 2 hours. Add remaining ingredients; simmer 1 hour longer. Remove bone.

10 servings.

   1 serving = 72 calories
                 13 mg cholesterol
                 1 gm fat

Note: Unsalted bouillon cubes may be used. If using dry herbs, tie in cheesecloth.

PIZZA MUFFIN

1 English Muffin (page 113), split and
  toasted
1 teaspoon margarine, softened
1 tablespoon tomato paste
1 tablespoon water
1 tablespoon finely chopped green pepper
⅛ teaspoon basil
⅛ teaspoon oregano
Dash each garlic powder and pepper
½ teaspoon parsley flakes
2 onion rings
1 fresh mushroom, sliced

Heat oven to 400°. Spread toasted side of
each muffin half with ½ teaspoon margarine.
Mix remaining ingredients except parsley
flakes, onion rings, and mushroom; spread on
muffin halves. Sprinkle with parsley flakes and
top each with an onion ring and mushroom
slices. Place on ungreased baking sheet.
Bake until bubbly, 3 to 5 minutes.

> 1 serving = 204 calories
>   trace cholesterol
>   5 gm fat

MACARONI VEGETABLE SOUP

¼ cup uncooked macaroni rings
1 cup cut-up, cooked, unsalted beef
2 cups unsalted beef broth
½ cup sliced carrot
¼ cup chopped celery
¼ cup finely chopped onion
2 medium tomatoes, peeled and cut up
1 teaspoon lemon juice
¼ teaspoon marjoram
¼ teaspoon thyme

Cook macaroni rings as directed on package, except omit salt.

Heat remaining ingredients to boiling, stirring occasionally. Reduce heat; cover and
simmer 15 minutes. Stir in macaroni rings and
heat.

> *8 servings (½ cup each).*
>   1 serving = 61 calories
>   16 mg cholesterol
>   1 gm fat

HEALTHFUL SANDWICHES

Spread each slice bread with softened margarine or low-fat mayonnaise. Add crisp lettuce leaves, spinach leaves, or alfalfa sprouts
topped with thin slices roast beef, roast
chicken, turkey, Chicken Salad (page 91), or
Tuna Salad (page 92) for filling; if you like,
add thin slices cucumber, tomato, radish, or
green pepper. Serve sandwich with carrot
curls.

Note: Check food groups and individual
recipes for calorie information.

SALMON SALAD SANDWICH

½ cup drained canned salmon
2 tablespoons Gourmet Dressing
  (page 95)
1 teaspoon chopped onion
2 slices pumpernickel or other dark bread
1 tablespoon snipped parsley

Mix salmon, Gourmet Dressing, and onion. Spread on bread slices and top with parsley.

2 servings.

    1 serving = 217 calories
                17 mg cholesterol
                10 gm fat

Note: Low-fat mayonnaise can be substituted for the Gourmet Dressing.

TOASTED CHICKEN and TOMATO SANDWICH

1 slice bread
1 teaspoon margarine
1 ounce sliced cooked chicken
2 tomato slices
½ teaspoon oregano
1 tablespoon dry bread crumbs
1 teaspoon margarine, melted

Set oven at broil and/or 550°. Toast bread on 1 side. Spread untoasted side of bread with 1 teaspoon margarine. Arrange chicken and tomato slices on bread. Sprinkle oregano and half of the bread crumbs on tomato slices. Drizzle melted margarine on top and sprinkle with remaining bread crumbs. Broil 5 inches from heat until crumbs are golden brown, 3 to 5 minutes.

    1 serving = 296 calories
                26 mg cholesterol
                19 gm fat

CHUCKWAGON EGG SANDWICH

1 tablespoon margarine
¼ cup chopped onion
2 tablespoons chopped green pepper
2 tablespoons chopped red pepper
½ cup egg substitute
4 slices whole-wheat bread, toasted

Melt margarine in small skillet. Cook and stir onion, green pepper, and red pepper in margarine until onion is tender. Pour egg substitute on vegetables. As egg mixture begins to set at bottom and side, gently lift cooked portion with spatula so that thin uncooked portion can flow to bottom. When almost set, cover skillet and cook until set, about 2 minutes. Cut egg mixture in half; place each half on piece of toast and top with remaining toast piece.

2 servings.

    1 serving = 242 calories
                trace cholesterol
                10 gm fat

12 Breads

PANCAKES

2 cups all-purpose flour
¼ cup sugar
1 tablespoon plus 1 teaspoon baking
** powder**
½ cup egg substitute
1½ cups skim milk
¼ cup vegetable oil

Measure flour, sugar, and baking powder into mixing bowl. Mix egg substitute, milk, and oil; stir into dry ingredients. Beat only until large lumps disappear.

Heat griddle, which has been sprayed with vegetable spray. Griddle is hot enough if a few drops of water sprinkled on griddle "skitter around." Pour batter from tip of large spoon or from pitcher onto hot griddle. Turn pancakes when bubbles break and edges are cooked. Bake other side until golden brown (total time 6 to 7 minutes). Serve immediately.

Sixteen 4-inch pancakes.

    1 pancake = 113 calories
                trace cholesterol
                4 gm fat

PANCAKE AND WAFFLE MIX

3¼ cups all-purpose flour
3 cups whole-wheat flour
4 tablespoons baking powder
½ cup sugar
3 teaspoons salt

Mix all ingredients. Store in tightly covered container.

For pancakes:
2 ounces egg substitute
1 cup skim milk
1 cup Pancake and Waffle Mix
2 tablespoons wheat germ

Combine egg substitute and milk. Stir in mix and wheat germ just until ingredients are moistened. (Batter will be lumpy.)

Heat nonstick skillet or griddle until a drop of water sprinkled in skillet sizzles. Pour batter by tablespoonsful onto hot skillet. Turn pancakes as soon as they are puffed and bubbled but before bubbles break. Bake other side until golden brown.

Twenty 3-inch pancakes.

    1 pancake = 29 calories
                trace cholesterol
                trace fat

For waffles:
Add 1 tablespoon vegetable oil to batter. Pour batter by ¼ cupsful onto center of heated waffle iron. Bake until steaming stops.

Seven 4½-inch waffles.

    1 waffle = 99 calories
               trace cholesterol
               2 gm fat

Variation: Add 1 tablespoon grated orange peel and 1 tablespoon cinnamon to batter.

CRÊPES

1 cup skim milk
1 cup water
2 egg whites
¼ teaspoon salt
1 cup all-purpose flour
2 tablespoons vegetable oil

Measure all ingredients into bowl; beat with rotary beater until smooth. Strain batter. It should be as thick as cream. If it is thicker, add water, a little at a time, to get desired consistency.

Heat crêpe pan or 6-inch skillet until a few drops water sprinkled in it sizzle. Brush pan with oil. For each crêpe, pour ⅛ cup batter into pan. Immediately rotate pan until batter covers bottom. Cook until top of crêpe has lost its glossiness. Loosen around edge with spatula; turn and cook other side until light brown. Repeat oiling pan and baking crêpes until all batter is used.

Stack crêpes, placing waxed paper or paper towel between them. Keep crêpes covered to prevent them from drying out.

Use crêpes at once or cool completely; then wrap in aluminum foil and place in freezer. Crêpes will keep for several weeks in the freezer.

To thaw crêpes, thaw in foil wrap at room temperature or in warm oven.

14 crêpes.

1 crêpe = 57 calories
trace cholesterol
2 gm fat

FRENCH TOAST

1 cup egg substitute
½ cup skim milk
1 loaf (1 pound) French bread or 12 slices
 day-old bread
2 tablespoons unsalted margarine
Syrup, jam, or honey

Mix egg substitute and milk in shallow dish. If using French bread, cut into 1-inch slices.

Melt margarine in large skillet. Dip bread slices into egg substitute mixture, coating both sides and arrange in skillet. Cook over medium heat until light brown. Turn and cook until light brown on other side. Serve with syrup.

6 servings.

1 serving = 262 calories
1 mg cholesterol
7 gm fat

Note: Salt-free bread can be used.

BAKING HINTS FOR WHOLE-GRAIN FLOURS

1. Always stir flours before measuring.
2. When using all-purpose flour recipes for whole-grain flour, increase the amounts of liquid and yeast, and knead the dough for a longer period.
3. Best temperature for yeast mix is 105°.
4. Best temperature for rising of dough is 85°.
5. Brush hot loaves with margarine immediately after removing from pans. This gives a soft crust.

FRUIT SYRUPS

Strawberry: Measure 1½ cups sliced strawberries and 1 cup light corn syrup into blender. Blend on high speed until smooth, about 10 seconds. Cover and refrigerate.

2 cups.

2 tablespoons = 62 calories
0 cholesterol
0 fat

Apricot: Cook ⅓ cup dried apricots (packed) and 1 cup water in covered saucepan until apricots are tender and water is absorbed, 10 to 15 minutes. Mash apricots and blend in 1 cup light corn syrup. Cover and refrigerate.

1⅔ cups.

2 tablespoons = 80 calories
0 cholesterol
0 fat

Pineapple: Place 1 can (8 ounces) crushed pineapple in unsweetened pineapple juice and 1 cup light corn syrup in blender. Blend on high speed until smooth, about 10 seconds. Cover and refrigerate.

1¾ cups.

2 tablespoons = 75 calories
0 cholesterol
0 fat

Blackberry: Place 1 package (10 ounces) frozen blackberries (no sugar added), partially thawed, and 1 cup light corn syrup in blender. Blend on high speed until smooth, about 10 seconds. Or mash berries and corn syrup in bowl with fork until fairly smooth.

2 cups.

2 tablespoons = 65 calories
0 cholesterol
0 fat

Raspberry: Substitute 1 package (10 ounces) frozen raspberries (no sugar added), partially thawed, for the blackberries in Blackberry Fruit Syrup.

2 tablespoons = 64 calories
0 cholesterol
0 fat

Peach: Substitute 1 package (10 ounces) frozen peach slices (no sugar added), partially thawed, for the blackberries in Blackberry Fruit Syrup, above.

2 tablespoons = 64 calories
0 cholesterol
0 fat

Cherry: Substitute 1 package (10 ounces) frozen cherries (no sugar added), partially thawed, for the blackberries in Blackberry Fruit Syrup, above.

2 tablespoons = 68 calories
0 cholesterol
0 fat

Note: 1½ cups sliced fresh fruit or berries can be substituted for the frozen fruit.

MUFFINS

¼ cup egg substitute
1 cup skim milk
¼ cup vegetable oil
2 cups all-purpose flour
¼ cup sugar
3 teaspoons baking powder
¼ teaspoon salt

Heat oven to 400°. Spray 12 medium muffin cups (2¾ inches in diameter) with vegetable spray. Beat egg substitute, milk, and vegetable oil. Mix in remaining ingredients just until flour is moistened. Batter will be lumpy. Fill muffin cups ²/₃ full.

Bake 20 to 25 minutes or until golden brown. Immediately remove from pan.
12 muffins.

> 1 muffin = 141 calories
> trace cholesterol
> 5 gm fat

Chive Muffins: Mix in ¼ cup snipped fresh chives with the flour.

> 1 muffin = 142 calories
> trace cholesterol
> 5 gm fat

Raisin Muffins: Mix in ½ cup cut-up raisins with the flour.

> 1 muffin = 160 calories
> trace cholesterol
> 5 gm fat

Bran Muffins: Stir ½ cup all-bran cereal into egg-milk mixture and let stand 5 minutes. Decrease flour to 1½ cups.

> 1 muffin = 132 calories
> trace cholesterol
> 5 gm fat

Whole-Wheat Muffins: Decrease flour to 1 cup and baking powder to 2 teaspoons; add 1 cup whole-wheat flour.

> 1 muffin = 139 calories
> trace cholesterol
> 5 gm fat

Blueberry Muffins: Fold 1 cup fresh blueberries or ¾ cup drained canned blueberries into batter.

> 1 muffin = 149 calories
> trace cholesterol
> 5 gm fat

BRAN MUFFINS

¼ cup egg substitute
1 cup skim milk
3 tablespoons vegetable oil
1½ cups all-bran cereal
1 cup all-purpose flour
2 teaspoons baking powder
2 tablespoons sugar

Heat oven to 400°. Spray 12 muffin cups (2¾ inches in diameter) with vegetable spray. Beat egg substitute, milk, and vegetable oil. Stir in bran cereal and let stand 5 minutes.

Add flour, baking powder, and sugar to bran mixture; mix just until flour is moistened. Batter will be lumpy. Fill muffin cups ½ full.

Bake 18 to 20 minutes. Immediately remove from pan.
12 muffins.

> 1 muffin = 112 calories
> trace cholesterol
> 4 gm fat

BAKING POWDER BISCUITS

2 cups all-purpose flour
3 teaspoons baking powder
¼ teaspoon salt
⅓ cup vegetable oil
⅔ cup skim milk
Unsalted margarine

Heat oven to 450°. Measure flour, baking powder, and salt into bowl. Pour oil and milk into measuring cup (do not stir); pour into flour mixture. Stir with fork until mixture cleans side of bowl and forms a ball.

To knead dough, turn onto waxed paper. Lift paper by one corner and fold dough in half; press down firmly and pull paper back. Repeat until dough looks smooth. Pat or roll dough ½ inch thick between 2 sheets of waxed paper. Cut with unfloured 2-inch biscuit cutter. Place on ungreased baking sheet.

Bake until golden brown, 10 to 12 minutes. Serve hot with margarine and, if desired, with jelly, honey, jam, or syrup.

16 biscuits.

1 biscuit = 99 calories
trace cholesterol
4 gm fat

Drop Biscuits: Increase skim milk to 1 cup. Omit kneading and drop dough by teaspoonfuls onto baking sheet sprayed with vegetable spray.

1 biscuit = 101 calories
trace cholesterol
4 gm fat

Baking Powder Biscuits (no salt): Substitute 1 tablespoon plus 1½ teaspoons low-sodium baking powder for the baking powder and omit salt.

Herb Biscuits: Add 1¼ teaspoons caraway seed, ½ teaspoon crumbled leaf sage, and ¼ teaspoon dry mustard to flour mixture.

BAGELS

1 package active dry yeast
1 cup warm water (105 to 115°)
2 tablespoons sugar
¼ teaspoon salt
2¾ cups all-purpose flour
2 quarts water

Dissolve yeast in 1 cup warm water in large mixing bowl. Stir in sugar, salt, and 1¼ cups of the flour. Beat until smooth. Mix in remaining flour.

Turn dough onto lightly floured board. Knead until smooth and elastic, about 10 minutes. Place in greased bowl; turn greased side up. Cover; let rise in warm place until double, about 15 minutes. (Dough is ready if an indentation remains when touched.)

Punch down dough; divide into 8 equal parts. Roll each part into a rope 6 inches long; moisten ends with water and pinch to form a bagel. Or shape each part into a smooth ball, punch hole in center and pull gently to enlarge hole and make uniform shape. Let rise 20 minutes.

Heat oven to 375°. Heat 2 quarts water to boiling in large kettle. Reduce heat; add 4 bagels. Simmer 2 minutes, turning once (1 minute on each side). Drain on kitchen towel. Repeat with remaining bagels. Bake on baking sheet sprayed with vegetable spray 30 to 35 minutes or until golden brown. Cool. To serve, toast and spread with marmalade.

8 bagels.

1 bagel = 168 calories
0 cholesterol
trace fat

REFRIGERATOR ROLLS

1 package active dry yeast
1 cup warm water (105 to 115°)
¼ cup sugar
¼ cup egg substitute
¼ cup margarine, softened
3 cups all-purpose flour

Dissolve yeast in warm water in large bowl. Stir in sugar, egg substitute, margarine, and 1 cup of the flour. Beat until smooth. Stir in remaining flour, mixing with hand until dough cleans side of bowl and forms a ball. Place in greased bowl; turn greased side up. Cover tightly and refrigerate at least 8 hours or until ready to use. (Dough can be kept up to 5 days in refrigerator at 45° or below. Keep covered.)

Punch down dough; shape into desired rolls (below). Cover and let rise until double.

Heat oven to 400°. Bake 12 to 15 minutes.

1½ dozen.

1 roll = 113 calories
0 cholesterol
3 gm fat

Traditional Rolls: Divide dough into 18 pieces. Shape into smooth balls; place on baking sheet sprayed with vegetable spray.

Cloverleaf Rolls: Spray 18 muffin cups (2¾ inches in diameter) with vegetable spray. Shape bits of dough into 1-inch balls. Place 3 balls in each muffin cup.

Crescents: Roll dough into 18-inch circle, about ¼ inch thick. Cut into 18 wedges. Roll up, beginning at rounded edge. Place rolls with point underneath on sprayed baking sheet. Curve slightly.

Parker House Rolls: Divide dough in half. Roll each half into rectangle, 13 x 9 inches, about ¼ inch thick. Cut into 3-inch circles.

Make crease across each circle; fold so top half overlaps slightly. Press edges together.

Place close together in sprayed baking pan, 13 x 9 x 3 inches.

Sesame Rolls: After shaping rolls, sprinkle with 2 tablespoons toasted sesame seed (see *Note*). Or, stir in 2 tablespoons toasted sesame seed with the 1 cup flour.

Note: To toast sesame seed, spread seed on baking sheet; toast in 350° oven until golden, about 10 minutes.

Poppy Seed Rolls: Substitute 2 tablespoons poppy seed for the toasted sesame seed.

ENGLISH MUFFINS

1 package active dry yeast
1 cup warm water (105 to 115°)
½ teaspoon salt
1 teaspoon sugar
¼ cup vegetable oil
3 cups all-purpose flour
2 tablespoons cornmeal

Dissolve yeast in warm water in large mixing bowl. Stir in salt, sugar, oil, and flour until smooth. Roll dough ¼ inch thick on floured board. Cut into 3½-inch circles.

Sprinkle ungreased baking sheet with 1 tablespoon cornmeal; place circles on baking sheet. Sprinkle remaining cornmeal on circles. Cover; let rise in warm place until light, about 35 minutes. (Dough is ready if an indentation remains when touched.)

Heat ungreased electric griddle or skillet to 375°. Transfer circles to griddle. Cook 7 minutes on each side. Cool. To serve, split, toast, and spread with margarine and marmalade.

10 to 12 muffins.

1 muffin = 173 calories
0 cholesterol
5 gm fat

COUNTRY-STYLE ROLLS

1 package active dry yeast
1 cup warm water (105 to 115°)
2 tablespoons sugar
½ teaspoon salt
¼ cup egg substitute
2 tablespoons vegetable oil
2¼ cups all-purpose flour

Dissolve yeast in warm water in large mixer bowl. Add sugar, salt, egg substitute, oil, and 1 cup of the flour; beat until smooth. Mix in remaining flour until smooth, scraping batter from side of bowl. Cover and let rise in warm place until double, about 30 minutes.

Grease 16 muffin cups. Stir down batter and spoon into muffin cups, filling each about ½ full. Let rise uncovered 20 minutes.

Heat oven to 400°. Bake until golden brown, about 15 minutes.

16 rolls.

1 roll = 88 calories
0 cholesterol
2 gm fat

DINNER ROLLS

1 package active dry yeast
¼ cup warm water (105 to 115°)
⅛ teaspoon salt
¾ cup lukewarm skim milk (scalded, then cooled)
¼ cup sugar
¼ cup egg substitute
¼ cup vegetable oil
3½ cups all-purpose flour

Dissolve yeast in warm water in large bowl. Stir in salt, milk, sugar, egg substitute, oil, and 2 cups of the flour. Beat until smooth. Mix in enough remaining flour to make dough easy to handle.

Turn dough onto lightly floured board; knead until smooth, about 5 minutes. Place in greased bowl; turn greased side up. Cover; let rise in warm place until double, about 50 minutes. (Dough is ready if an indentation remains when touched.)

Punch down dough; divide in half. Shape only half the dough at a time into desired rolls (below). Cover; let rise until double, about 20 minutes.

Heat oven to 400°. Bake rolls 12 to 15 minutes.

16 rolls.

1 roll = 147 calories
trace cholesterol
4 gm fat

Cloverleaf Rolls: Shape bits of dough into about 1-inch balls. Place 3 balls in each muffin cup sprayed with vegetable spray.

Crescents: Roll dough into 16-inch circle. Cut into 16 wedges. Roll up, beginning at rounded edge. Place rolls with point underneath on baking sheet sprayed with vegetable spray. Curve slightly.

BLUEBERRY-WINNER COFFEE CAKE

1 cup fresh or frozen blueberries
2 tablespoons sugar
1 tablespoon cornstarch
1 tablespoon lemon juice
1 recipe Sweet Dough (page 118)
Lemon Icing (below)

Mix blueberries, sugar, cornstarch, and lemon juice in small saucepan. Cook, stirring constantly, until mixture thickens and boils. Boil and stir 1 minute. Cool.

Roll dough into rectangle, 18 x 6 inches, on lightly floured board. Spread blueberry mixture on rectangle to within ½ inch of edges. Roll up, beginning at long side. Pinch edge of dough into roll to seal well. Stretch roll to make even. Place roll seam side down on lightly greased baking sheet to form horseshoe shape. Cover; let rise until double, about 30 minutes.

Bake until golden brown, about 20 minutes. While warm, frost with Lemon Icing.

18 servings.

    1 serving = 108 calories
                 0 cholesterol
                 2 gm fat

Lemon Icing: Mix ¼ cup powdered sugar, 1½ teaspoons grated lemon peel, and 1 teaspoon lemon juice until smooth.

LAYERED PECAN COFFEE CAKE

1½ cups all-purpose flour
¾ cup sugar
2¼ teaspoons baking powder
¼ cup margarine, softened
¾ cup skim milk
¼ cup egg substitute
Nut Mixture (below)

Heat oven to 375°. Spray round layer pan, 9 x 1½ inches, with vegetable spray. Measure all ingredients except Nut Mixture into large bowl. Blend thoroughly with fork; beat vigorously ½ minute. Spread half the batter in pan. Sprinkle half the Nut Mixture on batter in pan. Top with remaining batter and Nut Mixture. Bake 25 to 30 minutes of until wooden pick inserted in center comes out clean. Serve warm.

16 servings.

    1 serving = 148 calories
                 trace cholesterol
                 5 gm fat

Nut Mixture: Mix ¼ cup brown sugar (packed), 1 teaspoon cinnamon, ¼ cup finely chopped pecans, and 1 tablespoon margarine, melted.

PINEAPPLE-ALMOND COFFEE CRESCENT

1 can (8 ounces) crushed pineapple in unsweetened pineapple juice, drained (reserve juice)
2 tablespoons cornstarch
¼ cup brown sugar (packed)
¼ cup sliced almonds
2 tablespoons unsalted margarine
2 tablespoons brown sugar
¼ cup all-purpose flour
¼ cup sliced almonds
1 recipe Sweet Dough (page 118)

Mix pineapple, cornstarch, and ¼ cup sugar in small saucepan. Cook, stirring constantly, until mixture thickens and boils. Boil and stir 1 minute. Remove from heat; stir in ¼ cup almonds. Cool.

Mix margarine, 2 tablespoons sugar, and the flour until crumbly. Stir in ¼ cup almonds and set aside.

Roll dough into rectangle, 18 x 6 inches, on lightly floured board. Spread pineapple mixture on rectangle to within ½ inch of edges. Roll up, beginning at long side. Pinch edge of dough into roll to seal well. Stretch roll to make even. Place roll seam side down on lightly greased baking sheet to form horseshoe shape. With scissors, make lengthwise cut through top layers of dough. Fold back layers to completely expose filling and double width of coffee cake. Sprinkle with crumbly mixture. Cover; let rise until double, about 30 minutes.

Bake until golden brown, about 20 minutes.

18 servings.

> 1 serving = 158 calories
> 0 cholesterol
> 5 gm fat

Glazed Pineapple-Almond Coffee Crescent: While warm, drizzle coffee cake with Glaze: Mix ½ cup brown sugar (packed) and 1 tablespoon plus 1 teaspoon of the reserved pineapple juice until smooth.

> 1 serving = 182 calories
> 0 cholesterol
> 5 gm fat

ELEGANT-BUT-EASY TEA RING

1 recipe Sweet Dough (page 118)
2 tablespoons unsalted margarine, softened
½ cup brown sugar (packed)
2 teaspoons cinnamon
½ cup raisins
Powdered Sugar Icing (below)

Roll dough into rectangle, 15 x 9 inches. Spread with margarine and sprinkle with sugar, cinnamon, and raisins. Roll up, beginning at long side. Pinch edge of dough into roll to seal well. Stretch roll to make even. With sealed edge down, shape into ring on baking sheet sprayed with vegetable spray. Pinch ends together. With scissors, make cuts ⅔ of the way through ring at 1-inch intervals. Turn each section on its side. Cover and let rise until double, about 30 minutes.

Heat oven to 375°. Bake until golden brown, 20 to 25 minutes. While warm, frost with icing. Serve warm.

17 servings.

> 1 serving = 159 calories
> 0 cholesterol
> 3 gm fat

Powdered Sugar Icing: Mix ½ cup powdered sugar, 2 teaspoons skim milk, and ¼ teaspoon vanilla until smooth.

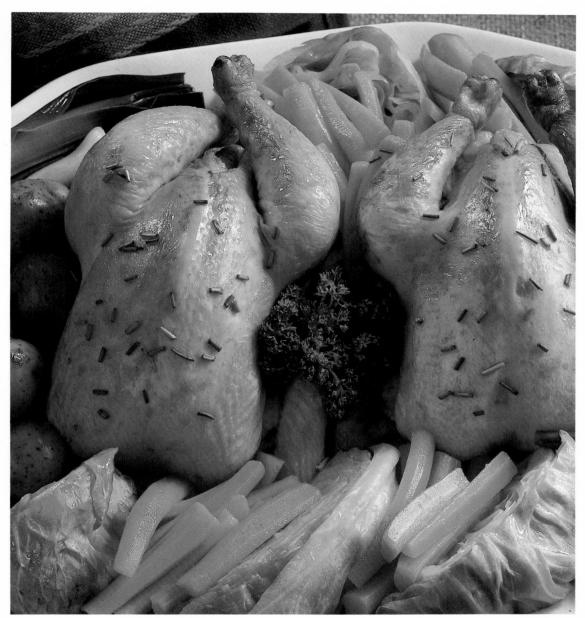

Poached Chicken and Vegetables.

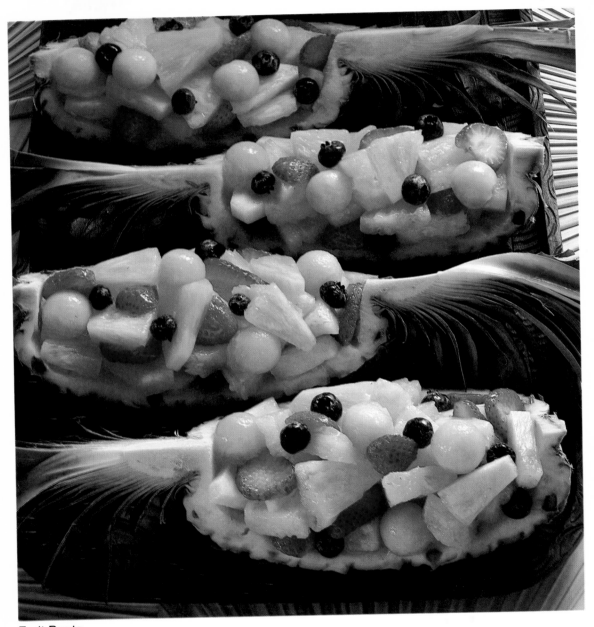

Fruit Boats.

POTECA

2 packages active dry yeast
¼ cup warm water (105 to 115°)
1 cup lukewarm milk (scalded then cooled)
¼ cup sugar
½ teaspoon salt
¼ cup unsalted margarine, softened
½ cup egg substitute
4½ cups all-purpose flour
Nut Filling (this page)
1 tablespoon unsalted margarine, softened

Dissolve yeast in warm water in large mixer bowl. Add milk, sugar, salt, ¼ cup margarine, the egg substitute, and 2½ cups of the flour. Blend on low speed ½ minute, scraping bowl constantly. Beat on high speed 2 minutes, scraping bowl occasionally. Stir in remaining flour with wooden spoon, mixing with hand until dough cleans side of bowl and forms ball. Place dough in greased bowl; turn greased side up. Cover and let rise in warm place until double, about 1 hour.

Punch down dough. Turn dough onto lightly floured board. Cover with bowl and let rest 10 minutes. Roll dough into rectangle, 30 x 20 inches. Spread Nut Filling over rectangle to within 1 inch of edge.

Roll up gently, beginning at one of the long sides. Moisten ends with water; pinch edge of dough into roll to seal. Stretch and shape even. On sprayed baking sheet, coil roll around to form snail shape. Cover and let rise until double, about 1 hour.

Heat oven to 350°. Bake 35 to 40 minutes or until golden brown. Brush top with 1 tablespoon margarine while warm. Cool on wire rack.

60 slices.

1 slice = 90 calories
trace cholesterol
4 gm fat

NUT FILLING

⅓ cup egg substitute
2 cups chopped walnuts
½ cup brown sugar (packed)
3 tablespoons unsalted margarine, softened
¾ teaspoon cinnamon
½ teaspoon vanilla

Mix all ingredients.

WALNUT COFFEE CAKE

¼ cup egg substitute
½ cup unsalted margarine, softened
⅔ cup skim milk
1 tablespoon lemon juice
1¾ cups all-purpose flour
½ cup sugar
2½ teaspoons baking powder
Walnut Filling (below)

Heat oven to 375°. Spray baking pan, 9 x 9 x 2 inches, with vegetable spray. Beat egg substitute, margarine, milk, and lemon juice until smooth. Mix in flour, sugar, and baking powder just until flour is moistened. Batter will be lumpy. Spread in pan. Spoon Walnut Filling on top; with knife, cut through batter several times for marbled effect.

Bake 20 to 25 minutes or until wooden pick inserted in center comes out clean.

12 servings.

1 serving = 219 calories
trace cholesterol
11 gm fat

Walnut Filling: Mix ¼ cup brown sugar (packed), ¼ cup chopped walnuts, and 1 tablespoon unsalted margarine, melted.

STOLLEN

1 package active dry yeast
¾ cup warm water (105 to 115°)
½ cup sugar
¼ teaspoon salt
¾ cup egg substitute
½ cup unsalted margarine, softened
3½ cups all-purpose flour
½ cup chopped blanched almonds
¼ cup cut-up citron
¼ cup raisins
1 tablespoon grated lemon peel
¼ cup plus 2 tablespoons unsalted
   margarine, softened
1 egg white
1 tablespoon water
Quick White Icing (below)
Blanched almond halves
Gumdrops

Dissolve yeast in warm water in large mixer bowl. Add sugar, salt, egg substitute, ½ cup margarine, and 1½ cups of the flour. Blend on low speed ½ minute, scraping bowl constantly. Beat on medium speed 10 minutes, scraping bowl occasionally.

Stir in remaining flour, the chopped almonds, citron, raisins, and lemon peel. Scrape batter from side of bowl. Cover; let rise in warm place until double, about 1 hour.

Stir down batter by beating 25 strokes. Cover bowl tightly; refrigerate at least 8 hours.

Turn dough onto well-floured board; turn to coat with flour. Divide dough in half. Press each half into oval, about 10 x 7 inches. Spread each with 3 tablespoons margarine. Fold lengthwise in half; press only folded edge firmly. Place on baking sheet that has been sprayed with vegetable spray. Beat egg white slightly; beat in 1 tablespoon water and brush on stollen. Let rise until double, about 35 minutes.

Heat oven to 375°. Bake 20 to 25 minutes or until golden brown. While warm, frost with Quick White Icing; decorate with almond halves and gumdrops. Or, if desired, dust stollen with powdered sugar.

32 slices.

> 1 slice = 167 calories
> 0 cholesterol
> 7 gm fat

Quick White Icing: Mix 1½ cups powdered sugar and 1½ tablespoons skim milk until smooth.

SWEET DOUGH

1 package active dry yeast
¼ cup warm water (105 to 115°)
¼ cup lukewarm skim milk (scalded then
   cooled)
¼ cup sugar
¼ cup egg substitute
2 tablespoons vegetable oil
2¼ to 2½ cups all-purpose flour

Dissolve yeast in warm water in bowl. Stir in milk, sugar, egg substitute, oil, and half the flour. Beat until smooth. Mix in enough remaining flour to make dough easy to handle. Turn onto lightly floured board. Knead until smooth and elastic, about 5 minutes. Place in greased bowl; turn greased side up. (At this point, dough can be refrigerated 2 to 3 days.) Cover; let rise in warm place until double, about 1 hour. (Dough is ready if an indentation remains when touched.)

Punch down dough. Shape dough for desired rolls or coffee cake. Cover; let rise until double. Heat oven to 375°. Bake as directed.

APRICOT COFFEE CAKE

1 package active dry yeast
¼ cup warm water (105 to 115°)
2 tablespoons unsalted margarine, softened
2 tablespoons sugar
¼ cup lukewarm milk (scalded then cooled)
¼ cup egg substitute
½ teaspoon vanilla
¼ teaspoon salt
2 to 2½ cups all-purpose flour
1 can (16 or 17 ounces) unsweetened apricot halves
Cheese Filling (this page)

Dissolve yeast in warm water in large mixer bowl. Add margarine, sugar, milk, egg substitute, vanilla, salt, and 1 cup of the flour. Beat on medium speed 2 minutes, scraping bowl frequently. Stir in enough remaining flour to make dough easy to handle.

Turn dough onto well-floured board; knead until smooth and elastic, 5 to 8 minutes. Place in greased bowl; turn greased side up. Cover and let rise in warm place until double, about 1 hour. (Dough is ready if an indentation remains when touched.)

Punch down dough; pat evenly in sprayed 9-inch springform pan, building up 2-inch ridge around edge. Cover and let rise 30 minutes.

Drain apricots; place halves on paper toweling to drain thoroughly.

Heat oven to 350°. Lightly pat down dough on bottom of pan only. Arrange apricot halves on dough in pan. Pour Cheese Filling on apricots. Bake 55 to 60 minutes or until filling is set. Cool 10 minutes before removing side of pan.

24 servings.

1 serving = 87 calories
1 mg cholesterol
1 gm fat

CHEESE FILLING

1 cup low-fat cottage cheese, strained
¼ cup sugar
¼ cup egg substitute
1 tablespoon flour
¼ teaspoon cinnamon

Mix all ingredients thoroughly.

DOUGHNUT BALLS

2 cups all-purpose flour
¼ cup sugar
3 teaspoons baking powder
1 teaspoon nutmeg or mace
¼ cup vegetable oil
¾ cup skim milk
¼ cup egg substitute
½ cup sugar
1 teaspoon cinnamon

Heat oil (3 to 4 inches) in deep fat fryer or heavy kettle to 375°. Measure flour, ¼ cup sugar, the baking powder, and nutmeg or mace into mixing bowl. Add oil, milk, and egg substitute; beat with fork until smooth.

Drop batter by teaspoonfuls (too large balls will not cook through) into hot oil. Fry until golden brown on both sides, about 3 minutes. Drain.

Mix ½ cup sugar and the cinnamon. Roll warm balls in sugar-cinnamon mixture or, if desired, glaze balls with a powdered sugar glaze.

2½ dozen balls.

1 ball = 70 calories
0 cholesterol
2 gm fat

BABKA

½ cup hot water
¼ cup unsalted margarine
½ cup sugar
¾ teaspoon cinnamon
1 tablespoon grated orange peel
1 package active dry yeast
¼ cup warm water (105 to 115°)
½ cup egg substitute
3½ to 4 cups all-purpose flour
2 tablespoons unsalted margarine, melted
Walnut-Raisin Filling (this page)

Mix ½ cup water, ¼ cup margarine, the sugar, cinnamon, and orange peel in large bowl. Dissolve yeast in ¼ cup warm water. Stir into margarine mixture. Add egg substitute and 1 cup of the flour; beat until smooth. Beat in enough remaining flour to make dough easy to handle.

Turn dough onto lightly floured board; knead until smooth and elastic, about 10 minutes. Place in greased bowl; turn greased side up. Cover and let rise in warm place until double, 1½ to 2 hours. (Dough is ready if an impression remains when touched.)

Punch down dough; allow to rise again, about 1 hour.

Punch down dough; divide in half. Roll each half into rectangle, 12 x 8 inches. Brush each with 1 tablespoon of the melted margarine and sprinkle with half the Walnut-Raisin Filling. Roll up, beginning at long side. Cut into ten 1-inch slices. Place 10 slices cut side up in single layer in well-greased 9-inch tube pan. Top with remaining slices and Filling. Let rise until double.

Heat oven to 350°. Bake 35 to 40 minutes or until golden brown. To serve, break rolls apart with 2 forks.

20 rolls.
1 roll = 181 calories
0 cholesterol
7 gm fat

WALNUT-RAISIN FILLING

½ cup chopped walnuts
½ cup raisins
2 tablespoons sugar
1 teaspoon cinnamon
2 tablespoons unsalted margarine, melted

Mix all ingredients.

WHOLE-WHEAT YOGURT BREAD

2 packages active dry yeast
¾ cup warm water (105 to 115°)
¼ cup unsalted margarine, softened
¼ cup brown sugar (packed)
1 teaspoon salt
1 teaspoon grated orange peel
1 cup wheat germ
4 cups whole-wheat flour
2 cups low-fat yogurt
1½ to 2 cups all-purpose flour

Dissolve yeast in warm water in large bowl. Stir in margarine, sugar, salt, orange peel, wheat germ, and 3 cups of the whole-wheat flour. Blend in yogurt. Mix in remaining whole-wheat flour and 1 cup of the all-purpose flour. Turn dough onto lightly floured board and knead in remaining flour; add sufficient flour and knead until dough is no longer sticky, about 10 minutes. Place in greased bowl; turn greased side up. Cover and let rise in warm place until double, about 2 hours.

Punch down dough. Place in 2½-quart casserole that has been sprayed with vegetable spray and shape. Cover; let rise until double, about 30 minutes.

Heat oven to 350°. Bake until loaf sounds hollow when tapped, about 1 hour.

18 slices.
1 slice = 225 calories
2 mg cholesterol
5 gm fat

WHOLE-WHEAT BREAD

1 package active dry yeast
¼ cup warm water (105 to 115°)
1 cup lukewarm skim milk (scalded then cooled)
2 tablespoons unsalted margarine, softened
2 tablespoons sugar
½ teaspoon salt
¼ cup egg substitute
1½ cups whole-wheat flour
2 to 2¼ cups all-purpose flour

Dissolve yeast in warm water in large bowl. Stir in milk, margarine, sugar, salt, egg substitute, and whole-wheat flour. Beat until smooth. Mix in enough all-purpose flour to make dough easy to handle.

Turn dough onto lightly floured board; knead until smooth and elastic, about 10 minutes. Place in greased bowl; turn greased side up. Cover and let rise in warm place until double, about 1 hour. (Dough is ready if an indentation remains when touched.)

Punch down dough. Place in sprayed loaf pan, 9 x 5 x 3 inches; shape into loaf with hand. Let rise until dough reaches top of pan, about 40 minutes.

Heat oven to 375°. Bake 35 to 40 minutes or until golden brown and loaf sounds hollow when tapped. Remove from pan and cool on wire rack.

16 slices.

1 slice = 125 calories
trace cholesterol
2 gm fat

CINNAMON ROLLS

1 package active dry yeast
¼ cup warm water (105 to 115°)
¼ cup plus 2 tablespoons lukewarm skim milk (scalded then cooled)
¼ cup granulated sugar
¼ cup unsalted margarine, softened
¼ cup egg substitute
¾ teaspoon grated lemon peel
2½ to 2¾ cups all-purpose flour
¼ cup unsalted margarine, softened
¼ cup brown sugar (packed)
1 teaspoon cinnamon
½ cup raisins

Dissolve yeast in warm water in large bowl. Stir in milk, granulated sugar, ¼ cup margarine, the egg substitute, lemon peel, and 1 cup of the flour. Beat until smooth. Stir in enough remaining flour to make dough easy to handle.

Turn dough onto lightly floured board; knead until smooth and elastic, 10 to 15 minutes. Place in greased bowl; turn greased side up. Cover and let rise in warm place until double, 2 to 2½ hours. (Dough is ready if an indentation remains when touched.)

Punch down dough. Roll dough on lightly floured board into rectangle, 16 x 8 inches. Spread with ¼ cup margarine; sprinkle with brown sugar, cinnamon, and raisins. Roll up, beginning at one of the long sides. Pinch edge of dough into roll to seal well. Stretch and shape even.

Cut roll into 12 slices. Place slices cut side down in sprayed 9-inch-round layer pan. Let rise until double, about 1½ hours.

Heat oven to 375°. Bake 25 to 30 minutes or until golden brown. Cool in pan 5 minutes before removing.

12 rolls.

1 roll = 226 calories
0 cholesterol
8 gm fat

WHOLESOME WHOLE-WHEAT BREAD

1 cup skim milk
¾ cup unsalted margarine
¼ cup honey
1 tablespoon grated orange peel
2 packages active dry yeast
¾ cup warm water (105 to 115°)
¾ cup egg substitute
4½ cups all-purpose flour
1½ cups whole-wheat flour

Heat milk to scalding. Remove from heat; stir in margarine, honey, and orange peel until margarine is melted. Cool to lukewarm.

Dissolve yeast in warm water in large mixer bowl. Add milk mixture and egg substitute. Mix all-purpose flour and whole-wheat flour; add ⅔ (4 cups) of the flour mixture to yeast mixture. Beat on low speed, scraping bowl frequently, until blended, about 1 minute. Beat on medium speed, scraping bowl occasionally, until smooth, about 2 minutes. With wooden spoon, beat in remaining flour. Mix dough in bowl by squeezing dough between fingers 20 to 30 times to develop gluten. (Dough is soft but manageable.) Cover bowl with waxed paper and towel; let rise in warm place until batter is above rim of bowl, about 1 hour.

Punch down batter; beat with spoon until smooth, about 30 seconds. Spray two 1½-quart casseroles, 2 loaf pans, 9¼ x 5¼ x 3 inches, or one 3-quart casserole with vegetable spray. Divide batter between casseroles and pat evenly. Let rise uncovered until double, 40 to 50 minutes. (Dough should rise slightly above rim of casserole.)

Heat oven to 375°. With sharp knife, cut 4-inch cross about ½ inch deep in top of batter. Bake 45 to 50 minutes or until deep golden brown and loaves sound hollow when tapped. Remove to wire rack. Serve warm, cut into wedges.

32 slices.
1 slice = 138 calories
0 cholesterol
5 gm fat

 Wholesome Whole-Wheat Rolls: After punching down batter, divide into thirds. Use one-third batter in each of the following variations. Brush with soft margarine. Let rise uncovered 30 to 40 minutes before baking.

Heat oven to 375°. Bake rolls 20 to 25 minutes or until golden brown.

Pan Rolls: Spray layer pan, 9 x 1½ inches, with vegetable spray. Cut dough into fourths; cut each into 6 pieces. Shape pieces of dough into smooth balls. Place in pan.

24 rolls.
1 roll = 184 calories
0 cholesterol
7 gm fat

Cloverleaf Rolls: Spray 16 muffin cups with vegetable spray. Cut dough into thirds; cut each third into 16 pieces. Shape pieces into smooth balls; place 3 balls in each muffin cup.

16 rolls.
1 roll = 277 calories
0 cholesterol
10 gm fat

Buns: Spray baking sheet with vegetable spray. Cut dough into 12 pieces. Shape pieces into smooth slightly flat ball. Place 1 inch apart on baking sheet.

12 buns.
1 bun = 369 calories
0 cholesterol
13 gm fat

GRANDMOTHER'S WHITE BREAD

2 packages active dry yeast
½ cup warm water (105 to 115°)
1¾ cups warm water
3 tablespoons sugar
1½ teaspoons salt
2 tablespoons vegetable oil
6 to 7 cups all-purpose flour
Unsalted margarine, softened

Dissolve yeast in ½ cup warm water in large bowl. Stir in 1¾ cups water, the sugar, salt, oil, and 3½ cups of the flour. Beat until smooth. Mix in enough remaining flour to make dough easy to handle.

Turn dough onto lightly floured board; knead until smooth and elastic, about 10 minutes. Place in greased bowl; turn greased side up. Cover and let rise in warm place until double, about 40 minutes. (Dough is ready if an indentation remains when touched.)

Punch down dough; divide in half. Roll each half into rectangle, 18 x 9 inches. Roll up, beginning at short side. Press each end with side of hand to seal. Fold ends under loaf. Place seam side down in sprayed loaf pan, 9 x 5 x 3 inches. Brush loaves lightly with margarine. Let rise until double, about 25 minutes.

Heat oven to 425°. Place loaves on low rack so that tops of pans are in center of oven. Pans should not touch each other or sides of oven. Bake 25 minutes or until deep golden brown and loaves sound hollow when tapped. Remove from pans and cool on wire rack.

32 slices.

1 slice = 105 calories
0 cholesterol
1 gm fat

Cinnamon-Raisin Bread: Stir in 1 cup raisins with the second addition of flour. Mix 2 tablespoons sugar and 2 teaspoons cinnamon. After rolling dough into rectangles, sprinkle each with 1 tablespoon water and half the sugar-cinnamon mixture.

1 slice = 123 calories

Swedish Orange Rye Bread: Decrease flour to 4 to 5 cups; stir in 2 cups rye flour, 2 tablespoons grated orange peel, and 1 tablespoon caraway, anise, or fennel seed with the first addition of flour.

1 slice = 116 calories

Rye Bread: Decrease flour to 4 to 5 cups and stir in 2 cups rye flour with first addition of flour.

1 slice = 115 calories

Herb Bread: Stir in 1 teaspoon caraway seed, ½ teaspoon nutmeg, and ½ teaspoon sage with the first addition of flour.

1 slice = 110 calories

Onion Bread: Stir in ¼ cup plus 1 tablespoon instant minced onion with first addition of flour.

1 slice = 105 calories

Garlic Bread: Stir in 1 teaspoon garlic powder with first addition of flour.

1 slice = 105 calories

WHEAT GERM CASSEROLE BREAD

2½ to 3 cups all-purpose flour
½ cup wheat germ
2 envelopes active dry yeast
2 teaspoons salt
1½ cups warm water (105 to 115°)
2 tablespoons unsalted margarine,
softened
2 tablespoons molasses

Measure 1 cup of the flour, the wheat germ, yeast, and salt into large mixer bowl. Add water, margarine, and molasses. Blend on low speed ½ minute, scraping bowl constantly. Beat on medium speed 2 minutes, scraping bowl occasionally. Add ½ cup of the remaining flour; beat on high speed 2 minutes, scraping bowl frequently. Stir in remaining flour until smooth. Scrape batter from side of bowl. Cover and let rise in warm place until double, about 45 minutes.

Heat oven to 375°. Stir down batter by beating with wooden spoon, about 30 seconds. Spread in sprayed 1½-quart casserole.

Bake 1 hour 15 minutes or until loaf sounds hollow when tapped. Remove loaf from casserole. Serve warm or cool on wire rack.

12 slices.

1 slice = 158 calories
0 mg cholesterol
3 gm fat

FRENCH BREAD

1 package active dry yeast
1¼ cups warm water (105 to 115°)
¾ teaspoon salt
1 tablespoon vegetable oil
3½ to 4 cups all-purpose flour
1 tablespoon cornmeal
1 egg white
2 tablespoons water

Dissolve yeast in warm water in large mixing bowl. Stir in salt, oil, and 1½ cups of the flour. Beat until smooth. Stir in enough remaining flour (first with spoon, then by hand) to make dough easy to handle.

Turn dough onto lightly floured board; knead until smooth and elastic, about 5 minutes. Place in greased bowl; turn greased side up. Cover with damp cloth; let rise in warm place until double, about 1 hour. (Dough is ready if an indentation remains when touched.)

Punch down dough; round up and let rise until almost double, about 20 minutes. Punch down; cover and let rest 15 minutes.

Lightly grease baking sheet; sprinkle with cornmeal. Roll dough into rectangle, 15 x 10 inches. Roll up tightly, beginning at long side. Pinch edge to seal. Roll gently back and forth to taper ends.

Place loaf on baking sheet. Make ¼-inch slashes across loaf at 2-inch intervals or make 1 slash lengthwise. Brush top of loaf with cold water.

Let rise uncovered about 35 minutes. Brush with cold water.

Heat oven to 375°. Bake 20 minutes. Beat egg white and 2 tablespoons cold water slightly; brush on loaf. Bake 25 minutes longer. Remove from baking sheet; cool on wire rack.

15 slices.

1 slice = 124 calories
0 cholesterol
1 gm fat

COTTAGE CHEESE-DILL BATTER BREAD

¼ cup chopped onion
1 tablespoon vegetable oil
1 package active dry yeast
¾ cup warm water (105 to 115°)
¼ cup egg substitute
2 tablespoons sugar
1 tablespoon dill seed
1 teaspoon salt
1½ cups low-fat cottage cheese
4 cups all-purpose flour

Sauté onion in oil until tender; set aside.

Dissolve yeast in warm water in large mixer bowl. Add onion, egg substitute, sugar, dill seed, salt, cottage cheese, and 2 cups of the flour. Blend on low speed, scraping bowl constantly. Beat on medium speed 2 minutes, scraping bowl occasionally. Stir in remaining flour with wooden spoon until smooth. Cover and let rise in warm place until double, about 1 hour.

Stir down dough by beating 25 strokes. Spread in sprayed 2½-quart casserole. Cover and let rise until double, about 30 minutes.

Heat oven to 350°. Bake 1 hour or until bread sounds hollow when tapped. Remove from casserole and cool on wire rack.

20 slices.

1 slice = 121 calories
1 mg cholesterol
1 gm fat

RYE BREAD

4 to 4½ cups all-purpose flour
2 packages active dry yeast
2 cups warm water (105 to 115°)
2 tablespoons sugar
¼ cup honey
1 teaspoon salt
2 cups rye flour

Measure 3 cups of the flour and the yeast into large mixer bowl. Add water, sugar, honey, and salt. Beat on low speed ½ minute, scraping bowl constantly. Beat on high speed 3 minutes. Stir in rye flour and enough remaining flour to make dough easy to handle. Turn out onto lightly floured board. Knead until smooth, 5 to 8 minutes. Place in greased bowl; turn greased side up. Cover and refrigerate 8 hours or overnight.

Spray three junior loaf pans, 7½ x 3½ x 2 inches, with vegetable spray. Punch down dough; divide in thirds. Shape each into loaf and place in pan. Let rise in warm place (85°) until double, about 1 hour 15 minutes.

Place loaves in unheated oven; turn on oven to 300°. Bake 15 minutes. Increase oven temperature to 325° and bake 30 minutes longer. Remove from pans and cool on wire rack.

42 slices.

1 slice = 75 calories
0 cholesterol
trace fat

CORN BREAD

1 cup yellow cornmeal
1 cup all-purpose flour
2 tablespoons sugar
3 teaspoons baking powder
¼ teaspoon salt
1 cup skim milk
¼ cup vegetable oil
¼ cup egg substitute

Heat oven to 425°. Spray baking pan, 8 x 8 x 2 inches, with vegetable spray. Blend all ingredients about 20 seconds. Beat vigorously by hand 1 minute. Pour into pan.

Bake 20 to 25 minutes or until golden brown.

12 servings.

1 serving = 136 calories
trace cholesterol
5 gm fat

Corn Bread Muffins: Fill sprayed muffin cups (2¾ inches in diameter) ½ full. Bake 15 minutes.

12 muffins.

CHALLAH

1 package active dry yeast
¼ cup warm water (105 to 115°)
¼ cup egg substitute
¼ cup sugar
¼ teaspoon salt
¼ cup unsalted margarine, softened
2½ to 3 cups all-purpose flour

Dissolve yeast in warm water in large bowl. Stir in egg substitute, sugar, salt, margarine, and 2 cups of the flour. Beat until smooth. Mix in enough remaining flour to make dough easy to handle.

Turn dough onto lightly floured board; knead until smooth and elastic, 5 minutes. Place in greased bowl; turn greased side up. Cover and let rise in warm place until double, 1½ to 2 hours.

Punch down dough; divide into 3 equal parts. Roll each part into rope 14 inches long. Place close together on sprayed baking sheet. Braid gently and loosely. Do not stretch. Pinch ends to seal; tuck ends under. Cover and let rise until double, about 1 hour.

Heat oven to 375°. Bake 30 to 35 minutes or until braid sounds hollow.

12 slices.

1 slice = 160 calories
0 cholesterol
4 gm fat

Note: For shiny crust, brush braid with slightly beaten egg white and 1 tablespoon water 10 minutes before end of baking time.

CARROT-RAISIN BREAD

1 cup skim milk
3 tablespoons margarine
2 packages active dry yeast
1 cup warm water (105 to 115°)
2 tablespoons brown sugar
1 teaspoon salt
1 tablespoon honey
3 tablespoons grated orange peel
½ teaspoon nutmeg
⅛ teaspoon ground cloves
¼ cup egg substitute
6½ to 7 cups all-purpose flour
1½ cups shredded carrot (about 2
 medium)
1 cup raisins

Heat milk and margarine in small saucepan over low heat until margarine is melted. Cool to lukewarm. Dissolve yeast in warm water in large mixing bowl. Stir in sugar, salt, honey, orange peel, nutmeg, cloves, egg substitute, and milk-margarine mixture with wooden spoon. Stir in 3 cups of the flour; beat until smooth. Mix in carrot and raisins. Mix in remaining flour until dough leaves side of bowl. Turn dough onto lightly floured, cloth-covered board. Knead until smooth and elastic. Place in greased bowl; turn greased side up. Cover and let rise in warm place until double, about 1 hour.

Punch down dough. Divide dough in half and shape into 2 loaves. Place each in loaf pan, 9½ x 5¼ x 3 inches, sprayed with vegetable spray. Cover and let rise until dough rises to top of pan, about 30 minutes.

Heat oven to 375°. Bake until brown and loaves sound hollow when tapped on bottom, 40 to 50 minutes.

2 loaves (32 slices).

1 slice = 133 calories
 trace cholesterol
 1 gm fat

BRAN DATE-NUT BREAD

1¼ cups boiling water
1 cup snipped dates
½ cup egg substitute
¼ cup vegetable oil
1 cup all-bran cereal
2¼ cups all-purpose flour
½ cup sugar
2½ teaspoons baking powder
½ teaspoon salt
½ teaspoon cinnamon
½ cup chopped walnuts
2 teaspoons grated orange peel

Pour boiling water over dates in mixing bowl; cool. Beat egg substitute and oil; stir in bran cereal and let stand 10 minutes.

Heat oven to 350°. Spray loaf pan, 9 x 5 x 3 inches, with vegetable spray. Mix bran mixture, flour, sugar, baking powder, salt, and cinnamon into date mixture just until flour is moistened. Stir in walnuts and orange peel. Spread in pan.

Bake 60 to 65 minutes or until wooden pick inserted in center comes out clean. Let cool in pan 10 minutes before turning onto wire rack.

16 slices.

1 slice = 195 calories
 0 cholesterol
 6 gm fat

BANANA BREAD

⅔ cup unsalted margarine, softened
½ cup sugar
½ cup egg substitute
1½ cups mashed ripe bananas
  (4 to 5 medium)
1 tablespoon lemon juice
2 cups all-purpose flour
1 teaspoon baking soda
½ teaspoon salt
½ cup snipped dates
1 tablespoon flour

Heat oven to 325°. Spray loaf pan, 9 x 5 x 3 inches, with vegetable spray. Cream margarine and sugar thoroughly. Add egg substitute, bananas, and lemon juice; beat until smooth. Mix in 2 cups flour, the baking soda, and salt just until flour is moistened. Mix dates and 1 tablespoon flour; stir into banana mixture. Spread in pan.

Bake 1 hour 10 to 20 minutes or until wooden pick inserted in center comes out clean. Remove from pan and cool on wire rack.

16 slices.

1 slice = 205 calories
          0 cholesterol
          8 gm fat

SPOON BREAD

2½ cups skim milk
¾ cup white cornmeal
¼ teaspoon salt
2 tablespoons unsalted margarine
2 tablespoons sugar
¼ cup egg substitute
2 egg whites

Heat oven to 350°. Heat milk in medium saucepan to scalding. Reduce heat; stirring constantly, sprinkle cornmeal slowly into hot milk. Cook, stirring constantly 5 minutes. Remove from heat; mix in margarine, sugar, salt, and egg substitute. Beat egg whites until stiff peaks form. Fold into cornmeal mixture. Pour into 1½-quart casserole. Bake 45 to 50 minutes. Serve hot.

6 servings.

1 serving = 128 calories
            2 mg cholesterol
            4 gm fat

GARLIC BREAD

Heat oven to 350°. Cut 1 loaf (1 pound) French bread horizontally in half. Mix ½ cup margarine, softened, and ¼ teaspoon garlic powder; spread generously on cut sides of loaf. Reassemble loaf; cut crosswise into 2-inch slices. Wrap securely in heavy-duty aluminum foil. Heat 15 to 20 minutes.

24 to 28 slices.

1 slice = 82 calories
          trace cholesterol
          4 gm fat

HOT SPICY BREAD IN FOIL

½ cup unsalted margarine
2 teaspoons minced onion
1 tablespoon snipped fresh tarragon
1 teaspoon snipped fresh thyme
2 tablespoons snipped parsley
¼ teaspoon sage
¼ teaspoon powdered rosemary
¼ teaspoon salt
¼ teaspoon freshly ground pepper
½ teaspoon Dijon-type mustard
1 loaf sliced snack rye bread

Heat oven to 350°. Beat margarine until light and fluffy. Mix in remaining ingredients except bread. Spread mixture evenly on slices. Reassemble loaf; wrap securely in heavy-duty aluminum foil. Heat in oven 10 minutes.

32 slices.

   1 slice = 46 calories
                trace cholesterol
                3 gm fat

TOAST CUPS

Remove crusts from 6 thin bread slices. Brush slices with 2 tablespoons melted margarine. Press buttered sides down into muffin cups. Bake until toasted, about 20 minutes.

6 cups.

   1 cup = 103 calories
              trace cholesterol
              5 gm fat

Note: For interesting flavor, add 1 teaspoon herbs, such as Italian seasoning, thyme, dill, or 1 teaspoon dry mustard.

SEASONED CROUTONS

4 cups ½-inch bread cubes
  (about 4 slices)
1 tablespoon thyme
2 teaspoons parsley flakes
¼ teaspoon freshly ground pepper
⅛ teaspoon dry mustard
⅛ teaspoon poultry seasoning
⅛ teaspoon garlic powder
⅛ teaspoon sage
½ cup unsalted margarine
½ cup finely chopped onion

Heat oven to 325°. Measure bread cubes and seasonings into bowl. Melt margarine in small skillet over low heat. Cook and stir onion in margarine until tender. Pour over bread cubes and toss. Spread in ungreased baking pan, 13 x 9 x 2 inches. Bake until golden brown, about 30 minutes.

4 cups.

   ¼ cup = 74 calories
              trace cholesterol
              6 gm fat

DUMPLINGS

1½ cups all-purpose flour
2 teaspoons baking powder
3 tablespoons vegetable oil
¾ cup skim milk

Measure flour and baking powder into mixing bowl. Mix in oil. Stir in milk. Drop dough by spoonfuls onto hot meat or vegetables in boiling stew. (Do not drop directly into liquid.) Cook uncovered 10 minutes; cover and cook 10 minutes longer.

10 dumplings.

   1 dumpling = 109 calories
                   trace cholesterol
                   4 gm fat

13 *Meat and Poultry*

EASY SKILLET DINNER

2 tablespoons vegetable oil
1- to 1½-pound flank steak, scored
½ cup chopped onion
½ cup water
2 cloves garlic, crushed
1 teaspoon Tabasco sauce
½ teaspoon oregano
½ teaspoon salt
1 bay leaf
½ pound green beans, cut into 1-inch
   pieces
8 to 10 new potatoes
2 tomatoes, peeled and cut up

Heat oil in large skillet; brown meat on both sides over medium heat. Add onion; cook and stir until tender. Stir in water, garlic, Tabasco sauce, oregano, salt, and bay leaf; heat to boiling. Reduce heat, cover and simmer 1 hour, adding water if necessary. Add beans, potatoes, and tomatoes; heat to boiling. Reduce heat; cover and cook over medium heat until potatoes are tender, about 30 minutes.

4 to 6 servings.

1 serving = 372 calories
             102 mg cholesterol
             14 gm fat

SAVORY BEEF STEW

1½ pounds extra lean boneless beef
   chuck, cut into 1-inch pieces
¼ cup all-purpose flour
¼ cup margarine
½ cup chopped onion
½ cup water
½ cup red wine
2 tablespoons snipped parsley
2 cloves garlic, minced
2 bay leaves
1½ teaspoons salt
½ teaspoon freshly ground pepper
2 teaspoons Italian seasoning or thyme,
   if desired
Dash Tabasco sauce
2 cups cubed pared potatoes
2 cups 1-inch pieces carrot
1 cup 1-inch pieces celery
10 small white onions

Coat meat with flour. Melt margarine in large saucepan; cook meat and chopped onion in margarine until meat is brown. Pour in water and cool. Chill several hours or overnight.

Remove fat from meat and stock. Add wine, parsley, garlic, bay leaves, salt, and pepper and heat to boiling. Reduce heat; cover and simmer until meat is tender, 1 to 1½ hours. Add potatoes, carrot, celery, and onions. Cook until vegetables are tender, about 30 minutes.

6 servings.

1 serving = 328 calories
             82 mg cholesterol
             14 gm fat

BEEF or LAMB SHISH KEBABS

Meat-Basting Sauce (below)
6 ounces lean beef or lamb cubes
2 small onions, each cut into quarters
6 cherry tomatoes
6 fresh mushroom caps
1 medium green pepper, cut into 1-inch
  pieces

Prepare Meat-Basting Sauce, except do not refrigerate sauce 24 hours. Place meat in deep bowl; pour sauce on meat and refrigerate at least 3 hours, turning meat occasionally. (Can be refrigerated up to 24 hours.)

Drain meat, reserving sauce. Alternate meat, onion quarters, tomatoes, mushrooms, and green pepper pieces on skewers.

Set oven at broil and/or 550°. Broil kebabs 3 inches from heat, turning and basting occasionally with reserved sauce, until desired doneness. Or kebabs can be grilled over hot coals.

4 servings.

1 serving = 224 calories
33 mg cholesterol
17 gm fat

MEAT-BASTING SAUCE

1 cup red wine
1 cup vegetable oil
¼ cup wine vinegar
2 medium onions, chopped
2 cloves garlic, peeled
⅛ teaspoon rosemary
⅛ teaspoon cayenne pepper

Shake all ingredients in tightly covered jar. Refrigerate 24 hours to blend flavors. Remove garlic. Use for basting meat or poultry while roasting or broiling.

About 2¼ cups.

HORSERADISH-STUFFED RIB ROAST

¼ cup prepared horseradish
2 cloves garlic, minced
5- to 6-pound rolled rib roast,
  well trimmed

Mix horseradish and garlic. Unroll rib roast; spread with horseradish mixture. Reroll roast and tie securely. Rub outside of roast with an additional clove of garlic.

To roast on rotisserie, insert spit rod lengthwise through center of roast. Secure meat on spit with holding forks. Insert meat thermometer in center of meat making sure it does not touch fat or spit. Cook roast on rotisserie in 500° oven 25 minutes. Reduce oven temperature to 325° and roast to desired doneness. For rare, allow 16 minutes per pound or until meat thermometer registers 150°. Or roast on rotisserie over medium coals 2½ to 3 hours or until desired doneness. Allow roast to stand for 15 minutes before slicing.

10 to 12 servings.

1 serving = 298 calories
149 mg cholesterol
10 gm fat

Note: This may also be oven-roasted without a rotisserie.

PIQUANT FLANK STEAK

1 cup vegetable juice
¼ cup minced onion or green onion
¼ cup minced green pepper
¼ cup minced celery
¼ cup olive oil
1 tablespoon vinegar
1 to 2 cloves garlic, minced
1 tablespoon chili powder
2-pound flank steak, scored

Heat vegetable juice, onion, green pepper, celery, olive oil, vinegar, garlic, and chili powder to boiling. Reduce heat; cover and simmer 15 minutes. Cool.

Place steak in shallow glass baking dish; pour marinade on meat. Cover and refrigerate at least 1 hour. Remove meat from marinade; reserve marinade. Place meat on grill 4 inches from hot coals. Cook 3 to 4 minutes for rare, basting with reserved marinade occasionally. Cut meat across grain at a slanted angle into thin slices.

4 to 6 servings.

1 serving = 292 calories
109 mg cholesterol
14 gm fat

HAMBURGERS DELUXE

1 pound ground lean beef
¼ cup finely chopped onion
1 tablespoon unsalted margarine, melted
1 tablespoon lemon juice
1½ teaspoons snipped parsley
1 teaspoon water
¼ teaspoon garlic powder
⅛ teaspoon marjoram leaves
⅛ teaspoon basil leaves

Mix all ingredients thoroughly. Shape mixture into 4 patties. Set oven at broil and/or 550°. Broil patties 3 inches from heat 3 to 4 minutes on each side for rare, 5 to 7 minutes for medium.

4 servings.

1 serving = 220 calories
95 mg cholesterol
9 gm fat

CONFETTI BURGERS

1 pound ground lean beef
¼ cup plus 2 tablespoons shredded carrot
2 tablespoons minced onion
1 tablespoon snipped parsley
2 tablespoons wheat germ
1 teaspoon dry mustard
¼ teaspoon salt
Freshly ground pepper

Mix all ingredients. Shape mixture into 4 patties, each about 3 inches in diameter and 1 inch thick.

Set oven at broil and/or 550°. Broil patties 3 inches from heat 3 to 4 minutes on each side for rare, 5 to 7 minutes for medium.

4 servings.

1 serving = 204 calories
91 mg cholesterol
7 gm fat

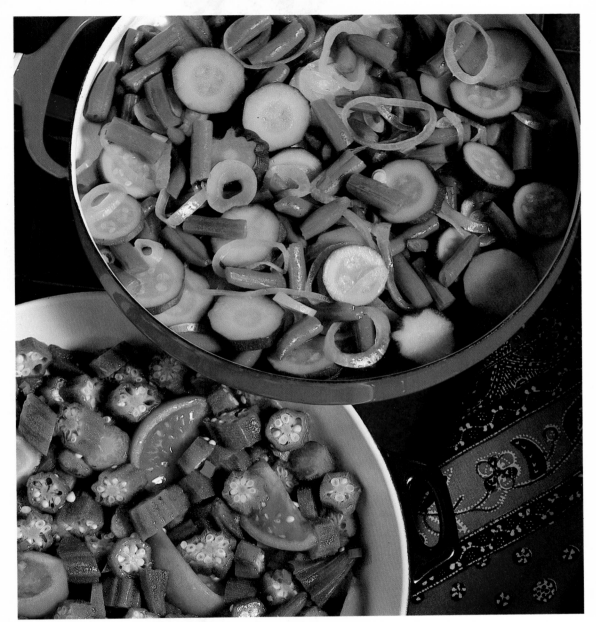

Okra Stir-Fry; Spicy Vegetable Combo

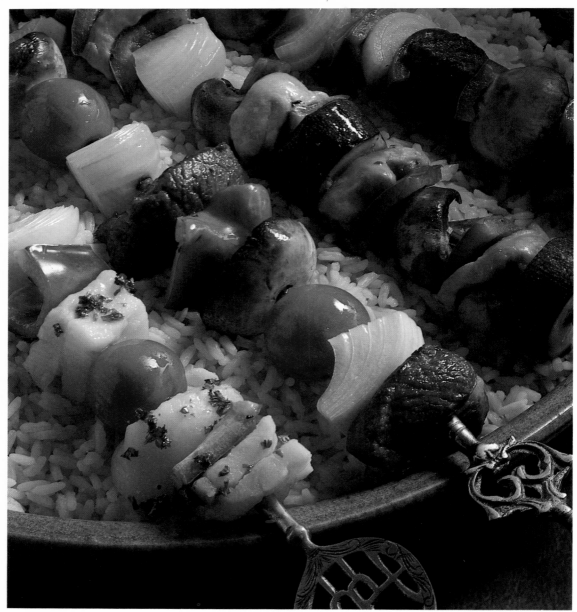

Shish Kebabs: Seafood, Beef, Lamb, and Chicken Brochette.

HAMBURGERS

1 pound ground lean beef
1 small onion, minced (¼ cup)
½ teaspoon freshly ground pepper
½ teaspoon dry mustard
¼ cup iced water
¼ teaspoon salt

Mix all ingredients. Shape mixture into 4 patties, each about 3 inches in diameter and 1 inch thick.

To Broil: Set oven at broil and/or 550°. Broil 3 inches from heat 3 to 4 minutes on each side for rare, 5 to 7 minutes for medium.

To Panfry: Fry in 1 to 2 teaspoons vegetable oil over medium heat, turning frequently, about 10 minutes.

To Grill: Place on grill 4 to 6 inches from hot coals. Cook, turning once, until done, about 12 minutes.

Italian-style Hamburgers: Before mixing, add ¼ teaspoon oregano.

4 servings.

> 1 serving = 223 calories
> 102 mg cholesterol
> 8 gm fat

HAMBURGER TOPPERS

Smothered Onions: Slice 2 large onions and separate into rings. Cook and stir onion rings in 1 tablespoon unsalted margarine until crisp-tender.

> 1 serving = 30 calories
> 0 cholesterol
> 1 gm fat

Pepper and Onion: Slice 1 medium onion. Cut ½ each red pepper and green pepper into thin strips. Cook and stir onion and pepper strips in 1 tablespoon vegetable oil until tender. Season with freshly ground pepper.

> 1 serving = 26 calories
> 0 cholesterol
> 1 gm fat

Mashed Potato: Top each hamburger with thin tomato slice and thin slice (½ ounce) low-sodium low-fat cheese. Spoon on ¼ cup mashed potatoes to which 1 tablespoon chopped onion has been added. Sprinkle with paprika.

> 1 serving = 18 calories
> trace cholesterol
> 0 fat

Hamburgers and Eggplant: Pare and slice eggplant into ¾-inch slices. Season with freshly ground pepper, then coat slices with flour. Cook in hot olive oil until tender. Keep hot while preparing hamburgers. Top each eggplant slice with hamburger, 3 tablespoons hot Tomato Sauce (page 167) and 1 tablespoon grated Parmesan cheese.

> 1 serving = 44 calories
> 2 mg cholesterol
> 3 gm fat

Horseradish and Onion: Before cooking hamburgers, heat 2 tablespoons water and 1 tablespoon horseradish powder over low heat. Spoon 1 teaspoon horseradish sauce in center of each hamburger patty. Top cooked patty with Smothered Onions (above).

> 1 serving = 30 calories
> 0 cholesterol
> 1 gm fat

MEAT LOAF

½ cup unprocessed bran
¼ cup wheat germ
½ cup water
2 egg whites or 1 egg
½ pound ground lean beef
½ pound ground veal
1½ cups minced onion (1 large)
½ cup thinly sliced celery
1 clove garlic, crushed
½ package onion soup mix (optional)
1 teaspoon dry mustard
1 teaspoon Italian seasoning
¼ teaspoon salt
Dash freshly ground pepper

Heat oven to 350°. Spray loaf pan, 9 x 5 x 3 inches, with vegetable spray. Measure bran and wheat germ into bowl; add water and allow to stand until softened. Mix in remaining ingredients. Turn into loaf pan. Bake 45 minutes or until brown.

6 servings.

1 serving = 194 calories
65 mg cholesterol
5 gm fat

MANICOTTI

1 carton (16 ounces) low-fat cottage cheese (2 cups)
8 ounces shredded part skim milk mozzarella cheese (2 cups)
1 teaspoon salt
1 cup low-fat mayonnaise
1 pound lean ground beef
2 cloves garlic, pressed
16 manicotti, cooked and drained
4 cups Tomato Sauce (page 167)
1 teaspoon oregano
⅔ cup grated Parmesan cheese

Mix cottage cheese, mozzarella cheese, salt, and mayonnaise in bowl. Cook and stir ground beef and garlic in skillet until meat is brown. Drain off fat. Stir ground beef into cottage-cheese mixture.

Heat oven to 325°. Fill each manicotti with about ¼ cup meat-cheese filling. Place 8 manicotti in each of 2 baking dishes, 11½ x 7½ x 1 inches. Sprinkle any remaining filling on filled manicotti. Pour 2 cups tomato sauce on manicotti in each baking dish and sprinkle with oregano and Parmesan cheese. Cover baking dishes with aluminum foil. Bake 15 minutes. Remove foil and bake 10 minutes longer.

8 servings.

1 serving = 551 calories
78 mg cholesterol
30 gm fat

BAKED LASAGNE

1 pound ground lean beef
2 tablespoons olive or vegetable oil
4 cups Tomato Sauce (page 167)
¼ teaspoon salt
Freshly ground pepper
1 package (8 ounces) lasagne noodles,
  cooked and drained
2 pounds ricotta cheese (Italian pot
  cheese)
½ pound part skim milk mozzarella
  cheese, shredded
3 tablespoons grated Parmesan cheese

Cook and stir ground beef in oil in large skillet until meat is brown. Stir in Tomato Sauce; reduce heat and simmer 15 minutes. Season with salt and pepper.

Heat oven to 375°. Reserve about ½ cup of tomato sauce mixture for thin top layer. Spread several tablespoons of remaining tomato sauce mixture in baking dish, 11¾ x 7½ x 1¾ inches. Layer ⅓ each of the noodles, remaining meat sauce, and the ricotta and mozzarella cheeses in baking dish. Repeat 2 times. Spread reserved tomato sauce mixture on top and sprinkle with Parmesan cheese. Cover tightly with aluminum foil and bake 20 minutes. Remove foil and bake 5 minutes longer.

8 servings.

1 serving = 540 calories
            103 mg cholesterol
            30 gm fat

BAKED STUFFED ACORN SQUASH

2 acorn squash
½ cup water
½ cup chopped onion
¼ cup chopped celery
½ clove garlic, crushed
½ pound ground beef
½ cup chopped peeled tomato
½ cup sliced mushrooms
⅓ cup cooked rice
1 tablespoon snipped parsley
½ teaspoon basil
⅛ teaspoon salt
¼ teaspoon freshly ground pepper
¼ cup shredded part skim milk mozzarella
  cheese

Heat oven to 400°. Cut squash lengthwise into halves; scoop out seeds and fibers. Place halves cut side down in shallow baking pan. Pour water into pan. Bake 45 minutes.

Cook and stir onion, celery, garlic, and ground beef in large skillet until meat is brown. Drain off fat. Stir in tomato, mushrooms, rice, parsley, basil, salt, and pepper and heat through. Divide mixture among squash halves. Sprinkle cheese on tops.

Reduce oven temperature to 350°. Bake filled squash until squash is tender, about 20 minutes.

4 servings.

1 serving = 272 calories
            50 mg cholesterol
            9 gm fat

SPICED LAMB BURGERS

2 pounds ground lamb
⅓ cup egg substitute
½ cup soft bread crumbs
½ cup chopped onion
1 teaspoon salt
2 teaspoons ground coriander
1½ teaspoons nutmeg
2 teaspoons curry powder
½ teaspoon freshly ground pepper
2 teaspoons grated lemon peel

Mix all ingredients thoroughly. Shape mixture into 16 patties, each about ¾ inch thick and 2½ inches in diameter.

To grill, place on grill about 3 inches from hot coals. Cook 5 minutes; turn patties and cook 5 minutes longer. (Patties may also be oven-broiled.) If desired, serve on curried rice and garnish with fresh mint sprigs.

8 servings.

1 serving = 181 calories
87 mg cholesterol
7 gm fat

MARINATED LEG OF LAMB

6- to 8-pound leg of lamb
⅔ cup olive oil or vegetable oil
3 tablespoons lemon juice
2 tablespoons snipped parsley
1 teaspoon oregano
3 bay leaves, crumbled
1 cup sliced onion
3 cloves garlic, thinly sliced
1 teaspoon salt

Have butcher remove fell from leg of lamb and most of the fat, then remove bone from leg. This will produce a fairly compact piece of meat with a large pocket. With a sharp knife, cut lengthwise through thinnest side of pocket and spread meat flat with fat side down. Remove any exposed fat, and separate thickest clump of meat with point of knife to make it lie flatter. Meat piece will be ragged and uneven.

Mix remaining ingredients except salt in shallow baking dish. Add meat, turning meat so both sides are coated with marinade. Cover and refrigerate at least 12 hours. If possible, allow 24 hours. Turn meat several times, spooning marinade on meat. Remove meat from refrigerator about 2 hours before broiling to come to room temperature.

Forty-five minutes before serving, set oven at broil and/or 550°. Allow oven to heat 15 minutes so broiler rack is very hot. Remove meat from marinade (do not dry) to hot broiler rack. Sprinkle with ½ teaspoon salt. Broil 15 minutes. Do not baste. If meat begins to burn around edge, lower heat. Turn meat with tongs; sprinkle with remaining salt and broil 15 minutes longer. Remove to hot platter and cut across the grain into ¼-inch slices. Serve immediately.

6 servings.

1 serving = 310 calories
120 mg cholesterol
18 gm fat

LAMB CHOPS L'ORANGE

6 shoulder lamb chops
1 cup orange juice
⅛ teaspoon salt
Freshly ground pepper
½ teaspoon ginger
½ teaspoon nutmeg
½ teaspoon dry mustard
½ teaspoon marjoram
1 teaspoon snipped chives
1 tablespoon slivered orange peel
1 tablespoon cornstarch
2 tablespoons water
1 orange, sliced

Arrange lamb chops in baking dish. Mix remaining ingredients except cornstarch, water, and sliced orange; pour on lamb chops. Cover and refrigerate 3 to 4 hours, turning chops occasionally.

Remove chops from marinade and drain on paper towels. Reserve marinade. Brown chops on both sides in large skillet. Pour reserved marinade on chops and heat to boiling. Reduce heat; cover and simmer until chops are tender, 35 to 40 minutes. Remove chops to platter and keep warm. Mix cornstarch and water until smooth. Stir into skillet. Cook, stirring constantly, until mixture thickens and boils. Boil and stir 1 minute. Add orange slices and heat. Spoon sauce on chops.

6 servings.
1 serving = 202 calories
90 mg cholesterol
7 gm fat

VEAL PICCATA

1½ pounds veal scallops
Freshly ground pepper
2 tablespoons margarine
1½ teaspoons tarragon
8 thin lemon slices
¼ cup white vermouth or dry white wine
2 tablespoons snipped parsley

Place scallops between sheets of waxed paper and pound, not roughly, to ¼-inch thickness. (A rolling pin or mallet can be used.) Season scallops with pepper. Melt margarine in large skillet. Brown 3 or 4 scallops at a time over medium-high heat. Turn and brown on other sides. Remove scallops to warm platter.

Return scallops to skillet; sprinkle with tarragon, arrange lemon slices on scallops and pour on wine. Cover and simmer until meat is hot, 3 to 4 minutes. Remove meat to warm platter; spoon sauce on top and sprinkle with parsley.

6 servings.
1 serving = 251 calories
99 mg cholesterol
15 gm fat

VEAL STEW with DILL

2 pounds boneless stewing veal, cubed
1 large onion
6 peppercorns
3 whole cloves
½ teaspoon salt
1 medium carrot, coarsely chopped
½ cup chopped celery (with leaves)
½ small lemon, sliced
2 stems dill
Water
2 tablespoons water
1 tablespoon flour
Juice of ¼ lemon
Salt and pepper
2 tablespoons snipped fresh dill

Place veal, onion, peppercorns, cloves, ½ teaspoon salt, the carrot, celery, lemon slices, and dill stems in Dutch oven; add enough water to cover meat. Heat to boiling; reduce heat and cover. Simmer until meat is tender, about 1 hour.

Remove meat to warm serving dish and keep warm. Strain cooking liquid into saucepan. Mix 2 tablespoons water and the flour until smooth. Stir into cooking liquid. Heat to boiling, stirring constantly. Boil and stir 1 minute. Stir in lemon juice and season with salt and pepper. Stir in snipped dill and pour sauce on meat.

6 servings.

1 serving = 273 calories
118 mg cholesterol
13 gm fat

VEAL MARSALA

1 tablespoon margarine
4 small veal cutlets
1 cup sliced mushrooms
½ clove garlic, minced
2 tomatoes, peeled and chopped
2 teaspoons snipped parsley
⅛ teaspoon sugar
⅛ teaspoon Italian seasoning
2 tablespoons Marsala
⅛ teaspoon salt
Freshly ground pepper

Melt margarine in skillet; brown cutlets on both sides and remove from skillet. Cook and stir mushrooms and garlic in skillet 5 minutes. Add cutlets and remaining ingredients; cover and cook over medium-low heat until cutlets are tender, about 45 minutes.

4 servings.

1 serving = 235 calories
89 mg cholesterol
13 gm fat

VEAL ROLLUPS

6 boneless veal cutlets (about 1½ pounds)
6 teaspoons Dijon-type mustard
1½ cups prepared bread stuffing
About 3 tablespoons flour
⅓ cup egg substitute
1 cup Italian bread crumbs
Vegetable oil
3 tablespoons snipped parsley

Pound meat until ¼ inch thick. Spread 1 teaspoon mustard on each cutlet, then top with about 3 tablespoons bread stuffing. Roll up and secure with wooden pick.

Coat rolls with flour, then dip into egg substitute and roll in bread crumbs. Heat enough oil in medium skillet to cover bottom; brown rolls, about 4 minutes. Cover and bake in 325° oven until rolls are tender, about 30 minutes. Sprinkle parsley on rolls and, if desired, serve with Mustard Sauce (page 70).

6 servings.

**1 serving = 352 calories
94 mg cholesterol
12 gm fat**

Chicken Rollups: Substitute chicken cutlets for the veal cutlets.

**1 serving = 240 calories
37 mg cholesterol
7 gm fat**

ESCALOPES DE VEAU AU CITRON

1½ pounds boneless veal cutlets
Freshly ground pepper
2 tablespoons flour
2 tablespoons margarine
¼ cup olive oil
¼ cup white wine
3 tablespoons lemon juice
2 lemons, thinly sliced
1 lemon, cut lengthwise into wedges
Snipped parsley

Pound meat until ¼ inch thick. Season with pepper and coat with flour. Melt margarine in oil in large skillet. Cook meat in oil over medium heat until brown, 3 to 4 minutes on each side. Pour wine and lemon juice on meat and cook over medium heat 3 to 4 minutes. Arrange meat with lemon slices between meat on heated serving dish. Pour sauce on meat. Arrange lemon wedges around meat and sprinkle with parsley.

6 servings.

**1 serving = 324 calories
99 mg cholesterol
19 gm fat**

SAUTÉED VEAL SCALLOPS à la DILLON

12 veal scallops (1 to 1½ ounces each)
3 tablespoons minced onion
½ clove garlic, minced
2 tablespoons margarine
1 tablespoon vegetable oil
⅓ cup white vermouth
1 tablespoon tarragon
1 cup Brown Sauce (this page)
1 tablespoon cornstarch
1 tablespoon water
Freshly ground pepper
Snipped parsley

Dry scallops thoroughly on paper towels. Cook and stir onion and garlic in margarine and oil in large skillet until onion is tender, 4 to 5 minutes. Arrange 3 or 4 scallops at a time in skillet and brown over medium-high heat. Turn and brown on other sides. Remove scallops to warm platter.

Add wine and tarragon to skillet; cook, stirring constantly, until liquid is reduced to 2 or 3 spoonfuls. Stir in Brown Sauce. Mix cornstarch and water until smooth. Stir into Brown Sauce mixture. Cook, stirring constantly until mixture thickens and boils. Boil and stir 1 minute.

Return scallops to skillet, basting each with sauce. Simmer until scallops are hot, 4 to 5 minutes. Season with pepper. Remove scallops to warm platter; spoon sauce on meat and sprinkle with parsley.

4 servings.

> 1 serving = 307 calories
> 89 mg cholesterol
> 20 gm fat

BROWN SAUCE

1 cup beef bouillon (see *Note*)
3 tablespoons minced onion
3 tablespoons diced carrot
1 tablespoon diced celery
½ cup white vermouth or dry white wine
½ bay leaf
⅛ teaspoon thyme

Measure all ingredients into saucepan. Heat to boiling; reduce heat and simmer 30 minutes. Strain; cool and refrigerate.

> *About 1½ cups.*
> ¼ cup = 9 calories
> 0 cholesterol
> 0 fat

Note: Beef bouillon can be made by dissolving 1 beef bouillon cube in 1 cup boiling water.

VEAL with FINES HERBES

3 tablespoons margarine
1 pound veal scallops
½ cup dry white wine
1 teaspoon snipped chives
½ teaspoon tarragon
1 tablespoon snipped parsley
1 tablespoon margarine

Melt 3 tablespoons margarine in large skillet. Cook meat in margarine until golden and tender. Remove to warm platter and keep warm.

Pour wine into skillet; cook over high heat until wine is reduced by half. Stir in chives, tarragon, parsley, and 1 tablespoon margarine. Heat to boiling and pour on meat.

4 servings.

> 1 serving = 300 calories
> 94 mg cholesterol
> 18 gm fat

VEAL CHOPS ITALIAN STYLE

6 veal loin chops ½ to ¾ inch thick (about 1¾ pounds)
½ cup vegetable oil
1 large clove garlic, crushed
1 tablespoon oregano leaves, crushed
4 ounces medium noodles, cooked and drained (about 3 cups)
2 tablespoons margarine, melted
2 tablespoons grated Parmesan cheese
2 tablespoons snipped parsley

Place veal chops in shallow dish. Mix oil, garlic, and oregano leaves; pour on chops. Cover and refrigerate 2 to 3 hours, turning chops several times.

Set oven at broil and/or 550°. Remove chops from marinade; place on broiler rack. Broil 3 inches from heat, turning once, until chops are brown and tender.

Toss hot noodles with margarine, cheese, and parsley. Place on warm serving platter and arrange chops on top.

6 servings.

    1 serving = 373 calories
                113 mg cholesterol
                18 gm fat

BROILED LEMON CHICKEN

3- to 3½-pound broiler-fryer, split into halves
½ cup lemon juice
1 clove garlic, crushed
¼ teaspoon salt
1 teaspoon rosemary leaves, crumbled
Freshly ground pepper

Place chicken halves skin side down in shallow dish. Mix remaining ingredients; pour on chicken. Cover and refrigerate 8 hours, turning chicken often.

Set oven at broil and/or 550°. Remove chicken from marinade; reserve marinade. Place chicken skin side down on rack in broiler pan. Broil 8 to 10 inches from heat 15 to 20 minutes, basting 2 or 3 times with marinade. Turn chicken; baste with marinade and broil until chicken is tender, about 15 minutes, basting with marinade occasionally.

Cut chicken halves into quarters; if desired, serve with rice. Remember to remove skin before eating.

4 servings.

    1 serving = 250 calories
                70 mg cholesterol
                7 gm fat

Note: When lowest setting for broiler rack is 5 to 6 inches from heat, lower heat to medium to prevent overbrowning.

POACHED CHICKEN and VEGETABLES

Two 2-pound broiler-fryers
¼ cup margarine
1 can (10½ ounces) condensed chicken
  broth
½ cup dry white wine
½ teaspoon thyme
Freshly ground pepper
1 pound small new potatoes
8 leeks, trimmed
Small green cabbage (1 pound), cut
  into 6 pieces
1 pound carrots, cut into strips
1 tablespoon snipped chives
Horseradish Sauce (this page)

Tuck wings under body; fasten skin at neck of chickens with skewers. Brown chickens in margarine in dutch oven, turning carefully with 2 wooden spoons. Turn chickens breast side up in pan; add broth, wine, and thyme. Season with pepper. Heat to boiling. Reduce heat; cover and simmer until chicken is tender, 45 to 60 minutes.

Cook potatoes in 1 inch boiling salted water (⅛ teaspoon salt) until tender, about 20 minutes. Drain; keep warm. Cook leeks in large skillet in 1 inch salted water (⅛ teaspoon salt) until tender, about 15 minutes. Drain. Cook cabbage and carrots in large saucepan in 1 inch salted water (⅛ teaspoon salt) until cabbage is tender, about 15 minutes. Drain.

Remove chickens to heated serving platter. Arrange hot cooked vegetables around chickens and sprinkle with chives. Serve with Horseradish Sauce.

6 servings.

> 1 serving = 285 calories
>   57 mg cholesterol
>   12 gm fat

HORSERADISH SAUCE

¼ cup margarine
2 tablespoons flour
¼ teaspoon salt
1½ cups skim milk
½ cup prepared horseradish, drained
Freshly ground pepper
Dash cayenne red pepper

Melt margarine in saucepan. Blend in flour and salt. Cook over low heat, stirring until mixture is smooth and bubbly. Remove from heat. Stir in milk. Heat to boiling, stirring constantly. Boil and stir 1 minute. Stir in horseradish; simmer 3 minutes. Season with pepper and cayenne pepper.

2 cups.

> 1 tablespoon = 21 calories
>   trace cholesterol
>   1 gm fat

ROSEMARY CHICKEN

6 chicken breast halves
1 teaspoon salt
Freshly ground pepper
3 tablespoons margarine, softened
2 teaspoons snipped rosemary leaves

Heat oven to 350°. Arrange chicken in shallow broiler-proof baking pan. Season with salt and pepper. Spread with margarine and sprinkle rosemary leaves on top. Pour water into pan to depth of ½ inch; cover with foil. Bake 1 hour 15 minutes, adding water if necessary.

Set oven at broil and/or 550°. Uncover chicken. Broil about 3 inches from heat until golden brown, about 15 minutes.

6 servings.

> 1 serving = 140 calories
>   72 mg cholesterol
>   7 gm fat

CHICKEN SCALOPPINE

8 chicken thighs or 4 chicken breast
  halves
1 clove garlic, pressed
2 tablespoons margarine
2 tablespoons olive oil
2 cups sliced fresh mushrooms
Freshly ground pepper
2 tablespoons snipped parsley or chives
¼ teaspoon marjoram
¼ teaspoon thyme
1 tablespoon lemon juice
¾ cup dry white wine
2 tablespoons pale dry sherry
Parsley sprigs

Remove skin and bone from chicken. Place chicken between sheets of waxed paper and pound, not roughly, to ¼-inch thickness. (A rolling pin or a mallet can be used.) Cut chicken into 3 x 1-inch pieces. Cook and stir garlic in margarine and oil in large skillet until hot. Brown chicken pieces on both sides in skillet over medium heat. Remove chicken to warm platter. Remove garlic and discard.

Cook and stir mushrooms in skillet until brown. Return chicken to skillet; season with pepper and stir in remaining ingredients except sherry, rice, and parsley. Cover; heat to simmering and simmer until chicken is tender, about 30 minutes. Stir in sherry. If desired, serve on rice. Garnish with parsley sprigs.

4 servings.

1 serving = 282 calories
               70 mg cholesterol
               17 gm fat

SPICY ORANGE CHICKEN

2 tablespoons margarine
3-pound broiler-fryer chicken, cut
  into 8 pieces
½ cup chopped onion
½ cup chopped celery
1 clove garlic, minced
1 teaspoon turmeric
1 teaspoon ground coriander
½ teaspoon fennel seed
¼ teaspoon ground ginger
¼ teaspoon cumin
⅛ teaspoon cayenne pepper
1 tablespoon flour
½ cup orange juice
½ cup water
1 cup chopped peeled tomato
1 green pepper, cut into strips
1 orange, pared and sectioned
¼ teaspoon salt
Hot cooked rice
Condiments (below)

Melt margarine in large skillet. Brown chicken in margarine on both sides. Remove chicken to platter. Cook and stir onion, celery, garlic, and spices in skillet until vegetables are tender. Stir in flour. Stir in orange juice and water. Heat to boiling, stirring constantly. Add chicken pieces, tomato, green pepper, and salt. Season with pepper; heat to boiling. Reduce heat; cover and simmer until chicken is tender, about 30 minutes. Serve with rice and choice of Condiments.

4 servings.

1 serving = 347 calories
               80 mg cholesterol
               11 gm fat

Condiments: Orange sections, flaked coconut, raisins, chutney, chopped unsalted peanuts.

SPICED OVEN-FRIED CHICKEN

½ cup dry bread crumbs
1 tablespoon minced onion
2 teaspoons curry powder
¼ teaspoon salt
¼ teaspoon garlic powder
¼ teaspoon paprika
½ teaspoon dry mustard
Dash cayenne pepper (optional)
2½-pound broiler-fryer, cut up
¼ cup skim milk

Heat oven to 375°. Mix all ingredients except chicken and milk. Dip chicken pieces in milk, then coat with crumb mixture. Arrange chicken skin side up in greased baking dish, 11¾ x 7½ x 1¾ inches. Bake until tender, about 1 hour. If served cold, cool; cover and refrigerate.

4 servings.

1 serving = 198 calories
103 mg cholesterol
7 gm fat

CHICKEN BROCHETTE

1 green pepper, cut into 1-inch pieces
1 large onion, cut into 1-inch pieces
1 medium zucchini, cut into 1-inch pieces
4 large mushroom caps, cut into fourths
½ cup vegetable oil
¼ teaspoon thyme
¼ teaspoon ground coriander
5 peppercorns, crushed
4 bay leaves
¾ pound chicken breasts, skinned and cut into 1-inch cubes
4 cherry tomatoes
Hot cooked rice

Cook separately green pepper, onion, zucchini, and mushrooms in oil 1 to 2 minutes. Remove to baking dish or casserole. Stir in thyme, coriander, peppercorns, and bay leaves. Cool. Add chicken and tomatoes; pour oil and juice from fry pan on mixture. Cover and refrigerate at least 12 hours, stirring occasionally.

On each of 4 skewers, alternate pieces of chicken, green pepper, onion, mushroom, and zucchini. Place tomato on end of each skewer. Reserve marinade. Set oven at broil and/or 550°. Broil skewers about 3 inches from heat to desired doneness, 10 to 12 minutes, turning and basting often with reserved marinade. Serve with rice.

4 servings.

1 serving = 219 calories
31 mg cholesterol
15 gm fat

CHICKEN-BEEF KEBABS

1 cup low-fat yogurt
¼ cup chopped onion
¼ cup skim milk
1 clove garlic, minced
1 teaspoon ground coriander
½ teaspoon salt
½ teaspoon ground cumin
½ pound boneless beef, cut into 1-inch cubes
1 large chicken breast, skinned, boned, and cut into 1-inch pieces
3 medium zucchini, cut into 1-inch pieces
8 small onions, cut into halves
16 cherry tomatoes
16 small mushrooms, trimmed

Mix yogurt, ¼ cup onion, the milk, garlic, coriander, salt, and cumin in bowl. Stir in beef and chicken pieces until coated. Cover and refrigerate at least 3 hours, stirring occasionally.

Set oven at broil and/or 550°. Drain meat, reserving marinade. Alternate pieces of beef, chicken, and zucchini on 8 skewers. Place in broiler pan. Broil 4 to 5 inches from heat 8 minutes. Brush kebabs with reserved marinade. Turn kebabs; brush with marinade and broil 8 minutes longer. Brush with marinade and to each skewer, add 2 onion halves, 2 cherry tomatoes, and 2 mushrooms. Turn kebabs and broil 6 minutes. Brush with marinade before serving.

8 servings.

1 serving = 115 calories
37 mg cholesterol
3 gm fat

ISLAND CHICKEN

2 tablespoons margarine
2 chicken breasts, halved
Freshly ground pepper
½ teaspoon tarragon
1 medium green pepper, cut into thin strips
1 can (8 ounces) pineapple chunks in unsweetened pineapple juice
2 tablespoons lime juice
½ teaspoon Tabasco sauce
Hot cooked rice

Melt margarine in skillet. Place chicken breasts skin side down in skillet; season with pepper and half of the tarragon. Brown chicken over medium heat, about 10 minutes. Turn chicken; season with pepper and remaining tarragon and brown. Add green pepper and pineapple chunks (with juice); heat to boiling. Mix lime juice and Tabasco sauce; pour on chicken. Cover and simmer until tender, about 10 minutes. Serve with rice.

4 servings.

1 serving = 206 calories
72 mg cholesterol
10 gm fat

CHICKEN with YOGURT

2½- to 3-pound broiler-fryer, cut up
1 cup low-fat yogurt
½ teaspoon salt
Freshly ground pepper
1 teaspoon turmeric
1 teaspoon curry powder
1 teaspoon dry mustard
1 clove garlic, crushed
1 tablespoon lemon juice
1 large onion, sliced
2 tablespoons vegetable oil
2 large carrots, sliced
3 small potatoes, pared and quartered, or
   5 small new red potatoes (unpared)
2 small zucchini, sliced
½ cup chopped red pepper (optional)
¼ cup snipped parsley

Place chicken in baking dish, 13 x 9 x 2 inches. Mix yogurt, salt, pepper, turmeric, curry powder, mustard, garlic, and lemon juice. Pour on chicken, turning pieces to coat thoroughly. Cover and refrigerate at least 8 hours, turning chicken occasionally.

Cook and stir onion in oil in large skillet until tender. Add chicken (with marinade), carrots, potatoes, and zucchini. Cover and cook over medium heat until chicken is fork-tender, about 30 minutes. Garnish with chopped red pepper and parsley.

4 servings.

  1 serving = 307 calories
                102 mg cholesterol
                13 gm fat

CHICKEN CACCIATORA

1 cup all-purpose flour
1 teaspoon salt
1 teaspoon paprika
1 teaspoon pepper
1 teaspoon tarragon
1 teaspoon thyme
¼ cup vegetable oil
3-pound broiler-fryer, cut up
2 medium onions, sliced
2 green peppers, cut into ¼-inch strips
8 ounces mushrooms, trimmed and sliced
3 cups cubed, unpared eggplant
  (see *Note*)
2 cloves garlic, minced
1 cup dry white wine
½ cup plus 1 tablespoon snipped parsley
2 cups Tomato Sauce (page 167)

Mix flour, salt, paprika, pepper, tarragon, and thyme. Heat oil in large skillet. Coat chicken with flour mixture. Cook chicken in oil over medium heat until light brown, 15 to 20 minutes. Remove chicken and set aside.

Cook and stir onion and green pepper in skillet until tender. Add mushrooms, eggplant, and garlic; cook and stir 2 to 3 minutes. Stir in wine, parsley, and Tomato Sauce and heat to boiling. Add chicken to skillet; cover tightly and simmer 30 minutes, basting chicken with sauce frequently, until thickest pieces are fork-tender.

8 servings.

  1 serving = 303 calories
                64 mg cholesterol
                15 gm fat

Note: Cut unpared eggplant into ½-inch slices; sprinkle with ½ teaspoon salt and cut into cubes.

CHICKEN PAPRIKA

3- to 3½-pound broiler-fryer, cut up
1 teaspoon salt
¼ teaspoon white pepper
Dash cayenne pepper
3 tablespoons olive or vegetable oil
1 medium onion, thinly sliced
1 clove garlic, minced
1 cup low-fat yogurt
3 to 4 teaspoons paprika

Season chicken with salt, pepper, and cayenne pepper. Heat oil in large skillet. Cook chicken in oil until brown. Remove chicken; set aside.

Cook and stir onion and garlic in skillet until onion is tender. Return chicken to skillet; spoon yogurt on chicken and sprinkle with paprika. Cover and simmer until chicken is fork-tender, 30 to 35 minutes. Serve sauce on chicken.

4 servings.

1 serving = 251 calories
84 mg cholesterol
16 gm fat

CHICKEN GOURMET

3 chicken breasts, boned and split
into halves
2 tablespoons margarine
¼ cup dry white wine
¼ teaspoon tarragon
Freshly ground pepper
1 teaspoon margarine
1 tablespoon flour
3 cups hot cooked rice
Snipped parsley

Heat oven to 350°. Arrange chicken breast halves in baking dish, 11¾ x 7½ x 1¾ inches. Melt 2 tablespoons margarine in small saucepan; stir in wine and tarragon. Pour on chicken and season with pepper. Bake 20 minutes.

Turn chicken and bake 15 minutes longer. Remove chicken to warm platter and reserve liquid in baking dish. Melt 1 teaspoon margarine in small saucepan; stir in flour until smooth. Stir in reserved liquid and heat to boiling, stirring constantly. If desired, arrange chicken on rice; pour sauce on chicken and garnish with parsley.

6 servings.

1 serving = 190 calories
70 mg cholesterol
8 gm fat

STUFFED ROCK CORNISH HENS

4 Rock Cornish hens (1 to 1¼ pounds
each)
2 cups toasted bread cubes
2 medium oranges, pared, sectioned,
and diced (1 cup)
1 small apple, pared and chopped (½ cup)
½ cup golden raisins
¼ cup chopped pecans
½ teaspoon salt
¼ teaspoon nutmeg
Melted margarine

Heat oven to 350°. Wash hens and pat dry. Measure bread cubes, orange sections, apple, raisins, pecans, salt, and nutmeg into bowl; toss. Stuff hens lightly with fruit stuffing. Close openings with skewers and lace with string. Place hens breast side up on rack in open shallow roasting pan; brush with melted margarine. Roast 1 hour, brushing hens often with margarine. Increase oven temperature to 400°; roast 10 minutes longer or until hens are brown.

4 servings.

1 serving = 387 calories
102 mg cholesterol
15 gm fat

ROAST TURKEY

When buying turkeys under 12 pounds, allow ¾ to 1 pound per serving. For heavier birds, 12 pounds and over, allow ½ to ¾ pound per serving.

Wash turkey and pat dry. If desired, rub cavity with lemon juice.

Stuff turkey just before roasting, not ahead of time. Fill wishbone area with stuffing first. Fasten neck skin to back with skewer. Fold wings across back with tips touching. Fill body cavity lightly. (Do not pack—stuffing will expand while cooking.) Tuck drumsticks under band of skin at tail or tie together with heavy string, then tie to tail.

Heat oven to 325°. Place turkey breast side up on rack in open shallow roasting pan. Brush with unsalted margarine. Insert meat thermometer so tip is in thickest part of inside thigh muscle or thickest part of breast meat and does not touch bone. Do not add water or cover.

Follow timetable below for approximate total cooking time. Place a tent of aluminum foil loosely over turkey when it starts to turn golden. When ⅔ done, cut band of skin or string holding legs.

Timetable for Roasting Turkey

Ready-to-Cook Weight	Approx. Total Cooking Time	Internal Temp.
6 to 8 pounds	3 to 3½ hours	185°
8 to 12 pounds	3½ to 4½ hours	185°
12 to 16 pounds	4½ to 5½ hours	185°
16 to 20 pounds	5½ to 6½ hours	185°
20 to 24 pounds	6½ to 7 hours	185°

This timetable is based on chilled or completely thawed turkeys at a temperature of about 40° and placed in preheated oven. Time will be slightly less for unstuffed turkeys. Differences in the shape and tenderness of individual turkeys can also necessitate increasing or decreasing the cooking time slightly. For best results, use a meat thermometer.

A thermometer placed in the thigh muscle should register 185° when the turkey is done. If the bird is stuffed, the point of the thermometer can register 165° when done. If a thermometer is not used, test for doneness about 30 minutes before the time in timetable. Move drumstick up and down; if done, the joint should give readily or break. Or press drumstick meat between fingers; the meat should be very soft.

When turkey is done, remove from oven and allow to stand about 20 minutes for easiest carving. As soon as possible after serving, remove every bit of stuffing from turkey. Cool stuffing, meat, and any gravy promptly; refrigerate separately. Use gravy or stuffing within 1 or 2 days; heat thoroughly before serving. Serve cooked turkey meat within 2 or 3 days after roasting. If frozen, it can be kept up to 1 month.

ROAST HALVES and QUARTERS of TURKEY

Prepare half and quarter turkeys according to the basic instructions for whole turkeys, except skewer skin to meat along cut edges to prevent meat shrinkage during roasting. Place skin side up on rack in open shallow roasting pan. Place meat thermometer in thickest part of inside thigh muscle or thickest part of breast. Be sure it does not touch bone.

Timetable for Roast Halves and Quarters

Ready-to-Cook Weight	Approx. Total Cooking Time	Internal Temp.
5 to 8 pounds	2½ to 3 hours	185°
8 to 10 pounds	3 to 3½ hours	185°
10 to 12 pounds	3½ to 4 hours	185°

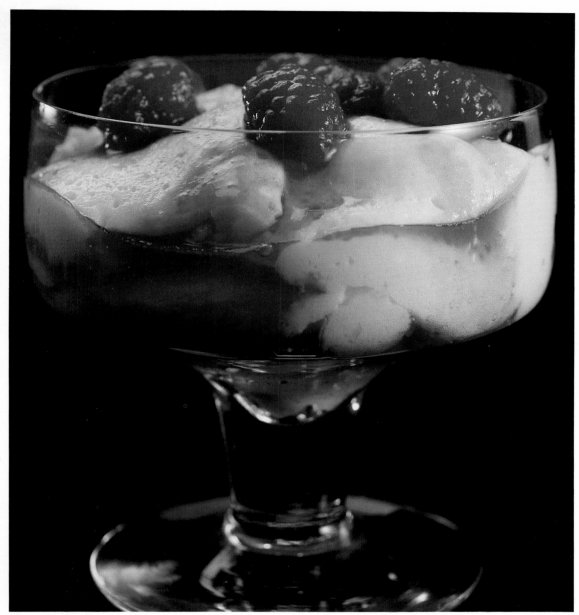

Snow Pudding.

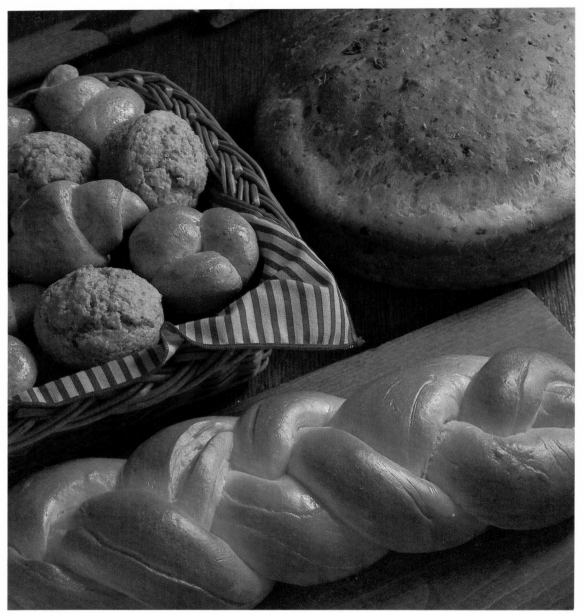

Cottage Cheese-Dill Batter Bread; Challah; Bran Muffins and
Wholesome Whole Wheat Dinner Rolls.

14 *Fish*

FISH are marketed in various forms for different uses. It is important to know these forms or "cuts" when you buy.

Whole: As the fish comes from the water. Before cooking it must be eviscerated and scaled; usually the head, tail, and fins are removed.

Drawn: Whole, eviscerated fish; usually the head, tail, scales, and fins are removed.

Dressed or Pan-dressed: Whole, eviscerated, and scaled fish; usually the head, tail, and fins are removed. Ready to use.

Steaks: Cross-section slices from large dressed fish. Ready to use.

Fillets: Sides of the fish cut lengthwise away from the backbone. Ready to use.

Sticks and Portions: Pieces of fish cut from blocks of frozen fillets and having uniform sizes ranging in weight from one to several ounces. Ready to use.

The amount of fish to buy depends on the size of the servings and amount of bone in the fish. This table can serve as a guide when buying fish.

Whole	1 pound per serving
Dressed	½ pound per serving
Fillets or steaks	½ pound per serving
Portions	⅓ pound per serving

Fish, unlike meat, is not cooked to tenderize it. It is already tender and is cooked only to develop flavor. Overcooking robs fish of its delicious natural juices, making it dry and tasteless. Good margarine, olive oil, herbs, spices, and wine enhance fish and give it added goodness.

The basic methods for cooking fish are baking, broiling, panfrying, deep frying, braising, and poaching. It is essential to control the time and temperature for each method. Cook fish for 10 minutes for every inch of thickness, measured at the thickest point. If fish is cooked from the frozen state (thawing is preferred), cooking time should be doubled, making it 20 minutes to the inch.

Because fish has very little connective tissue, it does not need long, slow cooking. Fish cooked quickly in the oven at very high temperature (450 to 500°) is especially delicious. When poaching fish, timing should start after the fish has been placed in the boiling poaching liquid. The liquid should be brought to a boil for the second time, the cooking utensil covered, the heat lowered, and the fish simmered for the time indicated in the recipe. Remove the fish immediately. With any cooking method, make the flake test to test for doneness.

Most cooked fish is extremely tender and will break easily, so it should be handled as little and as gently as possible after cooking. Wide metal spatulas are invaluable to use for lifting fish from the cooking utensil to serving dish.

When buying whole or dressed fresh fish, look for flesh that is firm and elastic to the touch and separates easily from the bones. Fresh fish has a mild characteristic odor, but not a strong or fishy odor. Its eyes are bright, clear, and full. The gills should be red and free from slime, and the skin should be shiny bright with tight-clinging scales.

When buying fresh fillets, steaks, and chunks, the flesh should have a fresh-cut appearance, firm in texture without any traces of browning around the edges. It should have a fresh and mild odor, and if wrapped, the wrappings should be of moisture-proof vapor-proof material with little or no air space between the fish and wrappings.

Fresh fish should be refrigerated in its original wrapper, and it should be cooked within 24 hours.

Frozen fish should be placed in a freezer at 0° temperature or lower to maintain quality. It should not be frozen for more than 6 months. If stored in a freezer compartment where the temperature is likely to be 10 to 25° above zero, do not store longer than 1 week.

In general, frozen fish should be thawed completely before cooking. To thaw, place the fish in its original wrapping in the refrigerator and allow 24 hours for thawing.

FISH STOCK

1 cup minced leek or 1½ cups minced onion
¼ cup olive oil
4 cloves garlic, peeled and crushed
4 tomatoes, chopped
3½ quarts (14 cups) water
8 sprigs parsley
2 bay leaves
½ teaspoon thyme
½ teaspoon basil
¼ teaspoon saffron (optional)
⅛ teaspoon freshly ground pepper
1 teaspoon salt
3 to 4 pounds lean fish (see *Note*), including heads, bones, and trimmings

Cook and stir leeks in olive oil until tender, about 5 minutes. Stir in garlic and tomatoes; cook over medium heat about 5 minutes. Add remaining ingredients and heat to boiling. Reduce heat and simmer at least 3 hours.

Strain soup into large saucepan, pressing juices out of ingredients. Stock can be made the day before serving, cooled and refrigerated, or it can be frozen up to 2 months.

6 to 8 servings.

1 serving = 74 calories
0 cholesterol
7 gm fat

Note: Sea bass, rock flounder, grouper, haddock, halibut, sole, perch, pollock, blue fish, spat, sea or lake trout, snapper, shellfish (clams, scallops, mussels, crab, lobster).

POACHED BASS

**4-pound striped bass, sea bass, or
  red snapper**
4 sprigs parsley
Green celery leaves
1 cup clam broth
1 stalk celery (with leaves), chopped
4 leeks (white part only), chopped
2 carrots, cut into julienne sticks
2 onions, finely chopped
3 cloves garlic, minced
2 tablespoons olive oil
**4 tomatoes, peeled, seeded, and coarsely
  chopped**
1 teaspoon basil
1 bay leaf
1 teaspoon thyme
Pinch saffron (optional)
1 cup dry white wine
Freshly ground pepper
1 tablespoon Pernod (optional)
12 small cherrystone clams, well scrubbed
1 cup snipped parsley

Have fish cleaned and filleted, reserving head and bones. Place head, bones, 4 sprigs parsley, and celery leaves in large kettle. Add water to cover and heat to boiling. Reduce heat and simmer 40 minutes.

Strain broth through sieve lined with several layers of dampened cheesecloth into bowl. Add clam broth and set aside.

Cook and stir celery, leeks, carrots, onion, and garlic in oil in large kettle until onion is tender. Add broth and remaining ingredients except clams, fish, and parsley. Heat to boiling. Reduce heat and simmer 20 minutes. Add clams and simmer 20 minutes longer.

Cut fish into bite-size pieces; add to soup and cook until fish flakes easily, 6 to 8 minutes. Serve in warm soup plates garnished with parsley. Serve with toasted garlic bread.

6 servings.

1 serving = 243 calories
              99 mg cholesterol
              6 gm fat

BROILED TURBOT

4 turbot fillets (about 1 pound)
2 tablespoons vegetable oil
2 tablespoons margarine, melted
¼ teaspoon salt
Freshly ground pepper
1 tablespoon snipped parsley
2 tablespoons lemon juice
Lemon wedges

Set oven at broil and/or 550°. Heat broiler pan 10 minutes. Brush hot broiler pan with oil. (Do not oil pan before; oil will burn and smoke.) Brush skin side of fillets with oil. Place skin side down in broiler pan. Brush with margarine; sprinkle with salt and season with pepper. Broil 4 inches from heat until fish flakes easily with fork, about 5 minutes, basting several times with juice in pan. Carefully remove fillets from pan with wide spatula to warm platter. Sprinkle with parsley and lemon juice. Garnish with lemon wedges.

4 servings.

1 serving = 206 calories
              59 mg cholesterol
              15 gm fat

BOUILLABAISSE

3 quarts (12 cups) Fish Stock (page 150)
2 dozen clams
2 pounds mussels
1 pound scallops
3 live lobsters (1½ pounds each)
2 pounds haddock
1 pound red snapper
1 pound flounder
1 pound sole
Parsley sprigs
Lemon wedges

Heat stock to boiling. Add clams, mussels, scallops, and lobsters; cover and heat to boiling. Boil 5 minutes. Add remaining fish; heat to boiling and simmer until fish is flaky and clams and mussels are open. (Discard any clams or mussels that do not open.) Remove fish immediately to serving platter and keep warm. Garnish with parsley and lemon wedges. Pour soup into tureen and serve immediately.

8 servings.

1 serving = 417 calories
205 mg cholesterol
17 gm fat

Note: This is a complete meal served with a salad and bread.

FISH POACHED in COURT BOUILLON

Court Bouillon (below)
3- to 4-pound lake trout, cleaned
(with head and tail on)

Prepare Court Bouillon. Wash fish quickly in cold water; pat dry. Wrap in double thickness of dampened cheesecloth (cheesecloth should be 12 inches wider than length of fish). Leave 6 inches at each end of fish; twist ends and tie with string. Place fish in bouillon. If liquid is not 1½ to 2 inches above fish, add water. Cover and simmer 15 minutes. Remove pan from heat; leave fish in liquid 15 minutes longer.

With tied ends lift fish to cutting board. Open cloth; skin fish with sharp knife, beginning at tail end. Pull skin from tail to gill. With cloth, turn fish and skin other side. Serve hot or cold. If fish is to be glazed, wrap in plastic wrap, then in aluminum foil, and chill. Reserve bouillon.

6 servings.

1 serving = 158 calories
92 mg cholesterol
6 gm fat

COURT BOUILLON

2 quarts water (8 cups)
2 cups dry white wine
¼ cup wine vinegar
3 onions, sliced
2 carrots, cut into 1-inch pieces
4 stalks celery, cut into 1-inch pieces
2 bay leaves
½ teaspoon tarragon
½ teaspoon thyme
1 tablespoon salt
10 peppercorns

Heat all ingredients in large saucepan to boiling. Reduce heat; simmer 30 minutes.

Strain through sieve into poaching utensil. Cool to lukewarm.

EPICUREAN TROUT

**6 trout (8 to 10 ounces each), cleaned
  and boned**
½ teaspoon salt
Freshly ground pepper
¼ cup all-purpose flour
½ cup margarine
2 tablespoons vegetable oil
1 lemon
½ cup dry white wine
24 seedless green grapes, cut into halves
2 tablespoons snipped parsley
¼ cup sliced almonds
2 lemons, each cut into 6 wedges
Watercress sprigs

Rinse fish quickly in cold water; pat dry. Open fish and flatten. Season with salt and pepper, then coat with flour.

Heat ¼ cup margarine and 1 tablespoon oil in each of two large skillets until bubbly. Place 3 fish open sides down in each skillet. Cook until golden brown, about 4 minutes. Carefully turn fish; squeeze juice from 1 lemon on fish.

Remove skillets from heat and cool slightly. Add ¼ cup wine and half the grape halves to each skillet. Simmer uncovered over low to medium heat (do not boil) until fish flakes easily with fork, 5 to 7 minutes.

Remove fish to warm serving platter. Pour sauce mixture from one skillet into the other; add parsley and almonds to sauce. Increase heat to medium-high and heat, stirring constantly, 1 minute to reduce sauce. Spoon sauce on fish and garnish with lemon wedges and watercress.

6 servings.

1 serving = 406 calories
            89 mg cholesterol
            29 gm fat

BROILED SHAD

2 pounds shad fillets
¼ cup vegetable oil
2 tablespoons lemon juice
1 tablespoon grated onion
1½ teaspoons salt
1 teaspoon paprika
½ teaspoon thyme
Dash freshly ground pepper
Snipped parsley
Lemon wedges

Spray broiler pan with vegetable spray. Cut fillets into serving-size pieces. Mix remaining ingredients, except parsley and lemon wedges. Place fish skin side up in broiler pan; brush with half the oil mixture.

Set oven at broil and/or 550°. Broil fish 3 inches from heat 5 minutes. Turn; brush with remaining oil mixture and broil until fish flakes easily with fork, 5 to 7 minutes. Sprinkle with parsley and garnish with lemon wedges.

6 servings.

1 serving = 206 calories
            79 mg cholesterol
            12 gm fat

SESAME RAINBOW TROUT

**6 rainbow trout or other small fish,
  pan-dressed**
¼ cup vegetable oil
¼ cup sesame seed
2 tablespoons lemon juice
½ teaspoon salt
Dash freshly ground pepper

Wash fish quickly in cold water; pat dry. Mix remaining ingredients. To grill, place fish in well-greased hinged wire grill. Baste fish with half the oil mixture. Cook fish about 4 inches from medium hot coals, 5 to 8 minutes. Baste fish with remaining oil mixture. Turn and cook until fish flakes easily with fork, 5 to 8 minutes longer.

6 servings.
1 serving = 240 calories
89 mg cholesterol
14 gm fat

Note: Fish may also be oven-broiled.

COQUILLES SAINT JACQUES

2 pounds sea scallops
1 cup dry sherry
½ cup water
1 bay leaf
1 pound mushrooms, trimmed and sliced
1 medium onion, chopped
½ cup margarine
3 tablespoons flour
2 tablespoons lemon juice
½ teaspoon paprika
⅛ teaspoon freshly ground pepper
Dash cayenne pepper
2 tablespoons dry bread crumbs
2 tablespoons grated Parmesan cheese

Wash scallops; remove any shell particles and cut each in half crosswise.

Heat oven to 325°. Heat scallops, sherry, water, and bay leaf to simmering. Cover and simmer 10 minutes. Remove scallops; drain and reserve broth. Cook and stir mushrooms and onion in margarine until onion is tender and mushrooms are brown. Stir in flour until bubbly. Stir in broth, lemon juice, ¼ teaspoon paprika, pepper, and cayenne pepper. Heat to boiling, stirring constantly until mixture thickens. Stir in scallops. Pour into 2-quart casserole or divide among 8 individual scallop shells. Sprinkle bread crumbs, cheese, and ¼ teaspoon paprika on top. Bake until golden brown, 15 to 20 minutes. Place under broiler last 2 to 3 minutes to melt cheese.

8 servings.
1 serving = 251 calories
49 mg cholesterol
14 gm fat

FILLETS of SOLE MEUNIÈRE

1½ pounds sole fillets (6 small)
¼ cup lemon juice
¼ cup all-purpose flour
White pepper
¼ cup margarine
1 tablespoon minced onion
¼ teaspoon minced garlic
1 tablespoon margarine
¼ cup white vermouth or dry white wine
1 tablespoon snipped parsley

Dip fillets in lemon juice and pat dry with paper towels. Sprinkle with flour and season with white pepper. Melt ¼ cup margarine in large skillet. Brown fillets on both sides in margarine, 3 to 4 minutes. Remove fish to warm serving platter. Cook and stir onion and garlic in 1 tablespoon margarine in skillet until hot. Stir in wine and simmer about 2 minutes. Spoon sauce on fish and sprinkle with parsley.

6 servings.

1 serving = 305 calories
76 mg cholesterol
22 gm fat

Note: Fresh dill or chervil leaves can be substituted for the parsley.

SEAFOOD SHISH KEBAB

1 clove garlic, peeled and crushed
¼ cup snipped parsley
¼ cup lemon juice
½ cup vegetable oil
Freshly ground pepper
½ teaspoon thyme
5 or 6 drops Tabasco sauce
1 pound swordfish, cubed
1 pound sea scallops, halved
12 cubes sweet onion
12 cubes green pepper
12 cherry tomatoes
2 lemons, cut into wedges

Mix garlic, parsley, lemon juice, oil, pepper, thyme, and Tabasco sauce in bowl or casserole. Add fish and scallops and turn to coat with marinade. Cover and refrigerate 1 to 2 hours, turning fish and scallops occasionally.

Remove fish from marinade and alternate cubes of fish, onion, green pepper, and cherry tomatoes on skewers. Grill, turning once, until fish flakes easily, about 10 minutes. Serve with lemon wedges.

4 servings.

1 serving = 388 calories
123 mg cholesterol
22 gm fat

Note: Kebabs can be oven-broiled but allow more cooking time.

BAKED STUFFED FISH

**3- to 6-pound fish (whitefish, pike),
  cleaned**
1 clove garlic, minced
½ teaspoon salt
¼ cup minced green onion (with tops)
½ cup chopped green pepper
½ cup chopped celery
2 tomatoes, peeled and chopped
3 tablespoons snipped parsley

Heat oven to 350°. Wash fish quickly in cold water; pat dry. Mix remaining ingredients. Stuff fish with mixture. Close opening with skewers and lace with string. Spray open shallow roasting pan with vegetable spray. Place fish in pan. Bake until fish flakes easily with fork, about 15 minutes per pound.

2 servings per pound.
1 serving = 222 calories
119 mg cholesterol
7 gm fat

Note: For crispy crust, roll fish in cornmeal before stuffing.

TURKISH BAKED FISH

**2 medium onions, sliced and separated
  into rings**
½ cup olive oil or vegetable oil
¼ cup tomato paste
1½ cups water
3 cloves garlic, crushed
½ teaspoon paprika
Juice of ½ lemon
3 stalks celery, chopped
4 small carrots, chopped
**3-pound striped bass, filleted and cut
  into 1-inch slices**
Snipped parsley
½ lemon, thinly sliced

Cook and stir onion rings in oil until tender. Stir in tomato paste, water, garlic, paprika, lemon juice, celery, and carrots. Heat to boiling, stirring constantly. Reduce heat; cover and simmer 25 minutes.

Heat oven to 350°. Arrange fish in baking dish. Pour sauce on fish. Bake until fish flakes easily with fork, about 25 minutes. Garnish with parsley and serve with lemon slices. If desired, serve with hot cooked rice.

4 servings.
1 serving = 289 calories
59 mg cholesterol
17 gm fat

FISH FILLETS

6 flounder fillets (about 1½ pounds)
Freshly ground pepper
⅓ cup dry white wine
Juice of ½ lemon
8 ounces mushrooms, trimmed and thinly
**   sliced**
2 tablespoons margarine, softened
¼ cup slivered almonds
1 tablespoon snipped parsley
⅛ teaspoon dry mustard
⅛ teaspoon nutmeg

Heat oven to 475°. Spray baking pan, 13 x 9 x 2 inches, with vegetable spray. Arrange fish in pan; season with pepper and pour wine on fish.

Sprinkle lemon juice on mushrooms in bowl. Stir in margarine, almonds, parsley, mustard, and nutmeg. Spread mushroom mixture on fillets. Bake 15 to 20 minutes or until fish flakes easily with fork.

6 servings.
   1 serving = 180 calories
                59 mg cholesterol
                10 gm fat

Fish Fillet Rollups: Delay pouring wine on fish until fillets have been rolled. After spreading mushroom mixture on fillets, roll up each fillet and secure with wooden pick. Place in pan and pour wine on rollups.

BAKED FISH FILLETS

1 pound fish fillets (sole, blue fish, pike,
**   sea bass, mackerel, haddock)**
¼ teaspoon salt
¼ cup margarine, melted
Freshly ground pepper
2 tablespoons margarine
2 tablespoons lemon juice
Watercress or snipped parsley
Lemon wedges

Heat oven to 350°. Spray shallow roasting pan with vegetable spray. Place fish in pan. Sprinkle with salt and the melted margarine. Season with pepper. Bake 20 minutes or until fish flakes easily with fork.

Heat 2 tablespoons margarine in small skillet until brown. Stir in lemon juice and pepper. Pour on fish. Garnish with watercress and lemon wedges.

4 servings.
   1 serving = 269 calories
                59 mg cholesterol
                22 gm fat

FISH STEAKS

Lemon Parsley Sauce (below)
3 pounds fresh or frozen ¾- to 1-inch-thick fish steaks (salmon, tuna, halibut, swordfish)

Prepare sauce.

Set oven at broil and/or 550°. Line broiler pan with aluminum foil and spread thin coating of sauce on foil. Place steaks in broiler pan. Broil 4 inches from heat, basting frequently with sauce, until fish flakes easily with fork, 6 to 8 minutes on each side. If desired, garnish with lemon wedges and parsley.

8 servings.

1 serving = 321 calories
105 mg cholesterol
23 gm fat

Note: Steaks also can be grilled on greased grill 4 inches from medium coals.

Lemon Parsley Sauce: Melt ½ cup margarine. Stir in ¼ cup lemon juice, 1 tablespoon plus 1½ teaspoons snipped parsley, ¼ teaspoon salt, and dash freshly ground pepper.

8 servings.

1 serving = 113 calories
0 cholesterol
12 gm fat

POACHED FISH

1 pound fish fillets
¼ teaspoon salt
½ teaspoon snipped parsley
1 bay leaf
1 tablespoon chopped onion
Parsley sprigs
Lemon wedges

Place fish in large skillet. Add salt and just enough water barely to cover fish. Add parsley, bay leaf, and onion; cover and simmer until fish flakes easily with fork, 5 to 10 minutes.

Remove fish to warm platter and garnish with parsley sprigs and lemon wedges.

3 or 4 servings.

1 serving = 103 calories
59 mg cholesterol
4 gm fat

Note: Poaching liquid is flavorful. If desired, reduce liquid by cooking; add thickening to make a sauce for fish.

POACHED FISH with CAPER SAUCE

Poached Fish (above)
1 cup low-fat yogurt
2 tablespoons minced capers
1 teaspoon grated lemon peel
1 tablespoon lemon juice
1 tablespoon snipped parsley
2 teaspoons minced onion

Prepare Poached Fish as described above, except cool fish and omit lemon wedges. Mix remaining ingredients for Caper Sauce, chill, and serve with fish.

About 1 cup.

1 serving = 146 calories
70 mg cholesterol
5 gm fat

GRILLED WHOLE SALMON

Hickory wood chips
8-pound salmon, cleaned (see *Note*)
¾ cup margarine, melted
2 tablespoons lemon juice
1 teaspoon oregano
½ teaspoon salt
Freshly ground pepper
Margarine, melted
Crisp lettuce leaves
Lime slices

Soak hickory wood chips in water about 30 minutes.

Wash fish quickly in cold water; pat dry. Mix ¾ cup margarine, the lemon juice, and oregano. Brush inside and outside of fish with margarine mixture; season with salt and pepper and let stand 30 minutes.

Brush large piece of heavy-duty aluminum foil with melted margarine. Place fish on foil and crimp edges of foil to form tray with ½-inch ridge.

Drain chips; add to hot coals. Place foil tray with fish on grill about 4 inches from coals. Cover grill with hood or aluminum foil. Cook fish, basting with melted margarine every 5 to 10 minutes, until fish barely flakes with fork, 40 to 45 minutes. Remove fish to warm platter and garnish with lettuce and lime slices.

6 servings.
1 serving = 267 calories
124 mg cholesterol
13 gm fat

Note: Four pounds fish fillets can be substituted for the whole fish. Arrange fillets in single layer on foil and reduce grilling time to 20 to 30 minutes.

LEMON SALMON STEAKS

½ cup margarine, melted
2 tablespoons lemon juice
1 tablespoon snipped parsley
1 tablespoon liquid smoke
Dash freshly ground pepper
2 pounds salmon steaks or other fish steaks

Mix all ingredients except fish. Brush fish with sauce. To grill, place fish in well-greased hinged wire grill. Cook about 4 inches from medium hot coals 8 minutes. Baste with sauce. Turn and cook until fish flakes easily with fork, 7 to 10 minutes.

6 servings.
1 serving = 211 calories
79 mg cholesterol
13 gm fat

Note: Fish steaks may also be oven-broiled.

FISH STEAK BROIL

4 fish steaks (salmon, swordfish, red snapper, halibut), 6-ounces each
⅓ cup margarine, melted
1 tablespoon lemon juice
½ teaspoon salt
¼ teaspoon paprika
Watercress or parsley sprigs
Lemon slices

Spray broiler pan with vegetable spray. Arrange fish steaks in pan. Mix margarine, lemon juice, salt, and paprika. Brush fish with half the margarine mixture.

Set oven at broil and/or 550°. Broil fish 2 inches from heat 5 to 8 minutes. Turn fish carefully; brush with remaining margarine mixture. Broil until fish flakes easily with fork, about 5 minutes. Remove to warm platter; garnish with watercress and lemon slices.

4 servings.
1 serving = 288 calories
92 mg cholesterol
20 gm fat

EASTERN SHORE CLAM BAKE

6 dozen soft shell clams
12 live blue crabs
12 small onions, peeled
6 medium baking potatoes, washed
6 ears corn (in husks), remove silk and
  replace husks
Lemon wedges
Melted margarine

Cut twelve 18 x 36-inch pieces of cheese-cloth and twelve 18 x 36-inch pieces of heavy-duty aluminum foil. Place 2 pieces of cheesecloth on each 2 pieces of foil.

Wash clams thoroughly. Have the fish retailer dress the crabs for eating. Rinse in cold water and drain.

Make 6 packages: Place 2 onions, 1 potato, 1 ear of corn, 12 clams, and 2 crabs on each double-layered cheesecloth. Tie corners of cheesecloth up over food. Bring foil up over package; pour in 1 cup water in package and securely seal edge of foil.

Place package on grill 4 inches from hot coals. Cover grill with hood or aluminum foil. Cook until onion and potato are tender, 45 to 60 minutes. Serve with lemon wedges and margarine.

6 servings.

1 serving = 339 calories
145 mg cholesterol
6 gm fat

SALMON BURGERS

1 can (16 ounces) salmon
⅓ cup dry bread crumbs
½ cup egg substitute
¼ cup snipped parsley
1 teaspoon dry mustard
¼ teaspoon salt
½ cup chopped onion
¼ cup margarine
½ cup dry bread crumbs
Lemon wedges

Drain salmon, reserving ⅓ cup liquid. Flake salmon in bowl. Add ⅓ cup bread crumbs, the egg substitute, parsley, mustard, salt, and reserved liquid.

Cook and stir onion in margarine in small skillet until tender. Mix onion into salmon mixture. Shape mixture into 6 patties; coat with ½ cup bread crumbs.

Set oven at broil and/or 550°. Broil patties on broiler rack 3 inches from heat until brown, 3 to 5 minutes. Carefully turn patties; broil until other side is brown, about 3 minutes. Remove to warm serving platter and serve with lemon wedges.

6 servings.

1 serving = 261 calories
28 mg cholesterol
14 gm fat

LINGUINE with WHITE CLAM SAUCE

48 small cherrystone clams
2 tablespoons minced garlic
½ cup snipped parsley
¼ teaspoon hot red pepper (see *Note*)
⅓ cup olive oil or vegetable oil
1½ pounds linguine
½ cup water
Freshly ground pepper
Snipped parsley

Wash clams thoroughly, discarding any broken shell or dead clams. Cook and stir garlic, parsley, and red pepper in oil about 5 minutes. Remove from heat and set aside.

Fill 8-quart kettle about ⅔ full with water; heat to boiling. Add linguine; heat to boiling and cook 4 minutes. Drain linguine into colander. Return linguine to kettle; stir in oil mixture, clams, and water. Cover and cook on high heat until clams are open. Divide linguine among 6 plates and serve 8 clams with each portion. Season with pepper and garnish with parsley.

6 servings.

1 serving = 441 calories
40 mg cholesterol
13 gm fat

Note: Use 1 dried red pepper, crushed. Caution: Wash hands immediately after handling pepper, and avoid touching eyes with fingers before washing hands.

MOULES à la MARINIÈRE

36 mussels
⅓ cup all-purpose flour
1 cup dry white wine or dry vermouth
¼ cup chopped shallots
¼ cup snipped parsley
2 cloves garlic, crushed
¼ teaspoon salt
½ teaspoon thyme
¼ teaspoon pepper
1 bay leaf

Examine mussels and discard any that are not tightly closed. Scrub under running cold water to remove sand. Trim off the "beard" around edges with scissors or sharp knife.

Place mussels in large bowl; cover with water. Stir in flour; allow mixture to stand 1 hour or longer. Remove mussels to colander and rinse under running cold water.

Heat remaining ingredients in large kettle to boiling. Add mussels; cover and heat to boiling. Cook until shells open, 5 to 6 minutes.

Remove mussels with slotted spoon or tongs to warm serving dish. Spoon some liquid on mussels. Serve remaining liquid in bowl.

6 servings.

1 serving = 162 calories
64 mg cholesterol
2 gm fat

Note: Mussels are available in the shell, packed in jars, or shucked, packed in jars or cans. Add mussels to pasta for a delicious main dish.

TUNA CASSEROLE

3 ounces medium noodles
1 can (6½ or 7 ounces) tuna packed in water,
  drained and flaked
½ cup cooked peas
1 tablespoon minced onion
¼ cup finely chopped celery
1 tablespoon margarine
1 tablespoon flour
¼ teaspoon salt
⅛ teaspoon garlic powder
1 cup skim milk
Freshly ground pepper
3 tablespoons whole-wheat bread crumbs
1 tablespoon wheat germ
Paprika

Cook noodles as directed on package, except omit salt. Turn noodles into 1½-quart casserole. Add tuna and peas.

Heat oven to 325°. Cook and stir onion and celery in margarine until tender. Stir in flour, salt, and garlic powder. Cook over low heat, stirring constantly, until bubbly. Remove from heat; stir in milk. Heat to boiling, stirring constantly. Season with pepper. Pour sauce on tuna mixture and carefully mix. Sprinkle bread crumbs, wheat germ and paprika on top. Bake until bubbly, about 40 minutes.

6 servings.

1 serving = 148 calories
            18 mg cholesterol
            3 gm fat

COUNTRY TUNA

¼ cup minced onion
1 cup diced celery
2 tablespoons unsalted margarine
2 cans (6½ or 7 ounces each), tuna packed
  in water, drained
¼ teaspoon thyme
½ teaspoon Tabasco sauce
¼ cup unsalted margarine
¼ cup all-purpose flour
2 cups skim milk
½ cup cornflake crumbs (see *Note*)
1 medium apple, finely chopped
2 tablespoons snipped parsley

Cook and stir onion and celery in 2 tablespoons margarine until onion is tender. Remove from heat; stir in tuna, thyme, and Tabasco sauce. Pour into 1½-quart casserole.

Heat oven to 425°. Melt ¼ cup margarine in saucepan. Blend in flour. Cook over low heat, stirring until mixture is smooth and bubbly. Remove from heat. Stir in milk. Heat to boiling, stirring constantly. Boil and stir 1 minute. Pour on vegetables and tuna in casserole and mix carefully. Sprinkle cornflake crumbs on top. Bake until bubbly, about 20 minutes. Garnish with apple and parsley.

4 servings.

1 serving = 376 calories
            54 mg cholesterol
            19 gm fat

Note: Unsalted cornflake crumbs can be used.

15 Non-Meat Main Dishes

BAKED STUFFED SUMMER SQUASH

4 small yellow summer squash
2 tablespoons chopped fresh mushrooms
2 tablespoons minced onion
1 tablespoon chopped celery
1 tablespoon margarine
1 cup dry bread crumbs
¼ teaspoon sage
⅛ teaspoon thyme
⅛ teaspoon freshly ground pepper

Cut off top ¼ of each squash. Cook squash pieces in boiling water 5 minutes. Drain and cool slightly.

Heat oven to 350°. For stuffing, cook and stir mushrooms, onion, and celery in margarine until onion is tender. Stir in remaining ingredients.

Scoop out pulp from squash with a teaspoon, leaving a ½-inch wall. Mix scooped-out pulp and stuffing; fill shells with mixture. Place top pieces on stuffing. Place filled squash in shallow baking dish sprayed with vegetable spray. Bake until squash is tender, 20 to 25 minutes.

4 servings.

1 serving = 146 calories
trace cholesterol
4 gm fat

TOMATO-ZUCCHINI PIE

Pastry for 9-inch One-Crust Pie (page 209)
3 cups sliced unpared zucchini
  (2 to 4 small)
2 medium onions, thinly sliced and
  separated into rings
2 tablespoons vegetable oil
1 medium tomato, sliced
¼ teaspoon salt
Freshly ground pepper
¼ cup plus 2 tablespoons egg substitute
1 cup skim milk
1 tablespoon Italian seasoning
1 teaspoon dry mustard
¼ teaspoon salt
½ cup shredded part skim milk mozzarella
  cheese
Freshly ground pepper

Prepare pastry. Cook and stir zucchini and onion in large skillet in oil until onion is tender and zucchini is light brown, about 5 minutes.

Heat oven to 350°. Layer zucchini-onion mixture and tomato slices in pastry-lined pie pan. Sprinkle ¼ teaspoon salt on vegetables and season with pepper. Beat egg substitute, milk, Italian seasoning, mustard, and ¼ teaspoon salt. Stir in cheese; season with pepper and pour on vegetables. Bake 40 to 45 minutes or until filling is set and crust is brown.

6 servings.

1 serving = 291 calories
8 mg cholesterol
18 gm fat

RAISIN-STUFFED EGGPLANT

**1 medium to large eggplant
(1½ to 2 pounds)
3 tablespoons vegetable oil
¾ cup cooked rice
½ cup raisins
¼ to ½ teaspoon cinnamon
¼ to ½ teaspoon nutmeg
¼ to ½ teaspoon curry powder
1 tablespoon honey
2 tablespoons margarine**

Wash eggplant. Cut lengthwise into halves. Remove and cube eggplant from shell. Sauté eggplant cubes in oil until tender. Heat oven to 350°. Stir in rice, raisins, cinnamon, nutmeg, curry powder, and honey. Cook over medium-low heat, stirring occasionally, about 10 minutes. Fill eggplant shells with mixture. Dot with margarine. Bake 20 to 25 minutes.

4 servings.

1 serving = 314 calories
0 cholesterol
16 gm fat

Note: Filled eggplant shells can be covered and refrigerated. To heat, bake in 350° oven 1 hour.

VEGETARIAN CASSEROLE

**2 tomatoes, cut into ½-inch pieces
5 mushrooms, trimmed and thinly sliced
3 small zucchini, cut into ¼-inch slices
½ teaspoon basil
½ teaspoon thyme
½ teaspoon oregano
½ teaspoon salt
Freshly ground pepper**

Cook tomatoes in saucepan over medium heat until almost liquid. Stir in remaining ingredients except salt and pepper. Cover and cook over medium heat until zucchini is tender, about 10 minutes. Season with salt and pepper.

4 servings.

1 serving = 33 calories
0 cholesterol
trace fat

LENTILS AND RICE

**3 large onions, chopped
2 tablespoons vegetable oil
2 quarts plus 1 cup water (9 cups)
2 cups red lentils
1 cup uncooked regular rice
1 teaspoon garlic powder
1 teaspoon cumin powder
1 teaspoon salt
Pinch saffron**

Cook and stir onions in oil in large kettle until brown. Add water and lentils; heat to boiling. Reduce heat; cover and simmer until lentils are almost tender, about 1 to 2 hours.

Cook and stir onions in oil in large kettle until brown. Add water and lentils; heat to boiling. Reduce heat; cover and simmer until lentils are almost tender, about 1 to 2 hours.

6 servings.

1 serving = 271 calories
0 cholesterol
5 gm fat

VEGETABLE CURRY

1 tablespoon vinegar
1 clove garlic, minced
1 tablespoon ground coriander
¼ teaspoon salt
1 teaspoon turmeric
½ teaspoon ground cumin
½ teaspoon dry mustard
¼ teaspoon ginger
¼ teaspoon pepper
3-inch cinnamon stick
2 cardamom seeds, peeled and pulverized
2 bay leaves
⅛ teaspoon cayenne pepper
2 cups sliced cauliflowerets
2 cups diagonally sliced carrot
½ pound green beans, cut into 1-inch
   pieces
½ cup chopped onion
½ cup chopped green pepper
¼ cup margarine
2 cups cubed, pared potatoes
2 teaspoons lemon juice
1 cup chicken broth
2 cartons (8 ounces each) low-fat yogurt

Mix vinegar, garlic, and seasonings in large bowl. Add cauliflowerets, carrot, and beans and toss. Cover and refrigerate at least 2 hours.

Cook and stir onion and green pepper in margarine in large skillet until tender. Stir in potatoes; cover and cook 5 minutes. Stir in seasoned vegetables, lemon juice, and chicken broth; heat to boiling. Reduce heat; cover and simmer, stirring occasionally, 25 minutes. Remove cinnamon stick and bay leaves. Serve curry with yogurt.

8 servings.

1 serving = 168 calories
            4 mg cholesterol
            8 gm fat

CHEESE-FILLED SHELLS

½ package (12 ounce size) jumbo shells
1 tablespoon minced onion
1 tablespoon minced green pepper
1 tablespoon margarine
1 to 2 tablespoons snipped parsley
½ teaspoon Italian seasoning
Freshly ground pepper
1 pound part skim milk ricotta cheese,
   diced
¼ pound part skim milk mozzarella
   cheese, diced
¼ cup grated Parmesan cheese
2 tablespoons egg substitute
2 cups Tomato Sauce (page 167)

Heat oven to 350°. Cook shells as directed on package, except omit salt.

Cook and stir onion and green pepper in margarine in small skillet until tender. Remove from heat; stir in parsley, Italian seasoning, and pepper. Mix cheeses and egg substitute in bowl. Stir in onion mixture. Fill shells with mixture, using butter knife or teaspoon. Pour half the Tomato Sauce in baking dish. Arrange filled shells in single layer on sauce. Pour remaining sauce on shells. Bake until bubbly, about 30 minutes.

6 servings.

1 serving = 396 calories
            40 mg cholesterol
            19 gm fat

FRESH VEGETABLE SOUFFLÉ

¼ **cup all-purpose flour**
⅛ **teaspoon freshly ground pepper**
½ **teaspoon dill weed**
¼ **teaspoon dry mustard**
½ **cup low-fat mayonnaise**
¼ **cup skim milk**
1 **cup finely chopped cooked vegetables (carrot, green beans, green pepper, corn)**
4 **egg whites**

Heat oven to 325°. Spray 1½-quart soufflé dish or casserole with vegetable spray. Mix flour, pepper, dill weed, mustard, and mayonnaise. Stir in milk and vegetables.

Beat egg whites until stiff peaks form. Fold vegetable mixture into egg whites. Pour into soufflé dish. Bake 40 minutes or until knife inserted in center comes out clean. Serve immediately.

4 servings.

1 serving = 168 calories
10 mg cholesterol
10 gm fat

EGGPLANT and TOMATO CASSEROLE

1 **medium eggplant**
1 **cup egg substitute**
1 **cup dry bread crumbs**
2 **tablespoons vegetable oil**
½ **cup chopped onion**
½ **cup chopped green pepper**
1 **medium zucchini, chopped**
1 **clove garlic, crushed**
3 **ripe medium tomatoes, peeled and chopped**
½ **teaspoon salt**
¼ **teaspoon freshly ground pepper**
1 **teaspoon basil**
8 **ounces part skim milk mozzarella cheese, cut into small cubes**

Heat oven to 350°. Pare eggplant and cut into thin slices. Dip slices in egg substitute, then in bread crumbs. Layer slices in baking dish, 11¾ x 7½ x 1½ inches. Bake until tender, 30 to 40 minutes.

Cook and stir onion, green pepper, zucchini, and garlic in oil until onion is tender. Stir in tomatoes, salt, pepper, and basil. Cook, stirring occasionally, until tomatoes are tender.

Remove half the eggplant from baking dish. Pour half the tomato sauce on eggplant in baking dish. Top with half the cheese cubes. Add remaining eggplant, sauce, and cheese cubes. Bake until bubbly and cheese is melted, about 15 minutes.

8 servings.

1 serving = 198 calories
20 mg cholesterol
9 gm fat

VEGETABLE and BROWN RICE CASSEROLE

1 cup brown rice
2½ cups water
2 medium carrots, sliced and cooked
1 medium zucchini, sliced and steamed
2 cups cooked cauliflowerets
2 cups cooked broccoli spears
½ cup shredded low-fat mozzarella cheese
½ teaspoon salt

Heat rice and water to boiling, stirring once or twice. Reduce heat to simmer; cover pan tightly and cook 30 to 40 minutes. (Do not lift cover or stir rice.) Remove from heat. Fluff rice lightly with fork; cover and let steam 5 minutes.

Turn rice into 1½-quart casserole and sprinkle with ⅛ teaspoon salt. Layer carrot slices, zucchini, cauliflowerets, and broccoli spears on rice, sprinkling each layer with ⅛ teaspoon salt. Sprinkle cheese on top.

Set oven at broil and/or 550°. Broil casserole 3 inches from heat until cheese is melted.

4 servings.
   1 serving = 232 calories
              10 mg cholesterol
              3 gm fat

TOMATO SAUCE for PASTA

1 medium onion, minced
1 clove garlic, minced
1 carrot, diced
1 stalk celery, diced
¼ cup margarine
¼ cup olive oil
4 pounds plum tomatoes, peeled and coarsely chopped
1 tablespoon sugar
¼ teaspoon salt
1 teaspoon oregano
1 teaspoon basil
1 tablespoon snipped parsley
Freshly ground pepper

Cook and stir onion, garlic, carrot, and celery in margarine and oil until vegetables are tender. Stir in tomatoes, sugar, salt, oregano, basil, and parsley. Season with pepper. Heat to boiling, stirring occasionally. Reduce heat; cover and simmer, stirring occasionally and breaking tomatoes, 2 to 3 hours. (For thicker sauce, remove cover last 1½ hours of cooking.) If desired, strain sauce.

Enough sauce for 1 pound pasta.
8 servings.
   1 serving = 183 calories
              0 cholesterol
              13 gm fat

Note: This recipe can be doubled. Sauce can be frozen in plastic containers and, at serving time, thawed and heated.

GARLIC-WINE PASTA SAUCE

½ cup margarine
½ cup white wine
½ cup chicken broth
1 teaspoon basil or 1 tablespoon snipped
   basil leaves
1 tablespoon snipped parsley
4 cloves garlic, crushed
½ teaspoon salt

Measure all ingredients into small saucepan. Heat to boiling; reduce heat and simmer 5 minutes.

About 1½ cups sauce (enough for 8 ounces pasta).
6 servings.

1 serving = 154 calories
0 cholesterol
16 mg fat

Note: When serving pasta with sauce, pass bowl of freshly grated Parmesan cheese to be sprinkled on top. This sauce is excellent alone or as an accompaniment to almost any meat dish.

VEGETARIAN PASTA SAUCE

2 medium onions, chopped
2 large garlic cloves, minced
2 tablespoons olive oil
2 tablespoons vegetable oil
1 can (28 ounces) Italian plum tomatoes
2 tablespoons basil
1 teaspoon oregano
1 teaspoon sugar
½ teaspoon salt
Freshly ground pepper
1 medium eggplant
2 tablespoons vegetable oil

Cook and stir onions and garlic in olive oil and 2 tablespoons vegetable oil in large saucepan until onion is tender. Stir in tomatoes (with liquid), basil, oregano, sugar, and salt. Break up tomatoes into small pieces. Season with pepper. Heat to boiling. Reduce heat and simmer uncovered 30 minutes.

Cut eggplant into 1-inch slices. Pare slices and cut into 1-inch pieces. Cut and stir eggplant in 2 tablespoons oil in large skillet until tender, 10 to 12 minutes. Stir into tomato sauce.

Enough sauce for 1 pound pasta.
6 servings.

1 serving = 200 calories
0 cholesterol
14 gm fat

Note: Cooked meatballs can be substituted for the eggplant. Two pounds tomatoes, peeled, seeded, and chopped, can be substituted for the canned tomatoes.

VEGETARIAN'S FANCY

1 cup uncooked brown rice
2 cups 2-inch pieces green beans
2 tablespoons margarine
¼ cup chopped onion
1¼ cups sliced mushrooms
¾ teaspoon paprika
½ teaspoon oregano
1 cup chopped peeled tomato
2 tablespoons sunflower seeds

Cook rice as directed on package. Fifteen minutes before rice is tender, cook and stir green beans in margarine in large skillet 8 minutes. Stir in onion, mushrooms, paprika, and oregano. Cook and stir 5 minutes. Add tomato and heat. Mix sunflower seeds into rice carefully. Spoon rice mixture onto serving dish and top with vegetable mixture.

4 servings.

1 serving = 266 calories
0 cholesterol
9 gm fat

PESTO (BASIL, GARLIC, and CHEESE SAUCE)

2 cups coarsely chopped fresh basil (see Note), or 2 cups coarsely chopped Italian parsley and 2 tablespoons dried basil

½ teaspoon freshly ground black pepper

1 to 2 teaspoons chopped peeled garlic

3 tablespoons chopped pine nuts or walnuts

1 cup olive oil

½ cup freshly grated imported Parmesan cheese

Cooked spaghetti or linguine

Measure all ingredients except cheese and spaghetti into blender. Blend on high speed until smooth. Turn off blender occasionally to scrape sides with rubber scraper. Pour sauce into saucepan and heat. Remove from heat; stir in cheese. Pour on spaghetti and toss.

8 or 9 servings.

1 serving = 272 calories
7 mg cholesterol
27 gm fat

Note: Strip leaves from stems of basil; chop coarsely and pack tightly in measuring cup. Pesto is best when it is freshly made. It can be partially made, excluding the cheese, and frozen in an ice-cube tray. When frozen, remove cubes, wrap in plastic, and return to freezer.

NOODLE-CHEESE BAKE

1 package (8 ounces) wide noodles

3 tablespoons margarine

1½ cups low-fat cottage cheese

1 cup low-fat yogurt

1 tablespoon plus 1 teaspoon flour

½ teaspoon salt

Freshly ground pepper

¼ teaspoon nutmeg

½ cup golden raisins

4 egg whites, stiffly beaten

3 tablespoons dry bread crumbs

Heat oven to 375°. Cook noodles as directed on package, except omit salt. Drain noodles and turn into large bowl. Add margarine; toss until noodles are coated. Mix cottage cheese, yogurt, flour, salt, pepper, nutmeg, and raisins; stir into noodles. Fold in egg whites.

Turn mixture into 2-quart casserole that has been sprayed with vegetable spray. Sprinkle bread crumbs on top. Bake until light brown, about 30 minutes. If desired, serve with yogurt.

8 servings.

1 serving = 226 calories
10 mg cholesterol
6 gm fat

16 *Vegetables*

VEGETABLES with their bright green, yellow, red, and while colors are so attractive that many an enterprising grocer helps to sell his stock by making a pleasing display of them. Vegetables probably do more than any other group of foods, except fruits, to add appetizing texture, color, and flavor to meals. It is wise to purchase vegetables on the days when they reach the store. Buy so you store them the least possible time before using. Leafy vegetables, peas, and green beans should be stored, unwashed, in plastic bags at about 45°. Thick-skinned vegetables, potatoes, rutabagas, and turnips should be stored, unwashed, in a cool, dry place about 55 to 60°. Cut the leaves from root vegetables.

Certain vegetables and fruits should not be stored together. For example, apples give off an ethylene gas that makes carrots bitter, and onions hasten the spoilage of potatoes.

Wash vegetables just before using. Most vegetables should not be soaked in water, because moisture will leach away the water-soluble vitamins. Vegetables that are scrubbed, scraped, or thinly pared should be cooked immediately to retain the greatest amount of nutrients.

Baking, boiling, steaming, and pressure steaming are the most common methods of cooking vegetables. The most important factor in cooking is the influence of the method on the retention of nutrients. Baking, steaming, pressure steaming, and cooking in the skins have been called "conservation methods" because they retain food values more than other methods.

Baking can be done by the direct heat of the oven, or the vegetable may be pared, sliced, or diced and placed in a covered casserole. Moderately hot oven temperature, which forms steam quickly within the vegetable, gives better texture to starchy vegetables than low temperatures. Prompt serving of baked vegetables as soon as they are done is recommended to lessen vitamin loss.

When vegetables are boiled, they are either partially or fully submerged in water, which means that soluble constituents are likely to be lost in the cooking water. These losses vary with the time of cooking and amount of surface exposed to the water. Tests have shown that cooking in a covered saucepan with small amounts of boiling water reduced the cooking time and resulted in less loss of valuable nutrients.

Steaming consists of cooking in steam either with or without pressure. Some tender young vegetables may cook rather quickly in steam, but some vegetables cooked in an ordinary steamer require longer to cook than when boiled. Because the vegetable is not actually in water more water-soluble constituents are retained, but many green vegetables may lose color and nutrients if a longer time is required to cook.

BASIC RULES FOR COOKING VEGETABLES

—Never overcook vegetables. Vegetables taste and look best and retain their nutrients when they are cooked "tender crisp"—barely tender, with a slightly crunchy texture.

—Use a small amount of cooking liquid, or simply margarine-steam vegetables. Too much water cooks out many of the vitamins and minerals. Invest in a steaming basket; they are inexpensive and easy to use, and they help retain many of the nutrients.

—Never throw out leftover vegetables. If not overcooked, they still retain much of their nutritional value, so add them to soups or casseroles to stretch a meal.

—Use herbs, spices, and other seasonings to enhance vegetables. Experiment with lemon juice, and consult a good herb cookbook or spice chart (see page 60). You will need less margarine to flavor your vegetables, so you will save calories.

—Think of vegetables as replacements for other foods. Instead of eating nutritionally empty, calorie-laden snacks, keep precut raw vegetables in refrigerator. Instead of a second starch in a meal, serve a vegetable, and instead of meat, serve a vegetable main dish.

STEAMING VEGETABLES

There are 3 basic types of steamers: bamboo, aluminum, and electric. Bamboo steamers have several tiers of racks and will fit a 14-inch wok. Aluminum steamers include complete pan and rack units or steamer racks that can be set in a saucepan. Electric steamers are usually multipurpose appliances.

To improvise a steamer, a large kettle or electric skillet with a domed lid can be used for the steamer container. Place a small can with bottom and top removed in the kettle. To support the cooking-serving dish, place a wire rack on the can.

To steam, heat water in a covered pan to boiling. The water should not touch the dish on the rack. Use a serving bowl to cook the vegetables. Steam heat is not hot enough to damage even good china. To maintain even steam, reduce heat once the steaming process starts. Cook vegetables just to "crisp-tender."

Remove the lid to check as little as possible, but check the water level and refill with boiling water if necessary. Remove the lid by tilting away from you because steam can burn. Use hot pads to remove dish. If steaming on several tiers, remember that the bottom layer cooks faster. Put large items on the bottom or rotate them.

VEGETABLES IN SOUP

Almost any vegetable is delicious in a creamed soup, served hot or cold. Tomatoes, onions, cucumbers, and bell peppers finely chopped and seasoned (or whirled in a blender) with garlic, vinegar, and chicken broth make the Spanish classic—cold gazpacho soup.

Perhaps the most flexible of all soups is minestrone; it welcomes any vegetable and always smells and tastes heavenly. Minestrone is at its best when hot, but you might try it as the Italians do in midsummer, at room temperature.

STUFFED VEGETABLES

Leftover meat can be used to stuff vegetables. Chop meat and mix with rice, bread crumbs, or chopped vegetables. Mix with a medium white sauce, egg substitute, or egg white and season to taste.

Vegetables such as artichokes, eggplant, green peppers, onions, and turnips should be parboiled before being stuffed. Tomatoes, mushrooms, and cucumbers should not be precooked. Place meat mixture in vegetable. Place vegetable in shallow baking dish. Pour in water, broth, or wine (¼-inch depth) and bake at 350° for 20 to 25 minutes.

VEGETABLE FILLINGS

Vegetables, whether fresh or cooked, can be used as fillings and flavorings in any number of dishes. With a little gravy or sauce to moisten them, they can stuff a turnover, meat pie, or crêpe. Diced leftover vegetables can stretch a small amount of meat loaf mix or can be combined with other ingredients in a quiche.

Approximate Cooking Time for Vegetables

Vegetable	Approximate quantity for 4 servings	Preparation for cooking	Approximate amount of water for boiling	Amount of water for pressure saucepan	Time (minutes)			
					Boiling	Steaming	Baking	Pressure saucepan (15 lb pressure)
Artichokes								
French	2 pounds	whole	to cover	1 cup	25 to 40			10
Jerusalem	1 pound	whole, pared	partially cover	1 cup	20 to 30	35	30 to 60	15
Asparagus	1 pound	woody ends broken off, scales removed	to cover	⅓ cup	tips 5 to 10 / butts 20 to 25	tips 10 to 15 / 25 to 30		tips to 1½ / large tips 2
Beans green or wax	¾ pound	whole or broken, strings removed	half the volume of beans	⅓ cup	10 to 20	20 to 30		3
lima	2 pounds	shelled	½- to 1-inch depth in pan, add as needed	⅓ cup	10 to 20			2 to 2½ (5-lb pressure)
Beets	1½ pounds	whole, 2 inches of stem left on	to cover	¾ cup	20 to 35	60 to 75		small 12 / large 18
Beet greens	1 to 1½ pounds	whole leaf with tender stem and mid-rib	partially cover	½ cup	15 to 20			2
Broccoli	1½ to 2 pounds	woody stems and coarse leaves removed, smaller stems pared and split	to cover stems	⅓ cup	flowerets 5 to 10 / stems 20 to 25			1½ to 2

Approximate Cooking Time for Vegetables—Continued

Vegetable	Approximate quantity for 4 servings	Preparation for cooking	Approximate amount of water for boiling	Amount of water for pressure saucepan	Time (minutes)			
					Boiling	Steaming	Baking	Pressure saucepan (15 lb pressure)
Brussels sprouts	¾ to 1 quart	whole, outer leaves removed; larger compact heads partially split	partially cover	½ cup	10 to 15			1 to 2
Cabbage	1 pound	outer leaves and stalk removed, shredded	partially cover	½ cup	6 to 9	9 to 10		1 to 1½
Carrots	1 pound	scraped, whole	partially cover	⅓ cup	15 to 20	20 to 25		4
		scraped and cut into pieces lengthwise or diced	partially cover	⅓ cup	10 to 15	15 to 20		2
Cauliflower	1½ to 2 pounds	outer leaves and stalk removed, whole or separated into flowerets	partially cover	½ cup	pieces 8 to 10 / whole 20 to 25	pieces 10 to 15 / whole 25 to 30		pieces 1½ / whole 3 to 4
Celery	1 bunch	cut into ½- to ¾-inch pieces	½ inch depth in pan, add water if needed	⅓ cup	10 to 15	20 to 25		2 to 3
Corn	4 ears	on cob	partially cover	½ cup	5 to 8			3
		cut off	to cover	⅓ cup	5 to 8			2
Okra	1 pound	sliced or whole	partially cover	⅓ cup	10 to 20	20 to 25		sliced 3

Approximate Cooking Time for Vegetables—Continued

Vegetable	Approximate quantity for 4 servings	Preparation for cooking	Approximate amount of water for boiling	Amount of water for pressure saucepan	Time (minutes)			
					Boiling	Steaming	Baking	Pressure saucepan (15 lb pressure)
Onions	1 pound	2 outer layers removed; whole, cut into halves, quarters, or slices	cover	½ cup	whole 20 to 35 / quarters 10 to 20			whole 6 to 7 / quarters 3
Parsnips	1 pound	scrape or pare; whole or cut lengthwise into halves	partially cover	½ cup	25 to 30	30 to 35		sliced, 2 whole, 7
Peas, fresh	2 pounds in pod; 2 cups shelled	shelled	2 cups	⅓ cup	15 to 25	20 to 40		2 to 3
Potatoes	1 to 1½ pounds	whole, with or without skins	cover	1 cup	30 to 35	30 to 40	40 to 60	15
		pared, cut into pieces	barely cover	¾ cup	20 to 30	30 to 35		8
Potatoes sweet	1 to 1½ pounds	whole with or without skins	cover	1 cup	30 to 35	35 to 40	45 to 60	15
		pared, halved	cover	½ cup	20 to 30	25 to 35		8 to 10
Rutabaga	1¼ pounds	pared and diced	barely cover	½ cup	20 to 30			4
Spinach	1 pound	roots removed, with or without coarse stems	1 cup per pound or none	½ cup	6 to 8			1 to 1½

Approximate Cooking Time for Vegetables—Continued

Vegetable	Approximate quantity for 4 servings	Preparation for cooking	Approximate amount of water for boiling	Amount of water for pressure saucepan	Time (minutes)				Pressure saucepan (15 lb pressure)
					Boiling	Steaming	Baking		
Squash Hubbard or winter	1½ to 2 pounds	pared, cut into 2x3-inch pieces cut into 1 portion, rind on	½- to 1-inch depth in pan	¾ cup	20 to 25	30 to 35	45 to 60		6 to 8
Squash summer	1½ to 2 pounds	sliced	½- to 1-inch depth in pan	⅓ cup	5 to 15	10 to 20	15 to 20		2
Tomatoes	1 pound	whole	little or none	¼ cup	5 to 10	10	20 to 30		1 to 2
Turnips	1 pound	pared, sliced or diced	barely cover	½ cup	15 to 20	20 to 25			1½ to 4
Turnip Greens	1 to 1½ pounds		1 to 2 cups		15 to 25				

ASPARAGUS

Break off tough ends of 1½ pounds asparagus as far down as stalks snap easily. Wash asparagus thoroughly. Remove scales if sandy or tough (if necessary, remove sand particles with vegetable brush). For spears, tie whole stalks in bundles with string or hold together with band of aluminum foil. Or cut stalks into 1-inch pieces.

To cook spears: In deep, narrow pan or coffeepot, heat 1 inch lightly salted water to boiling. Place asparagus upright in pan. Heat to boiling; cook uncovered 5 minutes. Cover and cook 7 to 10 minutes longer, or until stalk ends are crisp-tender. Drain.

To cook in skillet: Do not tie stalks in bundles. Fill 10-inch skillet half full with lightly salted water. Heat water to boiling; add asparagus and heat to boiling. Cover; cook until stalk ends are crisp-tender, 8 to 12 minutes. Drain.

4 servings.

1 serving = 30 calories
0 cholesterol
0 fat

HERBED ASPARAGUS WITH LEMON

Cook 1½ pounds asparagus as directed above. Drizzle with ¼ cup unsalted margarine, melted, and 3 tablespoons lemon juice. Season with freshly ground pepper or mace, allspice, dill weed, marjoram, or savory.

4 servings.

1 serving = 102 calories
0 cholesterol
6 gm fat

CREAMED FRESH BEANS and CELERY

½ pound wax beans, cut into 1-inch pieces
½ pound green beans, cut into 1-inch pieces
1 cup diagonally sliced celery
¼ cup water
⅛ teaspoon salt
2 tablespoons margarine
¼ cup chopped onion
2 tablespoons chopped celery leaves
⅛ teaspoon salt
⅛ teaspoon pepper
1 tablespoon caraway seed

Heat beans, celery, water, and ⅛ teaspoon salt in saucepan to boiling. Reduce heat; cover and simmer until beans are crisp-tender, about 10 minutes. Drain.

Cook and stir onion and celery leaves in margarine until onion is tender. Stir in ⅛ teaspoon salt, the pepper, caraway seed, and bean-celery mixture and heat.

5 servings.

1 serving = 92 calories
0 cholesterol
5 gm fat

BROCCOLI POLONAISE

1½ pounds broccoli
¼ cup margarine
1 tablespoon lemon juice
¼ cup dry bread crumbs
¼ cup chopped pimiento

Trim off large leaves of broccoli; remove tough ends of lower stems. Wash broccoli. If stems are thicker than 1 inch in diameter, make lengthwise gash in each stem.

Heat 1 inch water in saucepan to boiling. Add broccoli. Cover and heat to boiling; cook until stems are tender, 12 to 15 minutes. Drain.

Melt margarine; stir in lemon juice, bread crumbs, and pimiento. Sprinkle mixture on broccoli.

4 servings.

1 serving = 187 calories
trace cholesterol
13 gm fat

BROCCOLI with LEMON

Cook 1½ pounds broccoli as directed in Broccoli Polonaise (above) and omit bread-crumb topping. Mix 3 tablespoons margarine, melted, and 1 tablespoon lemon juice and pour on broccoli. If you wish, garnish with lemon slices.

6 to 8 servings.

1 serving = 69 calories
0 cholesterol
4 gm fat

BROCCOLI in CHERVIL MARGARINE

2 pounds broccoli
2 tablespoons margarine
¼ cup lemon juice
1 tablespoon chervil
½ teaspoon garlic powder
Freshly ground pepper

Trim off large leaves; remove tough ends of lower stems. Wash broccoli. If stems are thicker than 1 inch in diameter, make lengthwise gashes in each stem.

Heat 1 inch water to boiling. Add broccoli. Cover and heat to boiling. Cook about 10 minutes, or until broccoli is barely tender. Heat margarine, lemon juice, chervil, and garlic powder until margarine is melted. Stir and pour on broccoli.

6 servings.

1 serving = 86 calories
0 cholesterol
4 gm fat

BRUSSELS SPROUTS MEDLEY

1 pint brussels sprouts, trimmed
1 teaspoon margarine
1 tablespoon vegetable oil
¼ cup finely chopped green pepper
¼ cup finely chopped red pepper
3 green onions (with tops), thinly sliced
1 cup cherry tomatoes
Freshly ground pepper

Cook and stir brussels sprouts in margarine and oil over high heat 2 to 3 minutes. Reduce heat; cover and cook over low heat 15 minutes. Add green pepper, red pepper, onion, and tomatoes; cook and stir over medium heat until onion is tender, 3 to 4 minutes. Season with pepper.

4 to 6 servings.

1 serving = 64 calories
0 cholesterol
3 gm fat

PANNED RED CABBAGE

¼ cup chopped onion
2 tablespoons margarine
1 small red cabbage (about 1 pound),
  shredded
¼ teaspoon salt
1 teaspoon sugar
¼ teaspoon pepper
¼ teaspoon marjoram
Juice of ½ lemon
Freshly ground pepper

Cook and stir onion in margarine in large skillet 5 minutes. Add cabbage, salt, sugar, pepper, and marjoram; cook over medium heat, stirring occasionally, until cabbage is crisp-tender, 10 to 15 minutes. Sprinkle lemon juice on cabbage and stir. Season with pepper.

6 servings.

    1 serving = 64 calories
                0 cholesterol
                4 gm fat

STEAMED CARROTS

3 cups thinly sliced carrots (see *Note*)
1 teaspoon margarine
¼ teaspoon salt
Freshly ground pepper
2 tablespoons snipped parsley

Place carrots in steamer basket or cooking-serving dish over water in medium saucepan. Cover; heat to boiling and steam 4 to 5 minutes.

Turn carrots into serving bowl; stir in margarine. Season with salt and pepper and sprinkle with parsley.

6 servings.

    1 serving = 30 calories
                0 cholesterol
                trace fat

Note: If possible, purchase carrots with green tops. Remove tops, wash carrots, and slice in food processor.

LEMON DILL CARROTS

8 medium carrots
1 tablespoon plus 1½ teaspoons
  margarine
¼ teaspoon salt
¼ teaspoon sugar
2 tablespoons water
1 rounded tablespoon chopped fresh dill
  or 1 teaspoon dill weed
Juice of ½ lemon
Freshly ground pepper

Cut carrots into julienne strips. Melt margarine in heavy saucepan. Add carrots, stirring until coated. Sprinkle with salt, sugar, and water; cover tightly and cook over moderately low heat, shaking pan often, until carrots are crisp-tender, 4 to 7 minutes. Stir in dill and lemon juice and season with pepper.

6 servings.

    1 serving = 70 calories
                0 cholesterol
                3 gm fat

SHINY VICHY CARROTS

1 pound carrots, thinly sliced
2 tablespoons margarine
½ teaspoon salt
1 tablespoon snipped parsley

Heat ¾ inch water in saucepan to boiling. Add carrots, margarine, and salt; heat to boiling. Reduce heat; cover and simmer, shaking pan once or twice, until carrots are crisp-tender, about 6 minutes. Remove cover; cook over high heat until most of liquid has evaporated. Stir in parsley.

6 servings.

    1 serving = 71 calories
                0 cholesterol
                4 gm fat

CARROTS and GREEN BEANS

2 cups thinly sliced carrot (about ²/₃ pound)
1 cup one-inch pieces fresh green beans
1 tablespoon margarine
½ teaspoon salt
¼ cup water
Freshly ground pepper

Heat all ingredients except pepper to simmer. Stir; cover and cook, stirring once or twice, until vegetables are crisp-tender. Season with pepper.

6 servings.

1 serving = 43 calories
0 cholesterol
2 gm fat

LEMON-MINT CUCUMBERS

1 tablespoon margarine
1 large cucumber, pared and cut into 1-inch pieces
¼ teaspoon salt
1 teaspoon lemon juice
Pinch dried mint leaves or 1 teaspoon chopped fresh mint

Melt margarine in saucepan. Add cucumber; cover and cook over low heat, stirring occasionally, 5 minutes. Stir in salt, lemon juice, and mint leaves; cover and cook 2 minutes longer. Delicious served with salmon or lamb.

6 servings.

1 serving = 28 calories
3 mg cholesterol
trace fat

CUBAN EGGPLANT

1 medium onion, chopped
1 clove garlic, crushed
3 tablespoons olive oil
2 tomatoes, peeled and chopped
½ teaspoon freshly ground pepper
1 teaspoon oregano
1 medium eggplant (1½ to 2 pounds), pared and cut into 1-inch cubes

Cook and stir garlic and onion in oil in large skillet until onion is tender. Stir in tomatoes; heat to boiling. Cover; reduce heat and simmer until tomatoes are tender, about 10 minutes. Stir in pepper, oregano, and eggplant; simmer, stirring occasionally, until eggplant is crisp-tender, about 20 minutes.

4 servings.

1 serving = 149 calories
0 cholesterol
10 gm fat

Note: This vegetable can be served on cooked spaghetti.

GRILLED MELON

1 medium cantaloupe
2 tablespoons margarine

Pare melon and cut into ½-inch slices. Place slices on baking sheet; dot with margarine. Set oven at broil and/or 550°. Broil 2 to 3 inches from heat until slices begin to brown. Serve 3 or 4 slices per serving as a substitute for a vegetable.

6 servings.

1 serving = 69 calories
0 cholesterol
4 gm fat

BROILED HERBED EGGPLANT

2 tablespoons vegetable oil
2 tablespoons olive oil
¼ teaspoon basil
¼ teaspoon thyme
¼ teaspoon oregano
½ teaspoon salt
Freshly ground pepper
½ teaspoon minced garlic
1½-pound eggplant, cut into ¼-inch slices
2 tablespoons margarine
2 tablespoons snipped parsley
½ cup whole-wheat bread crumbs

Heat oven to 375°. Mix oils, basil, thyme, oregano, salt, pepper, and garlic in small skillet. Coat both sides of eggplant slices with oil-herb mixture. Place on ungreased baking sheet. Bake 15 minutes; turn slices and bake 15 minutes longer.

Melt margarine in small skillet; stir in parsley and bread crumbs. Spread mixture on eggplant slices.

Set oven at broil and/or 550°. Broil slices 2 to 3 inches from heat until topping is brown, 2 to 3 minutes.

6 servings.

1 serving = 158 calories
trace cholesterol
13 gm fat

OKRA STIR-FRY

2 tablespoons margarine
2 cups sliced okra
¼ cup chopped scallions
1 tomato, peeled and cut into eighths
1 teaspoon lemon juice
¼ teaspoon thyme
⅛ teaspoon salt
⅛ teaspoon pepper

Melt margarine in large skillet. Add remaining ingredients; cover and cook over medium heat, stirring occasionally, until vegetables are crisp-tender, 10 to 12 minutes.

6 servings.

1 serving = 69 calories
0 cholesterol
4 gm fat

STEAMED SUGAR PEAS

1 pound sugar peas, trimmed
1 teaspoon margarine
Freshly ground pepper

Place sugar peas in steamer basket or cooking-serving dish over water in medium saucepan. Cover; heat to boiling and steam 4 to 5 minutes.

Turn peas into serving bowl and toss with margarine. Season with pepper.

6 servings.

1 serving = 55 calories
0 cholesterol
trace fat

Note: Shelled fresh peas can be steamed in the same manner, except increase steaming time to 6 to 8 minutes.

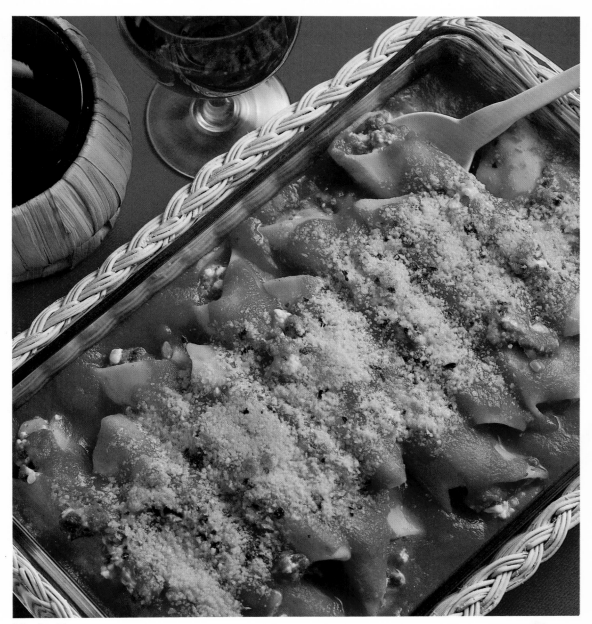
Manicotti.

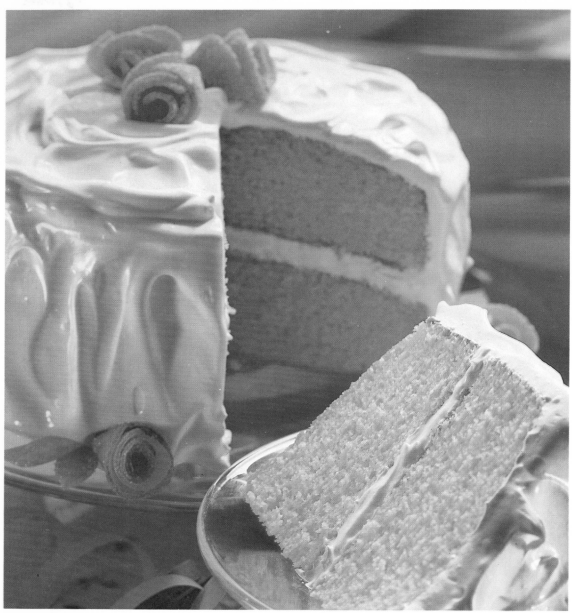
Yellow Cake.

INDIAN-STYLE STRING BEANS

1½ teaspoons mustard seed
2 tablespoons vegetable oil
¾ cup coarsely chopped onion
½ teaspoon ground cumin
½ teaspoon salt
½ teaspoon turmeric
2 tablespoons lemon juice
1 pound fresh green beans, cut into
    ¾-inch pieces

Cook and stir mustard seed in oil in 2-quart saucepan over medium heat until seed is black, about 3 minutes. Add onion; cook and stir until onion is tender. Stir in remaining ingredients; cover and cook over medium heat, stirring frequently, until beans are crisp-tender.

6 servings.

1 serving = 76 calories
            0 cholesterol
            5 gm fat

STEAMED NEW POTATOES

1 pound small new red potatoes
2 tablespoons margarine
¼ cup snipped chives

Wash potatoes, but do not pare. Place in steamer basket or cooking-serving dish over water in medium saucepan. Cover; heat to boiling and steam until tender, about 20 minutes.

Melt margarine in large skillet. Stir in chives. Add potatoes and toss until coated.

6 servings.

1 serving = 90 calories
            0 cholesterol
            3 gm fat

PARSLEYED POTATOES

1 pound potatoes (3 medium)
2 tablespoons unsalted margarine
⅔ cup snipped parsley
2 teaspoons finely chopped onion
¼ teaspoon grated lemon peel
¼ teaspoon sugar
Freshly ground pepper

Pare potatoes and cut into balls with melon-ball cutter, or cut into ¼-inch slices. Cook potatoes covered in 1 inch boiling water until tender, about 5 minutes. Drain.

Melt margarine in saucepan; stir in parsley, onion, lemon peel, and sugar. Season with pepper. Add potatoes and heat, stirring frequently, until potatoes are coated and hot.

4 servings.

1 serving = 142 calories
            0 cholesterol
            6 gm fat

PARSLEYED NEW POTATOES

¾ pound small new potatoes
2 tablespoons unsalted margarine, melted
2 tablespoons snipped parsley
1½ teaspoons lemon juice

Cook potatoes covered in 1 inch boiling water until tender, 10 to 15 minutes. Drain and, if desired, peel potatoes.

Mix margarine, parsley, and lemon juice and pour on hot potatoes.

4 servings.

1 serving = 114 calories
            0 cholesterol
            6 gm fat

SPINACH with YOGURT

1 package (10 ounces) frozen chopped spinach
½ medium onion, finely chopped
1 clove garlic, minced
1 tablespoon plus 1½ teaspoons margarine
1 tablespoon plus 1½ teaspoons safflower oil
½ teaspoon salt
½ teaspoon pepper
Scant ½ teaspoon cinnamon
1 cup low-fat yogurt

Cook spinach as directed on package. Drain, pressing out excess liquid; set spinach aside.

Cook and stir onion and garlic in margarine and oil until onion is tender, about 3 minutes. Stir in spinach, salt, pepper, and cinnamon; heat through. Remove from heat; mix in yogurt. Cool and refrigerate at least 2 hours. Serve as a first course or as a salad substitute.

3 or 4 servings.

1 serving = 154 calories
4 mg cholesterol
12 gm fat

SPANISH RICE

½ cup uncooked regular rice
½ cup chopped green pepper
½ cup chopped onion
¼ cup margarine
1 can (8 ounces) stewed tomatoes or dietetic low-sodium tomatoes
¼ teaspoon sweet basil
¼ teaspoon oregano
⅛ teaspoon pepper
½ cup water

Cook and stir rice, green pepper, and onion in margarine until onion is tender. Stir in tomatoes, seasonings and water; heat to boiling. Reduce heat to simmer; cover and cook until rice is tender, 25 to 30 minutes.

Five ½-cup servings.

1 serving = 174 calories
0 cholesterol
10 gm fat

SPINACH

2 pounds spinach
2 tablespoons olive oil or vegetable oil
1 medium onion, cut in half

Remove root ends and imperfect leaves of spinach. Wash spinach several times in water, lifting it out of water to allow sand to sink to bottom. Drain. Measure oil into large saucepan. Place onion halves cut sides down in oil; place damp spinach leaves on onion. Cover and cook until water has evaporated, 3 to 10 minutes.

4 servings.

1 serving = 139 calories
0 cholesterol
8 gm fat

STEWED TOMATOES

4 large tomatoes (about 2 pounds), peeled and cut up
½ cup finely chopped onion
¼ cup chopped green pepper
1 bay leaf
1 tablespoon sugar
¼ teaspoon salt
1 cup soft bread cubes
Freshly ground pepper

Combine tomatoes, onion, green pepper, bay leaf, sugar, and salt in saucepan. Heat to boiling, stirring occasionally. Cover; reduce heat and simmer 8 to 10 minutes. Stir in bread cubes and heat. Remove bay leaf and season with pepper.

6 servings.

1 serving = 63 calories
trace cholesterol
trace fat

FIESTA YELLOW SQUASH

½ cup chopped onion
½ cup chopped green pepper
½ cup chopped red pepper
2 tablespoons margarine
4 yellow squash, unpared and sliced
¼ teaspoon salt
⅛ teaspoon pepper
¼ teaspoon thyme
1 teaspoon lemon juice

Cook and stir onion, green pepper, and red pepper in margarine in large skillet until onion is tender. Stir in squash and remaining ingredients. Cover and cook over medium-low heat until squash is crisp-tender, 10 to 15 minutes.

4 to 6 servings.

1 serving = 93 calories
0 cholesterol
4 gm fat

RATATOUILLE

1 small onion, thinly sliced
¼ cup olive oil
3 small zucchini, cut into ⅛-inch slices
4 medium tomatoes, peeled and chopped
2 medium sweet red peppers, chopped
1 clove garlic, finely chopped
½ teaspoon salt
¼ teaspoon white pepper
⅛ teaspoon dry mustard
1 teaspoon lemon juice
¼ cup snipped parsley

Cook and stir onion slices in oil until tender. Stir in remaining ingredients, except parsley. Reduce heat; cover and simmer 3 minutes. Uncover and cook over medium heat, stirring constantly, until liquid has evaporated. (Watch carefully.) Turn into serving dish and sprinkle with parsley.

6 servings.

1 serving = 114 calories
0 cholesterol
9 gm fat

DILLED ZUCCHINI

1 pound zucchini, cut into ¾-inch slices
1 tablespoon vegetable oil
**2 tablespoons snipped fresh dill or 2
   teaspoons dried dill weed**
¼ cup water
⅛ teaspoon salt

Cook and stir zucchini in oil in skillet over medium heat 1 minute. Stir in dill and water; cover and cook over medium-high heat 8 minutes. Stir in salt; cover and cook 2 minutes longer.

6 servings.
   1 serving = 31 calories
                0 cholesterol
                2 gm fat

STEAMED VEGETABLE COMBO

1 cup diagonally sliced carrot
1 cup diagonally sliced zucchini
¼ cup diagonally sliced celery
4 green onions (with tops), sliced
⅛ teaspoon garlic salt
Freshly ground pepper

Place vegetables in steamer basket or cooking-serving dish over water in medium saucepan. Sprinkle with garlic salt and season with pepper. Cover; heat to boiling and steam 5 minutes.

4 servings.
   1 serving = 26 calories
                0 cholesterol
                trace fat

STEAMED ZUCCHINI and YELLOW SQUASH

1 pound small zucchini
1 pound yellow squash
1 tablespoon margarine
Freshly ground pepper
⅓ cup grated Parmesan cheese

Leave zucchini and yellow squash whole and unpared. Place in steamer or on trivet in saucepan with small amount of water. Cover tightly and steam until zucchini is crisp-tender. Remove zucchini; then cook squash until tender, about 12 minutes. Run cold water on zucchini and squash, then slice lengthwise.

Heat oven to 450°. Grease shallow baking dish with half the margarine. Arrange slices of zucchini and squash in dish; season with pepper and dot with remaining margarine. Sprinkle cheese on top. Bake until cheese is bubbly, about 7 minutes.

6 servings.
   1 serving = 75 calories
                5 mg cholesterol
                4 gm fat

EASY ZUCCHINI

⅓ cup chopped scallions
2 tablespoons margarine
2 large zucchini, sliced
⅛ teaspoon salt
⅛ teaspoon pepper
¼ teaspoon dill weed
1 teaspoon lemon juice

Cook and stir scallions in margarine in large skillet until tender. Add remaining ingredients; cover and cook over low heat, stirring occasionally, until zucchini is crisp-tender, about 20 minutes.

4 servings.
   1 serving = 79 calories
                0 cholesterol
                6 gm fat

BAKED TOMATOES PROVENÇAL

6 large tomatoes
Salt
Freshly ground pepper
⅓ cup dry bread crumbs
4 cloves garlic, minced
6 to 8 sprigs parsley, snipped
¼ cup plus 2 tablespoons olive oil

Heat oven to 350°. Cut thin slice from stem end of each tomato. Place tomatoes in oiled baking dish and season with salt and pepper.

Mix bread crumbs, garlic, and parsley. Stir in enough oil to moisten bread-crumb mixture. Spoon mixture on tomatoes. Bake until tomatoes are tender and crumb mixture is brown, about 15 minutes.

6 servings.

1 serving = 176 calories
trace cholesterol
13 gm fat

ZUCCHINI and CHERRY TOMATOES

2 zucchini (about ¾ pound)
2 large cloves garlic, crushed
3 tablespoons olive oil or vegetable oil
¼ teaspoon salt
Freshly ground pepper
¼ teaspoon garlic powder
16 cherry tomatoes

Cut zucchini lengthwise into 4 slices, then cut each into ½-inch pieces. Cook and stir zucchini until tender, about 5 minutes. Season with salt, pepper, and garlic powder. Add tomatoes; cook just until tomatoes are heated through, about 2 minutes.

4 servings.

1 serving = 71 calories
0 cholesterol
5 gm fat

SPICY VEGETABLE COMBO

¼ cup margarine
¼ teaspoon Tabasco sauce
2 small onions, thinly sliced
¾ cup crisp-cooked sliced zucchini (see Note)
¾ cup crisp-cooked cut green beans

Melt margarine in large skillet; add Tabasco sauce. Cook and stir onion slices in margarine until tender. Add zucchini; cook, stirring occasionally, until heated through, about 5 minutes. Add beans and heat through.

4 servings.

1 serving = 131 calories
0 cholesterol
12 gm fat

Note: Cook vegetables in boiling water and ¼ teaspoon Tabasco sauce just until crisp-tender. Substitute ¾ cup cooked cauliflowerets or ¾ cup cooked peas for the zucchini and green beans.

17 Sauces and Relishes

SALSA FRIA (Cold Sauce)

2 pounds tomatoes, peeled and chopped
1 cup finely chopped onion
1 to 4 canned green chilis, chopped
2 tablespoons vegetable oil
½ teaspoon salt
¼ teaspoon freshly ground pepper
1 teaspoon ground oregano or chopped
    fresh coriander to taste
1 to 2 tablespoons vinegar (optional)

Mix all ingredients in large bowl. Cover and refrigerate at least 2 hours. Serve with meats.

2 cups.

    1 tablespoon = 16 calories
                      0 cholesterol
                    trace fat

Note: Fresh coriander resembles parsley in appearance but has a distinctive flavor of its own. It is a popular herb in Mexican food and in California, and it is found in some supermarkets and specialty grocers.

LEMON RELISH

2 lemons
6 green onions with tops
¼ cup chopped green pepper
¼ cup snipped parsley
1 cup chopped celery
½ teaspoon dry mustard
¼ teaspoon cardamom
¼ teaspoon salt
1 small hot red pepper, seeded and
    chopped, or ½ teaspoon Tabasco sauce
1 tablespoon sugar

Grate peel from lemons. Remove remaining white peel of lemons and discard. Combine grated lemon peel, lemon pulp, and remaining ingredients in blender. Cover and blend at high speed ½ minute. Pour into bowl; cover and refrigerate at least 8 hours. Serve as an accompaniment to meats and poultry.

1½ cups.

    ¼ cup = 36 calories
              0 cholesterol
              0 fat

Note: Vegetables also can be prepared in food processor.

GAZPACHO RELISH

3 tomatoes, peeled and finely chopped
½ cup chopped green pepper
¼ cup chopped onion
⅓ cup vinegar
1 tablespoon sugar
¾ teaspoon celery seed
¾ teaspoon mustard seed
¼ teaspoon salt
Freshly ground pepper

Combine tomatoes, green pepper, and onion in glass bowl. Mix remaining ingredients; pour on vegetables. Cover and refrigerate at least 8 hours.

2½ to 3 cups.

¼ cup = 16 calories
0 cholesterol
0 fat

HOLLANDAISE SAUCE

¼ cup plus 2 tablespoons egg substitute
3 tablespoons lemon juice
½ cup margarine, melted

Measure egg substitute and lemon juice into blender. Mix on high speed until smooth. Slowly pour in hot melted margarine while mixing on low speed. Mix until smooth and creamy.

About 1 cup.

¼ cup = 229 calories
0 cholesterol
25 gm fat

SOUFFLÉED HOLLANDAISE

1 egg white
½ cup Hollandaise Sauce (this page)

Beat egg white until stiff. Pour Hollandaise Sauce on egg white and blend. Spoon on vegetables such as cooked asparagus or broccoli or on cooked fish. Place under broiler and broil until golden, 3 to 4 minutes. Serve immediately.

1 cup sauce (enough for 4 servings).

¼ cup = 118 calories
0 cholesterol
12 gm fat

DIJON-TYPE MUSTARD

1½ cups tarragon vinegar
½ cup water
2 tablespoons sugar
¼ stick cinnamon
5 whole cloves
5 white peppercorns
5 black peppercorns
1 bay leaf
5 cans (2 ounces each) dry English
mustard
¼ to ⅓ cup olive oil (optional)

Simmer vinegar, water, sugar, cinnamon stick, cloves, peppercorns, and bay leaf in medium saucepan, uncovered, 5 minutes. Strain and pour on mustard in medium bowl; stir and cover bowl.

Let stand in bowl at room temperature, stirring every other day for about 2 months. (If mustard becomes dry, stir in small amount boiling water or cream sherry.) Stir in olive oil. Pour into jar; cover and store in cool place.

2 cups.

1 tablespoon = 76 calories
0 cholesterol
5 gm fat

THIN WHITE SAUCE

For creamed vegetables and cream soups
1 tablespoon margarine
½ to 1 tablespoon flour (see *Note*)
⅛ teaspoon salt
⅛ teaspoon pepper
1 cup skim milk

Melt margarine in small saucepan over low heat. Stir in flour, salt, and pepper, stirring until mixture is smooth and bubbly. Remove from heat. Stir in milk. Heat to boiling, stirring constantly. Boil and stir 1 minute. The consistency should be like light cream.

> *1 cup.*
> ½ cup = 108 calories
> 2 mg cholesterol
> 6 gm fat

Note: Use small amount of flour with starch vegetables (peas, potatoes) and larger amount with nonstarch.

MEDIUM WHITE SAUCE

For creamed and scalloped dishes
2 tablespoons margarine
2 tablespoons flour
⅛ teaspoon pepper
⅛ teaspoon salt
1 cup skim milk

Melt margarine in small saucepan over low heat. Stir in flour, salt, and pepper, stirring until mixture is smooth and bubbly. Remove from heat. Stir in milk. Heat to boiling, stirring constantly. Boil and stir 1 minute. The consistency should be like heavy cream.

> *1 cup.*
> ½ cup = 181 calories
> 2 mg cholesterol
> 12 gm fat

Curry Sauce (For chicken, lamb, shrimp, and rice): Stir in ½ teaspoon curry powder with the flour.

Dill Sauce (For bland meat or fish): Stir in 1 teaspoon finely chopped fresh dill or ½ teaspoon dill weed and dash of nutmeg with the flour.

Cucumber Sauce (For salmon and other fish): Stir in ½ cup shredded or thinly sliced cucumber and dash cayenne pepper with the flour.

THICK WHITE SAUCE

For croquettes and soufflés
¼ cup margarine
¼ cup all-purpose flour
⅛ teaspoon salt
⅛ teaspoon pepper
1 cup skim milk

Melt margarine in small saucepan over low heat. Stir in flour, salt, and pepper. Cook over low heat, stirring until mixture is smooth and bubbly. Remove from heat. Stir in milk. Heat to boiling, stirring constantly. Boil and stir 1 minute. The consistency should be like batter.

> *1 cup.*
> ½ cup = 318 calories
> 2 mg cholesterol
> 24 gm fat

18 *Fresh Fruits and Desserts*

FRUIT is a good source of vitamins as well as a natural source of sugar in its purest, most digestible form. The skin of the fruit contains many vitamins, so to get the most out of a piece of fruit, it should be eaten fresh. Spraying is now so universal that unless you buy organically grown fruit, you should wash the peel very thoroughly (some recommend that only hot water and soap will remove all the spray). If you are in doubt, remove the peel altogether.

BUYING FRUIT

Know what fruit is in season so you can buy it when it is freshest and cheapest. When selecting fruit, call upon your senses: your eyes to spot good color and notice shriveling or decay, your nose to recognize fragrant freshness, and your touch to judge ripeness. As with vegetables, test gently for firmness. Press fruit between your palms rather than poking it.

Size is no indication of quality. Medium size is generally preferred for most purposes. Fruit that is too large or particularly small is usually undesirable. Overlarge fruit may be coarse or overripe. Extremely small fruit may be immature and will have too much waste in relation to edible portion.

Shape is also important. Grossly misshapen fruit is usually inferior in texture and taste. It can also be difficult to prepare.

Canned fruit are graded:

    Grade A or U.S. Fancy
    Grade B or U.S. Choice
    Grade C or U.S. Standard.

These grades are based on color, flavor, texture, shape and freedom from defects. The higher grades look more attractive but their nutritive value is the same as that of the lower grades.

STORING FRUIT

Fresh fruit should be used within a short time after purchase. It does not keep well and should be refrigerated and stored for only a few days. Bananas, however, should not be refrigerated because they will turn black. Some fruit must be held to soften and to ripen. To hasten ripening, keep fruit at room temperature and away from direct sunlight. Depending upon the variety and the degree of ripeness at purchase, fruits will keep from overnight to a whole winter. However, long storage at home is generally not recommended.

All fruit must be covered after cutting; plastic wrap is most effective. Most fruits darken when cut surfaces are exposed to air. Apples, bananas, pears, peaches and avocados react almost immediately. (This darkening does not interfere with edibility; simply slice off the discolored portion.) If fruit must be sliced or peeled ahead, dip it in pineapple or citrus juice or use a commercial antioxidant to retard discoloration. For best flavor, serve fruit at room temperature. Hot or warm fruit requires less sugar than chilled fruit.

Freezing robs fruit of its texture. Fresh fruit in season is cheaper than frozen fruit. If you buy frozen fruit, make sure the package is hard, clean, frost-free and that the store has a fairly constant turnover of frozen goods.

FRUIT BOATS

1 pineapple
1 cup strawberries, sliced
½ cup blueberries
½ cup honeydew melon balls
¼ cup port
2 tablespoons orange juice
1 teaspoon lemon juice
1 tablespoon sugar
¼ teaspoon cinnamon

Select a pineapple with fresh green leaves. Cut pineapple lengthwise in half through green top; then cut each in half again, making 4 pieces. Cut core from each pineapple quarter and cut along curved edges with grapefruit knife to remove fruit from shells. Drain shells. Remove "eyes" from fruit and cut into bite-size pieces. Combine pineapple, strawberries, blueberries, and melon balls in bowl. Stir wine, orange juice, lemon juice, sugar, and cinnamon until sugar is dissolved. Pour on fruit and toss. Divide fruit among shells.

4 servings.

1 serving = 159 calories
0 cholesterol
trace fat

CANTALOUPE CUPS

3 cantaloupes
3 cups grapefruit sections
1 cup honeydew melon balls
1 cup watermelon balls
Mint sprigs

Cut cantaloupes crosswise into halves; remove seeds. Remove cantaloupe from halves with melon-ball cutter. Combine grapefruit sections and all melon balls and mix carefully. Divide mixture among shells and garnish each with a sprig of mint.

6 servings.

1 serving = 130 calories
0 cholesterol
trace fat

HONEYED GRAPEFRUIT

Remove seeds from ½ grapefruit. Cut around edge and sections to loosen; remove center. Drizzle 1½ teaspoons honey on grapefruit; place 1 strawberry in center and refrigerate until serving time.

1 serving = 82 calories
0 cholesterol
0 fat

TO SECTION AN ORANGE
OR GRAPEFRUIT

Wash and dry fruit. Hold the fruit over a bowl to catch all the juice. With a sharp knife, cut around and around the fruit to remove the peel and white skin. (The removed peel will be a long curl). Cut down along the membrane on each side of sections to loosen. Lift out the section in one piece and remove any seeds.

WATERMELON BASKET

One 10-pound, long watermelon, chilled
2 cups sliced strawberries
2 cups unsweetened pineapple chunks
3 cups honeydew melon balls
2 cups cantaloupe balls
2 bananas, sliced
1 pound seedless grapes
1 cup cut-up apple
1 cup cut-up peaches
1 cup orange juice

Chill all ingredients. Cut watermelon lengthwise and slice off top third. Use larger part for basket. Remove watermelon from shell with melon-ball cutter. With teacup as guide, mark scalloped edge on shell and cut on markings. Cover shell and refrigerate.

Fill shell just before serving. Add fruits to shell; pour orange juice on fruits and mix carefully.

24 servings.

1 serving = 91 calories
0 cholesterol
trace fat

Note: Ginger ale, sherry, or brandy can be substituted for orange juice, but this will add calories.

GRAPES AND YOGURT

½ cup brown sugar (packed)
1 cup low-fat yogurt
4 cups seedless green grapes, cut into halves

Mix sugar and yogurt; pour on grapes and toss. Cover and refrigerate at least 2 hours. Serve in champagne glasses.

8 servings.

1 serving = 121 calories
2 mg cholesterol
trace fat

SPICED CITRUS SECTIONS

2 cups orange sections (4 medium oranges)
2 cups grapefruit sections (2 large grapefruit)
2 tablespoons brown sugar
½ teaspoon whole cloves
½ teaspoon nutmeg

Reserve juice when cutting sections from oranges and grapefruit. Heat reserved juice, sugar, cloves, and nutmeg to boiling, stirring until sugar is dissolved. Reduce heat and simmer 5 minutes. Remove from heat; remove whole cloves and pour syrup on orange and grapefruit sections. Serve warm or cold.

6 servings.

1 serving = 87 calories
0 cholesterol
trace fat

BAKED APPLE SURPRISE

1 baking apple
1½ teaspoons sugar
1 teaspoon raisins
½ teaspoon margarine
Dash cinnamon

Heat oven to 350°. Core apple; pare upper ⅓ to prevent skin from splitting. Place apple upright in baking dish. Fill center of apple with sugar, raisins, margarine, and cinnamon. Pour water (¼ inch deep) into dish.

Bake until apple is tender, 30 to 45 minutes. Serve hot or cold.

        1 serving = 108 calories
                       0 cholesterol
                       2 gm fat

Note: 1 tablespoon orange-flavored liqueur can be added to water in baking dish if desired.

FRUIT KEBABS GRAND MARNIER

1 tablespoon margarine
½ cup light corn syrup
3 tablespoons Grand Marnier
2 teaspoons grated lemon peel
1 tablespoon lemon juice
2 small bananas
3 red plums, pitted and cut into 8 slices each
1 cup seedless grapes

Heat oven to 350°. Melt margarine in small skillet over low heat. Stir in syrup, Grand Marnier, lemon peel, and juice. Remove from heat. Cut bananas into 1-inch chunks; place in syrup mixture, turning to coat all sides.

On 8 skewers, alternate fruits. Place kebabs in baking dish and spoon syrup mixture on fruits. Bake until just heated through, about 10 minutes.

        8 servings.
        1 serving =   70 calories
                        0 cholesterol
                        1 gm fat

MARINATED FRUIT

2 cans (8 ounces each) pineapple chunks in unsweetened pineapple juice
4 navel oranges, pared and sectioned
2 large pieces crystallized ginger, finely chopped
4 bananas

Place pineapple chunks (with juice), orange sections, and ginger in bowl. Cover and refrigerate 8 hours.

Slice ½ banana into each sherbet dish. Spoon pineapple mixture and juice on slices.

        8 servings.
        1 serving = 110 calories
                       0 cholesterol
                       trace fat

GRAPEFRUIT SIZZLE

1 medium grapefruit
2 teaspoons margarine
2 teaspoons sugar
¼ teaspoon cinnamon
1 strawberry, cut into halves

Cut grapefruit in half; remove seeds. Cut around edges and membranes of halves to loosen fruit; remove centers. Dot halves with margarine. Mix sugar and cinnamon and sprinkle on grapefruit.

Set oven at broil and/or 550°. Place grapefruit in shallow baking pan. Broil with tops 4 to 6 inches from heat until juice bubbles and edge of peel turns light brown, about 8 minutes. Serve hot, topped with strawberry halves.

        2 servings.
        1 serving = 102 calories
                       0 cholesterol
                       4 gm fat

MIXED MELON COOLER

2 small cantaloupes
1 large honeydew melon
1 tablespoon plus 1 teaspoon sugar
1 tablespoon plus 1 teaspoon white crème de menthe
Mint sprigs

Cut each cantaloupe into quarters. Remove seeds; cover quarters and chill.

Scoop balls with melon ball cutter from honeydew melon. Place in bowl; sprinkle with sugar and liqueur and toss. Let stand to blend flavors.

To serve, arrange melon balls in cantaloupe quarters and garnish with mint sprigs.

8 servings.
    1 serving = 71 calories
                  trace cholesterol
                  trace fat

CITRUS SURPRISE POPS

4 cups orange juice
1 cup grapefruit juice
1 banana

Mix orange and grapefruit juices. Fill twelve 5-ounce paper or plastic cups halfway with juice and place in freezer.

When partially frozen, remove from freezer. Cut banana into 12 pieces and place piece in center of each cup. Insert popsicle stick in banana. Fill cups with remaining juice, leaving ¼-inch space at top. Freeze until firm.

To serve, push up on bottom of cup until popsicle comes out.

12 servings.
    1 serving = 36 calories
                  0 cholesterol
                  0 fat

Note: Fresh strawberries, pineapple chunks, or melon pieces can be substituted for the banana.

FRESH MELON SHERBET

1 envelope unflavored gelatin
¼ cup sugar
½ cup water
¼ cup lemon juice
1 cup water
4 cups fresh cantaloupe or honeydew melon cubes

Mix gelatin and sugar in small saucepan. Stir in ½ cup water and heat to boiling, stirring until sugar is dissolved. Remove from heat; stir in lemon juice and cool.

Pour 1 cup water into blender; add melon cubes and blend until smooth. Mix in gelatin mixture. Pour into loaf pan, 9 x 5 x 3 inches. Freeze until almost firm.

Remove from freezer. Place melon mixture in bowl and beat until mushy and thick. Return to loaf pan and freeze until firm.

12 servings.
    1 serving = 38 calories
                  0 cholesterol
                  0 fat

Note: If using watermelon and casaba melon cubes, omit 1 cup water.

Variation: Pour mixture into ice cube tray and freeze. Serve cubes in dessert dishes, or, for an attractive dessert, fill melon halves with melon cubes. For popsicles, insert popsicle stick in each ice cube compartment when mixture is partially frozen.

LAYERED ICE

1 can (6 ounces) frozen orange juice
**   concentrate**
3 cans water
1 egg white
2 tablespoons honey

Measure all ingredients into blender. Cover and blend on high speed until smooth. Pour into 6 individual molds or into popsicle molds. Freeze until firm. If using popsicle molds, insert popsicle sticks in mixture when partially frozen.

6 servings.
    1 serving = 66 calories
                0 cholesterol
                0 fat

LIME SNOW

2 envelopes unflavored gelatin
½ cup sugar
1 cup water
1 can (6 ounces) frozen limeade
**   concentrate**
½ cup water
3 egg whites

Mix gelatin and sugar in small saucepan. Stir in 1 cup water and heat to boiling, stirring until sugar is dissolved. Remove from heat; stir in frozen limeade concentrate and ½ cup water. Refrigerate until mixture is thickened but not set.

Place gelatin mixture and egg whites in large mixer bowl. Beat on high speed until mixture holds its shape, about 7 minutes. If desired, stir in few drops green food coloring. Turn into 2-quart mold or into individual molds and chill until set.

8 servings.
    1 serving = 86 calories
                0 cholesterol
                trace fat

BANANA FREEZE

1 envelope unflavored gelatin
¼ cup sugar
1½ cups plus 3 tablespoons nonfat
**   dry milk**
1¾ cups plus 2 tablespoons water
3 medium bananas
1 teaspoon vanilla

Mix gelatin, sugar, and dry milk in small saucepan. Stir in water. Heat over medium heat, stirring constantly, until gelatin and dry milk are dissolved, about 5 minutes. Cool.

Pour about half the milk mixture into blender and slice bananas into it. Blend until smooth. Add vanilla and remaining milk mixture and blend. Pour into loaf pan, 9 x 5 x 3 inches; freeze until mushy. Pour into small mixer bowl; beat until smooth. Return mixture to loaf pan; freeze until firm.

16 servings.
    1 serving = 87 calories
                3 mg cholesterol
                trace fat

STRAWBERRY ICE

1 quart strawberries
¾ cup orange juice
½ cup honey
¼ teaspoon lemon juice
Fresh mint sprigs

Reserve 6 strawberries for garnish. Mix remaining strawberries, the orange juice, honey, and lemon juice in blender on high speed until smooth, scraping sides occasionally. Pour into baking pan, 8 x 8 x 2 inches. Freeze until firm. Let stand 5 minutes at room temperature before serving. Garnish servings with reserved strawberries and mint sprigs.

6 servings.
    1 serving = 102 calories
                0 cholesterol
                trace fat

ORANGE SNOW

1 envelope unflavored gelatin
2 tablespoons sugar
½ cup water
1 cup orange juice
3 medium oranges, sectioned and cut into
  small pieces (about 3 cups)
1 tablespoon lime juice
2 egg whites

Mix gelatin and sugar in small saucepan. Stir in water and heat to boiling, stirring until sugar is dissolved. Remove from heat; stir in orange juice, orange pieces, and lime juice. Refrigerate until thickened.

Beat egg whites until stiff peaks form. Beat gelatin until frothy. Fold gelatin mixture into egg whites. Pour into 5-cup mold. Refrigerate until set. Unmold and, if desired, garnish with orange slices and whole strawberries.

8 servings.

  1 serving = 54 calories
              0 cholesterol
              trace fat

PARFAITS

Alternate fruit and yogurt in parfait glasses.

Strawberry Parfait: For each parfait, use 3 large strawberries, sliced, and ½ cup frozen strawberry low-fat yogurt.

  1 serving = 139 calories
              5 mg cholesterol
              1 gm fat

Peach Parfait: For each parfait, use ½ peach, sliced, and ½ cup frozen peach low-fat yogurt.

  1 serving = 145 calories
              5 mg cholesterol
              1 gm fat

Orange Parfait: For each parfait, use ½ orange, pared, sectioned, and cubed, and ½ cup frozen orange-pineapple low-fat yogurt.

  1 serving = 151 calories
              5 mg cholesterol
              1 gm fat

Raspberry Parfait: For each parfait, use 2 tablespoons frozen raspberries, thawed, and ½ cup frozen vanilla low-fat yogurt.

  1 serving = 133 calories
              5 mg cholesterol
              1 gm fat

FRUIT CLOUDS

3 egg whites (⅓ to ½ cup)
¼ teaspoon cream of tartar
¼ teaspoon salt
¾ cup sugar
1 teaspoon vanilla
4 cups fruit (or 1 quart fruit ice)

Heat oven to 425°. Cover baking sheet with heavy brown paper. Beat egg whites, cream of tartar, and salt until foamy. Beat in sugar, 1 tablespoon at a time; continue beating until stiff and glossy. Do not underbeat. Make 8 meringues by dropping ⅓ cup mixture for each onto paper. Shape into circles, building up edges.

Place in oven; immediately turn off oven and leave meringues in oven at least 12 hours or until oven is completely cool.

Just before serving, fill each meringue with ½ cup fruit.

8 servings.

  1 serving = 111 calories
              0 cholesterol
              trace fat

Note: If using fruit ice instead of fruit, each serving contains approximately 135 calories.

FRUIT WHIP

1 envelope unflavored gelatin
1 cup canned unsweetened pineapple juice
½ teaspoon grated lemon peel
3 tablespoons honey
2 cups unsweetened applesauce
Cinnamon or nutmeg

Sprinkle gelatin on pineapple juice to soften. Stir over low heat until gelatin is dissolved. Stir in lemon peel, honey, and applesauce. Refrigerate, stirring occasionally, until mixture mounds slightly when dropped from spoon.

Beat until fluffy. Divide among 8 dessert dishes. Refrigerate until firm. Sprinkle each with cinnamon.

8 servings.

> 1 serving = 71 calories
> 0 cholesterol
> trace fat

ORANGE GEL

1 envelope unflavored gelatin
¼ cup sugar
¾ cup water
1 can (6 ounces) frozen orange juice concentrate
½ cup water

Mix gelatin and sugar into small saucepan. Stir in ¾ cup water. Stir over low heat until gelatin is dissolved. Remove from heat. Stir in frozen orange juice concentrate until melted. Stir in ½ cup water. Pour into 6 dessert dishes or individual molds; chill until set. Serve with whole or sliced strawberries on top if desired.

6 servings.

> 1 serving = 79 calories
> 0 cholesterol
> 0 fat

SNOW PUDDING

1 envelope unflavored gelatin
¾ cup sugar
1 cup water
1 tablespoon grated lemon peel
¼ cup lemon juice
2 egg whites
1 package (10 ounces) frozen raspberries, thawed

Mix gelatin and sugar in small saucepan. Stir in water and heat to boiling, stirring until sugar is dissolved. Remove from heat; stir in lemon peel and juice. Refrigerate until mixture is thickened but not set.

Beat egg whites in small mixer bowl until stiff peaks form. Beat gelatin mixture until frothy. Add gelatin mixture to egg whites and beat until mixture holds its shape. Divide among 6 dessert dishes; refrigerate until set. Serve with raspberries.

6 servings.

> 1 serving = 146 calories
> 0 cholesterol
> trace fat

APPLE SNOW

1 pound apples (3 medium)
1 tablespoon sugar
2 egg whites

Pare, core, and slice apples into saucepan. Add a small amount of water and the sugar; cover and cook over low heat until apples are soft. Turn mixture into blender and blend on high speed until smooth. Cool.

Beat egg whites until stiff. Fold in apple mixture and chill.

4 servings.

> 1 serving = 80 calories
> 0 cholesterol
> trace fat

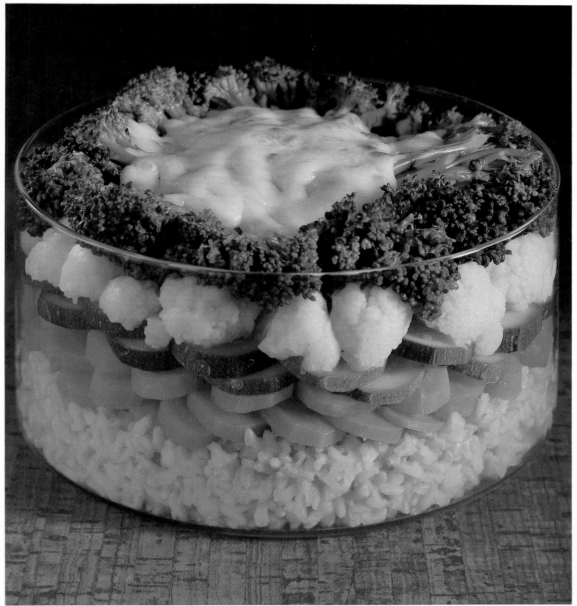

Vegetable and Brown Rice Casserole.

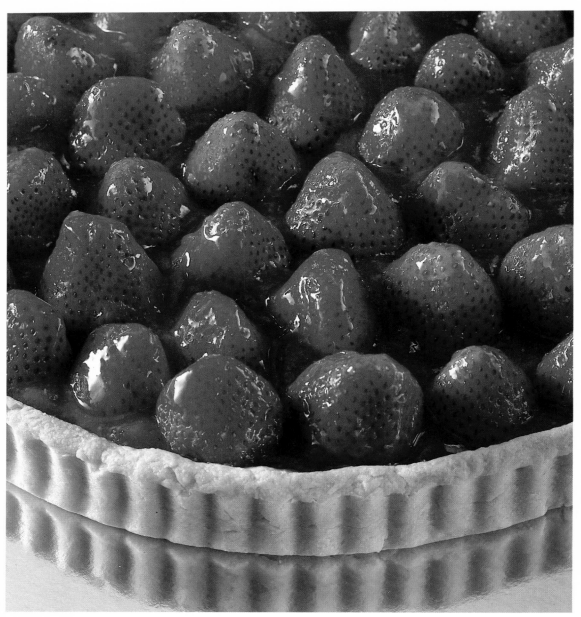

Strawberry Tart.

BAKED APPLE RICE PUDDING

⅓ **cup egg substitute**
2 cups finely chopped pared apple
  (2 medium)
1½ cups cooked rice
½ cup pitted dates, snipped
¼ cup sugar
½ teaspoon cinnamon
2 tablespoons unsalted margarine,
  softened
1 teaspoon vanilla
2 egg whites
¼ teaspoon cinnamon

Heat oven to 325°. Mix egg substitute, apple, rice, dates, sugar, ½ teaspoon cinnamon, the margarine, and the vanilla in 1½-quart casserole or soufflé dish. Beat egg whites until stiff peaks form; fold into rice mixture. Sprinkle ¼ teaspoon cinnamon on top.

Place casserole in pan of very hot water (1 inch deep). Bake about 1 hour 10 minutes. Serve warm or chilled. If desired, garnish with fresh apple slices dipped in lemon juice.

6 servings.
  1 serving = 195 calories
              0 cholesterol
              5 gm fat

FRUIT JEWELLED MELON

2 small cantaloupes
1 envelope unflavored gelatin
2 tablespoons sugar
1¾ cups reconstituted frozen
  unsweetened lime juice
2 drops green food coloring
1 cup blueberries

Cut cantaloupes lengthwise into halves; remove seeds. Using curved grapefruit knife, remove cantaloupe, leaving a ¾-inch-thick shell. Drain shells; cover and refrigerate. (Reserve scooped-out cantaloupe for future use. Wrap in plastic wrap and refrigerate.)

Mix gelatin and sugar in small saucepan. Stir in ½ cup of the lime juice and heat to boiling, stirring until sugar is dissolved. Remove from heat; stir in remaining 1¼ cups lime juice and the food coloring. Refrigerate until thickened.

Fold blueberries into gelatin mixture. Spoon mixture into cantaloupe shells. Cover and refrigerate until gelatin is set. Cut each shell lengthwise in half.

4 servings.
  1 serving = 160 calories
              0 cholesterol
              trace fat

QUICK CONCENTRATE GELS

1 envelope unflavored gelatin
1 tablespoon sugar
½ cup water
1 can (6 ounces) frozen juice concentrate
  or punch (see *Note***)**
¾ cup water

Mix gelatin and sugar in small saucepan. Stir in ½ cup water. Stir over low heat until gelatin is dissolved, about 3 minutes. Remove from heat; stir in frozen concentrate until melted. Stir in ¾ cup water. Pour into dessert dishes or 2-cup mold. Chill until set.

  4 servings.
    1 serving = 81 calories
               0 cholesterol
               trace fat

Note: Choose orange, orange-grapefruit, tangerine, grape or apple juice concentrates. Do not use frozen pineapple juice or punches containing pineapple juice.

ZABAGLIONE

¾ cup egg substitute
2 tablespoons sugar
½ cup Marsala

Beat egg substitute and sugar in top of double boiler until light and fluffy. Continue beating and slowly add wine. Place top of double boiler over simmering water. Cook, beating constantly, until thick and fluffy, about 20 minutes. Mixture will form soft peaks. Serve in sherbet dishes or, if desired, serve as a sauce for fresh fruits.

  8 servings.
    1 serving = 50 calories
               0 cholesterol
               1 gm fat

CAFE DIABLE MOLD

2 envelopes unflavored gelatin
½ cup water
2¾ cups water
¼ cup instant coffee
2 sticks cinnamon
6 whole cloves
½ cup sugar
½ cup rum (see *Note***)**
Whipped Topping (below)

Sprinkle gelatin on ½ cup water to soften. Heat 2¾ cups water, the instant coffee, cinnamon sticks, and cloves to boiling. Reduce heat and simmer 5 minutes. Remove cinnamon sticks and cloves. Stir in gelatin and sugar until dissolved. Stir in rum. Pour into 4-cup mold and chill until set. Unmold and serve with Whipped Topping.

  8 servings.
    1 serving = 79 calories
               0 cholesterol
               0 fat

Note: If rum is not available, use 2 teaspoons rum flavoring and ¼ cup water.

WHIPPED TOPPING

Pour 1 can (6½ ounces) evaporated skim milk into small mixer bowl. Place in freezer with the beater until crystals form around edge of milk in bowl, 15 to 20 minutes.

Beat on high speed until stiff. Add 2 tablespoons sugar and 1 teaspoon vanilla and continue beating 1 to 2 minutes.

  About 1½ cups.
    2 tablespoons = 22 calories
                   0 cholesterol
                   0 fat

Note: If topping is not used immediately, place in freezer up to 30 minutes. Beat 1 minute before serving.

VANILLA CUSTARD

⅓ cup sugar
2 tablespoons flour
1 tablespoon cornstarch
1½ cups skim milk
⅓ cup egg substitute
1¼ teaspoons vanilla

Mix sugar, flour, and cornstarch in saucepan. Stir in milk. Cook over medium heat, stirring constantly, until mixture thickens and boils. Boil and stir 1 minute. Stir about half the hot mixture into egg substitute. Blend egg mixture into remaining hot mixture. Cook and stir 1 minute. Remove from heat and stir in vanilla. Press plastic wrap onto filling and refrigerate.

6 servings.
1 serving = 92 calories
1 mg cholesterol
trace fat

Note: This custard will fill an 8-inch baked pie shell, or it can be used as a filling for an 8- or 9-inch cake.

DESSERT CRÊPES

1½ cups all-purpose flour
1 tablespoon sugar
½ teaspoon baking powder
2 cups skim milk
⅓ cup egg substitute
½ teaspoon vanilla
2 tablespoons unsalted margarine, melted

Measure all ingredients into bowl; beat with rotary beater until smooth.

Lightly grease 7- or 8-inch skillet with margarine; heat over medium heat until margarine is bubbly. For each crêpe, pour scant ¼ cup batter into skillet; immediately rotate skillet until batter covers bottom. Cook until light brown. Loosen around edge with wide spatula; turn and cook other side until light brown. Stack crêpes, placing waxed paper or paper towel between them. Keep crêpes covered to prevent them from drying out.

If desired, spread applesauce, sweetened strawberries, currant jelly, or raspberry jam on each crêpe and roll up. (Roll crêpes so most attractive side is on the outside.) Sprinkle with powdered sugar.

12 to 16 crêpes.
1 crêpe = 83 calories
trace cholesterol
2 gm fat

19 Cakes, Pies, and Cookies

ANGEL FOOD CAKE

1 cup cake flour
¾ cup plus 2 tablespoons sugar
12 egg whites (1½ cups)
1½ teaspoons cream of tartar
¾ cup sugar
1½ teaspoons vanilla
½ teaspoon almond extract

Heat oven to 375°. Mix flour and first amount of sugar; set aside. Beat egg whites and cream of tartar in large mixer bowl until foamy. Add second amount of sugar, 2 tablespoons at a time, beating on high speed until meringue holds stiff points. Fold in flavorings. Sprinkle flour-sugar mixture ¼ cup at a time over meringue, folding in gently just until flour-sugar mixture disappears. Push batter into ungreased tube pan, 10 x 4 inches.

Bake 30 to 35 minutes or until top springs back when touched lightly with finger. Invert tube pan on funnel; let hang until cake is completely cool.

16 servings.

1 slice = 114 calories
0 cholesterol
0 fat

BLUEBERRY CRUMB CAKE

1½ cups all-purpose flour
2 teaspoons baking powder
¼ teaspoon salt
2 cups blueberries
¼ cup unsalted margarine, softened
¼ cup sugar
¼ cup egg substitute
½ cup skim milk
Crumb Topping (below)

Heat oven to 375°. Spray baking pan, 8 x 8 x 2 inches, with vegetable spray. Stir together flour, baking powder, salt, and blueberries. Cream margarine and sugar thoroughly. Beat in egg substitute. Mix in milk and flour mixture. Pour into pan. Sprinkle Crumb Topping on top. Bake 30 minutes.

12 servings.

1 serving = 163 calories
trace cholesterol
6 gm fat

Crumb Topping: Mix 2 tablespoons sugar, 2 tablespoons flour, ¼ teaspoon cinnamon, and 2 tablespoons unsalted margarine until crumbly.

POUND CAKE

2 cups all-purpose flour
1 cup sugar
3 teaspoons baking powder
¾ cup skim milk
½ cup unsalted margarine, softened
½ cup egg substitute
1 teaspoon vanilla

Heat oven to 350°. Spray loaf pan, 9 x 5 x 3 inches, with vegetable spray. Measure all ingredients into large mixer bowl. Blend on low speed, scraping bowl constantly. Beat on high speed 3 minutes, scraping bowl occasionally. Pour into pan. Bake about 65 minutes, or until wooden pick inserted in center comes out clean.

16 servings.
    1 serving = 170 calories
                trace cholesterol
                6 gm fat

LEMON POUND CAKE

½ cup unsalted margarine, softened
1 cup sugar
¾ cup egg substitute
1 teaspoon vanilla
3 cups all-purpose flour
1½ teaspoons baking powder
½ teaspoon mace
⅛ teaspoon salt
1 tablespoon grated lemon peel
½ cup skim milk

Heat oven to 350°. Spray loaf pan, 9 x 5 x 3 inches, with vegetable spray. Beat margarine, sugar, egg substitute, and vanilla in large mixer bowl until light. Mix in remaining ingredients until smooth. Pour into pan.

Bake 1 hour, or until cake has pulled away from side and springs back when touched lightly. Cool in pan 10 minutes before turning onto wire rack.

16 servings.
    1 serving = 200 calories
                trace cholesterol
                7 gm fat

ORANGE PETITE CAKE

1 tablespoon chopped orange peel
¼ cup egg substitute
⅓ cup unsalted margarine, softened
¾ cup skim milk
1 teaspoon vanilla
1¼ cups all-purpose flour
1 cup sugar
1½ teaspoons baking powder
½ cup walnuts
½ cup raisins

Heat oven to 350°. Spray 2 round layer pans, 8 x 1½ inches, or 1 baking pan, 8 x 8 x 2 inches or 9 x 9 x 2 inches, with vegetable spray. Measure all ingredients in the order listed into blender. Mix on high speed 30 seconds or just until ingredients are mixed, stopping blender occasionally to scrape sides with rubber spatula. (Batter may be slightly lumpy.) Pour into pan. Bake layers about 25 minutes, 8-inch cake about 40 minutes, 9-inch cake about 35 minutes, or until wooden pick inserted in center comes out clean. Cool. Frost cake if desired.

12 servings.
    1 serving = 231 calories
                trace cholesterol
                9 gm fat

HONEY LEMON CAKE

½ cup unsalted margarine, softened
½ cup sugar
⅓ cup honey
½ cup egg substitute
2 cups all-purpose flour
3 teaspoons baking powder
⅔ cup skim milk
1 tablespoon grated lemon peel
1 tablespoon lemon juice

Heat oven to 350°. Spray baking pan, 9 x 9 x 2 inches, with vegetable spray. Cream margarine and sugar thoroughly. Blend in honey and egg substitute. Mix in flour and baking powder alternately with milk. Stir in lemon peel and juice. Pour into pan.

Bake about 40 minutes, or until wooden pick inserted in center comes out clean.

12 servings.

1 serving = 221 calories
trace cholesterol
8 gm fat

Honey Orange Cake: Substitute orange peel and orange juice for the lemon peel and juice.

OLD-FASHIONED POPPY SEED CAKE

½ cup poppy seed
1 cup skim milk
2¼ cups all-purpose flour
1½ cups sugar
3½ teaspoons baking powder
½ cup unsalted margarine, softened
1½ teaspoons vanilla
4 egg whites (½ cup)

Soak poppy seed in skim milk 1 hour.

Heat oven to 350°. Spray two layer pans, 8 or 9 x 1½ inches, or baking pan, 13 x 9 x 2 inches, with vegetable spray. Measure flour, sugar, and baking powder into large mixer bowl. Add margarine, a little more than half the poppy seed-milk mixture, and the vanilla. Beat on medium speed 2 minutes, scraping bowl constantly. Add remaining poppy seed-milk mixture and the egg whites; beat on high speed 2 minutes, scraping bowl frequently. Pour into pan(s). Bake layers 30 to 35 minutes, oblong about 35 minutes, or until wooden pick inserted in center comes out clean.

16 servings.

1 serving = 209 calories
trace cholesterol
6 gm fat

BANANA/YOGURT CAKE

¼ cup unsalted margarine, softened
½ cup sugar
½ cup egg substitute
½ cup mashed ripe banana (1 medium)
1 teaspoon vanilla
2¼ cups all-purpose flour
1 teaspoon baking powder
1 teaspoon baking soda
⅛ teaspoon salt
1 cup low-fat yogurt
Walnut-Raisin Filling (below)

Heat oven to 350°. Spray 9-inch tube pan or 6-cup Bundt pan with vegetable spray. Measure margarine, sugar, egg substitute, banana, and vanilla into large mixer bowl. Beat on medium speed 2 minutes, scraping bowl frequently. Mix in flour, baking powder, baking soda, and salt alternately with yogurt.

Sprinkle ¼ cup Walnut-Raisin Filling in pan. Spread about ⅓ batter on filling. Repeat 2 times, using half of the remaining Filling each time.

Bake about 1 hour 15 minutes, or until wooden pick inserted in center comes out clean. Cool cake in pan 20 minutes before turning onto wire rack.

20 servings.

1 serving = 163 calories
trace cholesterol
6 gm fat

WALNUT-RAISIN FILLING

1 cup chopped walnuts
½ cup golden raisins
3 tablespoons sugar
1 teaspoon cinnamon

Mix all ingredients.

HONEY CAKE

½ cup egg substitute
¼ cup sugar
¼ cup coffee
¼ cup honey
1 tablespoon vegetable oil
1¾ cups all-purpose flour
¼ teaspoon salt
½ teaspoon baking powder
½ teaspoon baking soda
1 cup coarsely chopped walnuts

Heat oven to 325°. Brush oil on 7¾ x 3⅝ x 2¼ inch loaf pan, then line with waxed paper and brush oil on paper. In a large bowl, beat egg substitute and sugar at high speed 5 minutes. On medium speed mix in coffee, honey, and oil. Mix in flour, salt, baking powder, and baking soda, scraping bowl occasionally, until batter is smooth. Stir in nuts. Pour into loaf pan.

Bake 1 hour and 10 to 20 minutes or until wooden pick inserted in center comes out clean. Turn cake out of pan; remove waxed paper and cool cake. Wrap securely and store 2 days before serving.

14 slices.

1 serving = 154 calories
0 cholesterol
6 gm fat

CREATIVE CAKES

COOKIE CUTTER CAKE

Frost cake with white frosting. Dip a cookie cutter into liquid food color; press into frosting, making an imprint on top of cake. Repeat around top of cake, dipping cutter into food color each time.

BALLOON CAKE

Frost cake with white frosting or one that has been delicately tinted with food color. On top of cake, arrange pastel mint-wafer "balloons." Use shoestring licorice for the ballon strings.

CARNIVAL CAKE

Frost cake with White Swirl Frosting. Mark top into 8 equal wedges. Sprinkle confetti candy on every other wedge.

GUMDROP ROSE CAKE

Frost cake with white frosting. Arrange gumdrop roses on top. For each rose, roll 4 large gumdrops on well-sugared board into ⅛-inch ovals. Sprinkle sugar on gumdrops. Cut each oval in half. Roll one half-oval tightly to form center of rose. Place remaining half-ovals around center, overlapping slightly. Press together at base and trim base. Cut leaves from rolled green gumdrops.

YELLOW CAKE

⅔ **cup unsalted margarine, softened**
1¾ **cups sugar**
½ **cup egg substitute**
1½ **teaspoons vanilla**
2¾ **cups all-purpose flour**
2½ **teaspoons baking powder**
1¼ **cups skim milk**

Heat oven to 350°. Spray baking pan, 13 x 9 x 2 inches, or two 9-inch layer pans with vegetable spray. Mix margarine, sugar, egg substitute, and vanilla in large mixer bowl until fluffy. Beat on high speed 5 minutes, scraping bowl occasionally. On low speed, mix in flour and baking powder alternately with milk. Pour into pan(s).

Bake oblong 45 to 50 minutes, layers 30 to 35 minutes, or until wooden pick inserted in center comes out clean. Cool.

15 servings.

1 serving = 264 calories
trace cholesterol
9 gm fat

WHITE CAKE

2 cups all-purpose flour
1½ cups sugar
3½ teaspoons baking powder
½ cup unsalted margarine
1 cup skim milk
1 teaspoon vanilla
4 egg whites

Heat oven to 350°. Spray baking pan, 13 x 9 x 2 inches, or 2 round layer pans, 8 or 9 x 1½ inches, with vegetable spray. Measure all ingredients except egg whites into large mixer bowl. Blend on low speed ½ minute, scraping bowl constantly. Beat on high speed 2 minutes, scraping bowl occasionally. Add egg whites; beat on high speed 2 minutes, scraping bowl occasionally. Pour into pan(s). Bake oblong 35 to 40 minutes, layers 30 to 35 minutes, or until wooden pick inserted in center comes out clean.

16 servings.

1 serving = 195 calories
trace cholesterol
6 gm fat

DEVILS FOOD CAKE

1¾ cups all-purpose flour
2 cups sugar
2 teaspoons baking powder
¼ cup unsalted margarine, softened
1½ cups skim milk
1 teaspoon vanilla
½ cup egg substitute
4 ounces sweet cooking chocolate, melted and cooled
1 cup chopped walnuts

Heat oven to 350°. Spray baking pan, 13 x 9 x 2 inches, with vegetable spray. Measure flour, sugar, baking powder, margarine, milk, and vanilla into large mixer bowl. Blend 2 minutes on medium speed, scraping bowl constantly. Add egg substitute and chocolate; beat on high speed 2 minutes, scraping bowl frequently. Stir in nuts. Pour into pan.

Bake 35 to 40 minutes, or until wooden pick inserted in center comes out clean.

16 servings.

1 serving = 285 calories
trace cholesterol
11 gm fat

FILLING AND FROSTING A TWO-LAYER CAKE

1. Before frosting cake, remove loose crumbs from side and edges of cooled layers. Support cake firmly with one hand and brush gently but thoroughly with the other.
2. Place one layer upside down on plate; spread about ½ cup of frosting to within ¼ inch of edge. (Use a spatula with a flexible blade; a stiff blade may dig into cake.)
3. Place second layer right side up on filling. Coat side with thin layer of frosting; swirl more frosting on side, forming a ¼-inch ridge above top of cake.
4. Spread remaining frosting over top of cake, just meeting the built-up ridge around side. Make attractive swirls or leave top smooth for decoration.

RICH HOLIDAY FRUITCAKE

1 cup dried apricots (4 ounces)
2 cups pitted dates (8 ounces)
**1 cup drained red and green maraschino
   cherries**
1½ cups Brazil nuts (¾ pound)
¾ cup all-purpose flour
¾ cup sugar
½ teaspoon baking powder
¾ cup egg substitute
1½ teaspoons vanilla

Heat oven to 300°. Line loaf pan, 9 x 5 x 3 or 8½ x 4½ x 2½ inches, with aluminum foil; grease. Leaving apricots, dates, cherries, and nuts whole, combine all ingredients in large bowl; mix thoroughly. Spread mixture evenly in pan.

Bake 1 hour 45 minutes, or until wooden pick inserted in center comes out clean. If cake becomes too dark, cover with aluminum foil last 30 minutes of baking. Remove from pan; cool. Wrap in plastic wrap or aluminum foil; store in cool place.

12 servings.

1 serving = 327 calories
0 cholesterol
13 gm fat

NUT AND RAISIN LOAF

¼ cup margarine, softened
¼ cup egg substitute
1 cup skim milk
2 cups all-purpose flour
¼ cup sugar
3 teaspoons baking powder
½ cup chopped walnuts
½ cup raisins

Heat oven to 350°. Spray loaf pan, 8½ x 4½ x 2½ inches, with vegetable spray. Beat margarine, egg substitute, and milk until smooth. Mix in flour, sugar, and baking powder just until flour is moistened. Batter will be lumpy. Stir in nuts and raisins. Spread in pan.

Bake 45 minutes, or until wooden pick inserted in center comes out clean. Let cool in pan 10 minutes before turning onto wire rack.

16 servings.

1 serving = 149 calories
trace cholesterol
6 gm fat

CARROT TEA CAKE

¾ cup plus 2 tablespoons vegetable oil
2 cups sugar
¾ cup egg substitute
2 cups finely shredded carrot
2 cups all-purpose flour
2 teaspoons baking soda
1 tablespoon cinnamon
1 teaspoon nutmeg

Heat oven to 350°. Spray 9-inch springform pan with vegetable spray. Mix oil, sugar, egg substitute, and carrot. Stir in flour, baking soda, cinnamon, and nutmeg. Pour into pan. Bake 1 hour.

16 servings.

1 serving = 277 calories
0 cholesterol
12 gm fat

PETITS FOURS

Prepare White Cake (page 205), except pour batter into greased and floured jelly-roll pan, 15½ x 10½ x 1 inch. Bake 25 minutes. Cool. Cut cake into small squares, rounds, diamonds, hearts, or other fancy shapes.

Glaze cake pieces by placing upside down, a few at a time, on wire rack over large bowl or baking dish. Pour Petits Fours Icing (below) over top so that entire cake piece is covered at one time. (Glaze that drips off cakes into bowl can be reheated and used again.) Decorate top with candy flowers, gumdrop roses, or with Decorators' Icing (below).

About thirty-five 2-inch squares.

1 serving = 260 calories
trace cholesterol
3 gm fat

Note: Petits Fours can also be glazed by placing each cake piece on a fork over icing in double boiler and spooning the glaze on each. With spatula or another fork, push cake off onto wire rack to set glaze.

PETITS FOURS ICING

9 cups powdered sugar (about 2 pounds)
½ cup water
½ cup light corn syrup
1 teaspoon vanilla
½ teaspoon almond extract

Combine all ingredients in top of double boiler and heat over boiling water just to lukewarm. (Do not overheat icing or it will become dull.) Remove from heat, leaving icing over hot water to keep it thin. If desired, tint parts of icing pastel colors with food coloring. If necessary, add hot water, just a few drops at a time, until of spreading consistency.

DECORATORS' ICING

Mix 2 cups powdered sugar and 1 tablespoon water. Add more water, 1 teaspoon at a time, until icing is of the consistency that can be used easily in a decorators' tube and yet hold its shape.

¾ cup.

WHITE SWIRL FROSTING

½ cup sugar
¼ cup light corn syrup
2 tablespoons water
2 egg whites (¼ cup)
1 teaspoon vanilla

Mix sugar, corn syrup, and water in small saucepan. Cover; heat to rolling boil over medium heat. Uncover; boil rapidly without stirring to 243° on candy thermometer (or until small amount of mixture spins 6- to 8-inch thread when dropped from spoon).

As mixture boils, beat egg whites until stiff peaks form. Pour hot syrup very slowly in a thin stream into egg whites, beating constantly on medium speed. Beat on high speed until stiff peaks form. Stir in vanilla during last minute of beating.

Fills and frosts two 8- or 9-inch layers or frosts a 13 x 9 x 2-inch cake.

Frosting for 1 serving of cake = 44 calories
0 cholesterol
0 fat

MARGARINE FROSTING

⅓ cup unsalted margarine, softened
3 cups powdered sugar
1½ teaspoons vanilla
About 2 tablespoons skim milk

Mix margarine and sugar. Stir in vanilla and milk; beat until smooth and of spreading consistency.

Fills and frosts two 8- or 9-inch layers or frosts a 13 x 9 x 2-inch cake.

> Frosting for 1 serv-
> ing of cake = 139 calories
> 0 cholesterol
> 4 gm fat

Note: To fill and frost three 8-inch layers, use ½ cup unsalted margarine, softened, 4½ cups powdered sugar, 2 teaspoons vanilla, and about 3 tablespoons skim milk.

Orange or Lemon Frosting: Omit vanilla and substitute orange or lemon juice for the milk. Stir in 2 teaspoons grated orange peel or ½ teaspoon grated lemon peel.

> Frosting for 1 serv-
> ing of cake = 139 calories
> 0 cholesterol
> 4 gm fat

Cherry Frosting: Stir in 2 tablespoons drained chopped maraschino cherries and 2 drops red food coloring.

> Frosting for 1 serv-
> ing of cake = 141 calories
> 0 cholesterol
> 4 gm fat

Maple Nut Frosting: Omit vanilla and substitute ½ cup maple-flavored syrup for the milk. Stir in ¼ cup finely chopped walnuts.

> Frosting for 1 serv-
> ing of cake = 183 calories
> 0 cholesterol
> 5 gm fat

Browned Margarine Frosting: Before mixing margarine and sugar, heat margarine in saucepan over medium heat until a delicate brown. (Margarine browns very slowly.)

Pineapple Frosting: Omit vanilla and substitute ⅓ cup well-drained crushed pineapple for the milk.

> Frosting for 1 serv-
> ing of cake = 141 calories
> 0 cholesterol
> 4 gm fat

LEMON FILLING

¾ cup sugar
3 tablespoons cornstarch
¾ cup water
1 teaspoon grated lemon peel
1 tablespoon margarine
⅓ cup lemon juice
4 drops yellow food coloring (optional)

Mix sugar and cornstarch in small saucepan. Stir in water gradually. Cook, stirring constantly, until mixture thickens and boils. Boil and stir 1 minute. Remove from heat; add lemon peel and margarine. Stir in lemon juice and food coloring. Cool thoroughly. If filling is too soft, refrigerate until set.

Fills an 8- or 9-inch two-layer cake.

> 1 serving = 55 calories
> 0 cholesterol
> trace fat

OIL PASTRY

8- or 9-inch One-Crust Pie
1 cup plus 2 tablespoons all-purpose flour
⅓ cup vegetable oil
2 to 3 tablespoons cold water

8- or 9-inch Lattice-Topped Pie or 10-inch One-Crust Pie
1¼ cups plus 1 tablespoon all-purpose flour
⅓ cup vegetable oil
2 to 3 tablespoons cold water

Measure flour into mixing bowl. Add oil; stir with fork until mixture looks like meal. Sprinkle water over mixture, 1 tablespoon at a time, mixing with fork until flour is moistened. Mix thoroughly until dough almost cleans side of bowl. (If dough seems dry, add 1 to 2 tablespoons oil. Do not add water.) Gather dough together with hands. Press into ball.

For One-Crust Pie: Shape dough into a flattened round. Roll out 2 inches larger than inverted pie pan between 2 long strips of waxed paper crossed in center. (Wipe table with damp cloth to prevent paper from slipping.) Peel off top paper; place pastry paper side up in pan. Peel off paper; fit pastry loosely into pan. If necessary, trim overhanging pastry 1 inch from edge of pie pan. Fold and roll pastry under, even with pan. Flute or fork edge. Fill and bake as directed in recipe. For baked pie shell, flute edge, and prick bottom and side well. Bake at 475° for 12 to 15 minutes. Cool. Fill as directed in recipe.

8 servings.
1 serving = 138 calories
0 cholesterol
9 gm fat

For Lattice-Topped Pie: Shape ⅔ of dough into a flattened round. Roll out 1½ inches larger than inverted pie pan between 2 long strips of waxed paper. Peel off paper; fit pastry loosely into pan, leaving a 1-inch overhang.

Roll ⅓ of the dough into circle about the size of inverted pie pan. Peel off top paper. Cut circle into strips, about ½ inch wide. Place 5 to 7 strips paper side up (depending on size of pie) across filling in pie pan. Peel off paper. Lay second half of strips across first strips. Remove paper; trim ends of strips. Fold trimmed edge of lower crust over ends of strips, building up a high edge. (A juicy fruit pie is more likely to bubble over when topped by lattice than when the juices are held in by a top crust. Be sure to build up a high pastry edge.) Seal and flute. Cover edge with 2- to 3-inch strip of aluminum foil to prevent excessive browning; remove foil last 15 minutes of baking. Bake as directed in recipe.

Note: For 9- and 10-inch pies, tape 2 pieces of waxed paper together.

8 servings.
1 serving = 152 calories
0 cholesterol
9 gm fat

STRAWBERRY TART

Pastry Shell (this page)
1 package (3 ounces) imitation cream cheese, softened
1 tablespoon plus 1½ teaspoons low-fat sour cream
1 tablespoon plus 1½ teaspoons low-fat yogurt
1 to 1½ quarts strawberries
¾ cup sugar
3 tablespoons cornstarch
½ cup water
Red food coloring (optional)

Bake Pastry Shell.

Beat cream cheese in small mixer bowl until fluffy. Add sour cream and yogurt; continue beating until smooth. Spread on pastry shell and refrigerate.

Mash enough strawberries to measure 1 cup. Force through sieve and add enough water to measure 1 cup.

Mix sugar and cornstarch in small saucepan. Stir in ½ cup water and the sieved strawberries. Cook, stirring constantly, until mixture thickens and boils. Boil and stir 1 minute. Remove from heat and cool slightly, stirring occasionally. Stir in red food coloring.

Arrange whole strawberries with tips up in pastry shell. Pour cooked strawberry mixture on top. Refrigerate at least 1 hour.

10 servings.

1 serving = 230 calories
3 mg cholesterol
9 gm fat

PASTRY SHELL

1 cup all-purpose flour
1 tablespoon sugar
¼ cup plus 2 tablespoons margarine, softened
1 tablespoon plus 1½ teaspoons egg substitute
1 tablespoon cold water

Mix flour, sugar, and margarine with fork or fingers until crumbly. Add egg substitute and water; mix until dough holds together. Pat into flat round; wrap in plastic wrap and refrigerate until firm enough to roll.

Place flattened round between two 15-inch strips of waxed paper. (Tape two pieces of paper together to make wider strips.) Wipe table with damp cloth to prevent paper from slipping. Roll pastry 2 inches larger than inverted 9-inch tart pan or pie pan. Peel off top paper. Place pastry paper side up in pan. Peel off paper. Press pastry gently in pan; trim edge of pastry even with rim of pan. Refrigerate 1 hour.

Heat oven to 375°. Bake until light brown, about 15 minutes, pricking shell with fork whenever it begins to bubble.

STANDARD PIE PASTRY

8- or 9-inch One-Crust Pie
1 cup all-purpose flour
⅓ cup plus 1 tablespoon unsalted margarine
2 to 3 tablespoons cold water

10-inch One-Crust Pie
1⅓ cups all-purpose flour
½ cup unsalted margarine
3 to 4 tablespoons cold water

8- or 9-inch Lattice-Topped Pie
1½ cups all-purpose flour
½ cup plus 1 tablespoon unsalted margarine
3 to 4 tablespoons cold water

Measure flour into mixing bowl. Cut in margarine thoroughly. Sprinkle in water, 1 tablespoon at a time, mixing until all flour is moistened and dough almost cleans side of bowl (1 to 2 teaspoons water can be added if needed).

Gather dough into ball; shape into flattened round on lightly floured cloth-covered board.

For One-Crust Pie: Roll dough with floured stockinet-covered rolling pin 2 inches larger than inverted pie pan. Fold pastry into quarters; unfold and ease into pan. Trim overhanging edge of pastry 1 inch from rim of pan. Fold and roll pastry under, even with pan; flute. Fill and bake as directed in recipe.

For Baked Pie Shell: Prick bottom and side thoroughly with fork. Bake at 475° for 8 to 10 minutes.

For Lattice-Topped Pie: Use ⅔ of dough; roll with floured stockinet-covered rolling pin 2 inches larger than inverted pie pan. Fold pastry into quarters; unfold and ease into pie pan. Trim overhanging edge of pastry 1 inch from rim or pan. Turn desired filling into pastry-lined pie pan. Roll one-third dough into circle about the size of inverted pie pan. Cut circle into strips, about ½ inch wide. Place 5 to 7 strips (depending on size of pie) across filling in pie pan. Lay second half of strips across first strips. Fold trimmed edge of lower crust over ends of strips building up a high edge. (A juicy fruit pie is more likely to bubble over when topped by lattice than when the juices are held in by a top crust. Be sure to build up a high pastry edge.) Seal and flute. Cover edge with 2- to 3-inch strip of aluminum foil to prevent excessive browning; remove foil last 15 minutes of baking. Bake as directed in recipe.

8 servings.

1 serving
(10-inch) = 181 calories
0 cholesterol
12 gm fat

1 serving
(8- or 9-inch) = 140 calories
0 cholesterol
10 gm fat

1 serving
(lattice-topped) = 204 calories
0 cholesterol
14 gm fat

FLUFFY MERINGUE PIE SHELL

4 egg whites
¼ teaspoon cream of tartar
1 cup sugar

Heat oven to 275°. Grease two 9-inch pie pans with unsalted margarine. Beat egg whites and cream of tartar in large mixer bowl until foamy. Beat in sugar, 1 tablespoon at a time; beat until stiff and glossy. Do not underbeat. Divide meringue between pie pans; press meringue against side of pan. Bake 45 minutes. Turn off oven; leave meringue shells in oven with door closed 45 minutes. Remove from oven; cool away from draft.

2 shells (8 servings each).

1 serving = 54 calories
0 cholesterol
0 fat

Note: Meringue shell can be frozen. Wrap carefully in aluminum foil and freeze. To serve, thaw in wrapper at room temperature 15 minutes.

SERVING IDEAS

Fill Meringue Pie Shell with fruit ice and fruit:
1. Raspberry ice; fresh raspberries.
2. Lemon ice; strawberries.
3. Lime ice; fresh lime slices and strawberries.
4. Orange ice; orange slices.

BASIC MERINGUE TOPPING

8-inch Pie
2 egg whites
¼ teaspoon cream of tartar
2 tablespoons sugar
¼ teaspoon vanilla

9-inch Pie
3 egg whites
¼ teaspoon cream of tartar
3 tablespoons sugar
½ teaspoon vanilla

Beat egg whites and cream of tartar until foamy. Beat in sugar, 1 tablespoon at a time; beat until stiff and glossy. Do not underbeat. Beat in vanilla.

Heap meringue onto hot pie filling; spread on filling, carefully sealing meringue to edge of crust to prevent shrinking or weeping. Bake in 400° oven until delicate brown, about 10 minutes. Cool away from draft.

1 serving = 17 calories (8-inch pie)
25 calories (9-inch pie)
0 cholesterol
0 fat

Note: A few drops lemon or almond extract or rum or maple flavoring can be added to meringue.

BLUEBERRY PIE

8-inch Pie
**Pastry for 8- or 9-inch Lattice-Topped Pie
   (page 209)**
3 tablespoons sugar
¼ cup all-purpose flour
½ teaspoon cinnamon
3 cups blueberries
1 teaspoon lemon juice
2 teaspoons unsalted margarine

9-inch Pie
**Pastry for 8- or 9-inch Lattice-Topped Pie
   (page 209)**
¼ cup sugar
⅓ cup all-purpose flour
½ teaspoon cinnamon
4 cups blueberries
1 tablespoon lemon juice
1 tablespoon unsalted margarine

Heat oven to 425°. Prepare pastry. Stir together sugar, flour, and cinnamon. Mix lightly with berries. Pour into pastry-lined pie pan. Sprinkle fruit with lemon juice and dot with margarine. Cover with Lattice Top (page 209). Cover edge with 2- to 3-inch strip of aluminum foil to prevent excessive browning; remove foil last 15 minutes of baking. Bake 8- and 9-inch pies 35 to 45 minutes, or until crust is brown and juice begins to bubble.

Frozen Blueberry Pie: Substitute unsweetened frozen blueberries, partially thawed, for the fresh blueberries. One package (12 ounces) frozen blueberries yields 2½ cups berries.

8 servings.

   1 serving
      (8-inch) = 284 calories
                     0 cholesterol
                     15 gm fat
   1 serving
      (9-inch) = 310 calories
                     0 cholesterol
                     16 gm fat

RHUBARB STRAWBERRY PIE

8-inch Pie
**Pastry for 8- or 9-inch Lattice-Topped Pie
   (page 209)**
⅓ cup sugar
¼ cup all-purpose flour
¼ teaspoon grated orange peel
1½ cups frozen rhubarb, thawed
1½ cups frozen strawberries, thawed
2 teaspoons unsalted margarine

9-inch Pie
**Pastry for 8- or 9-inch Lattice-Topped Pie
   (page 209)**
⅔ cup sugar
⅓ cup all-purpose flour
½ teaspoon grated orange peel
2 cups frozen rhubarb, thawed
2 cups frozen strawberries, thawed
1 tablespoon unsalted margarine

Heat oven to 425°. Mix sugar, flour, and orange peel. Pour half the rhubarb and strawberries into pastry-lined pie pan; sprinkle with half the sugar mixture. Repeat with remaining rhubarb, strawberries, and sugar mixture. Dot with margarine. Cover with Lattice Top (page 209). Sprinkle with sugar. Cover edge with 2- to 3-inch strip of aluminum foil to prevent excessive browning; remove foil last 15 minutes of baking. Bake 40 to 50 minutes, or until crust is brown and filling begins to bubble. Serve warm.

   8 servings.

   1 serving
      (8-inch) = 274 calories
                     0 cholesterol
                     15 gm fat
   1 serving
      (9-inch) = 321 calories
                     0 cholesterol
                     15 gm fat

PUMPKIN PIE

Pastry for 9-inch One-Crust Pie (page 209)
3 egg whites
⅔ cup sugar
½ teaspoon salt
½ teaspoon cinnamon
½ teaspoon ginger
½ teaspoon nutmeg
Dash cloves
1½ cups cooked pumpkin
1 teaspoon vanilla
1½ cups evaporated skim milk
½ teaspoon grated orange peel

Prepare pastry. Heat oven to 450°. Beat egg whites slightly in large mixer bowl. Add remaining ingredients and beat until smooth. Pour into pastry-lined pie pan. Bake 10 minutes.

Reduce oven temperature to 325°. Bake about 45 minutes longer, or until knife inserted in center comes out clean.

8 servings.

1 serving = 235 calories
trace cholesterol
10 gm fat

LEMON MERINGUE PIE

8-inch One-Crust Pie (page 209)
½ cup sugar
¼ cup cornstarch
1 cup water
¼ cup egg substitute
1 tablespoon unsalted margarine
1 teaspoon grated lemon peel
⅓ cup lemon juice
2 drops yellow food coloring (optional)
Basic Meringue Topping (page 212)

Bake pie shell. Heat oven to 400°. Mix sugar and cornstarch in medium saucepan. Stir in water. Cook over medium heat, stirring constantly, until mixture thickens and boils. Boil and stir 1 minute. Stir at least half the hot mixture into egg substitute, then blend into mixture in pan. Boil and stir 1 minute. Remove from heat; stir in margarine, lemon peel, juice, and food coloring. Pour into pie shell.

Heap meringue onto hot pie filling; spread over filling, carefully sealing meringue to edge of crust to prevent shrinking or weeping. Bake about 10 minutes or until delicate brown. Cool away from draft.

8 servings.

1 serving = 244 calories
0 cholesterol
11 gm fat

PERFECT PEACH PIE

8-inch Pie
**Pastry for 8- or 9-inch Lattice-Topped Pie
(page 209)**
**4 cups sliced fresh peaches (about 1¾
pounds)**
1 teaspoon lemon juice
⅓ cup sugar
3 tablespoons flour
¼ teaspoon cinnamon
2 teaspoons unsalted margarine
9-inch Pie
**Pastry for 8- or 9-inch Lattice-Topped Pie
(page 209)**
**5 cups sliced fresh peaches (about 2½
pounds)**
1 teaspoon lemon juice
½ cup sugar
¼ cup all-purpose flour
¼ teaspoon cinnamon
1 tablespoon unsalted margarine

Heat oven to 425°. Prepare pastry. Mix peaches and lemon juice. Stir together sugar, flour and cinnamon; mix with peaches. Pour into pastry-lined pie pan. Dot with margarine. Cover with Lattice Top (page 209). Cover edge with 2- to 3-inch strip of aluminum foil to prevent excessive browning; remove foil last 15 minutes of baking.

Bake 35 to 45 minutes, or until crust is brown and filling begins to bubble. Serve warm.

8 servings.

1 serving
(8-inch) = 294 calories
0 cholesterol
15 gm fat

1 serving
(9-inch) = 328 calories
0 cholesterol
15 gm fat

Note: 5 cups apricot halves may be substituted for the peaches.

CHERRY PIE

**Pastry for 8- or 9-inch Lattice-Topped Pie
(page 209)**
⅔ cup sugar
2 tablespoons flour
**2 cups frozen pitted sweet cherries,
thawed**
¼ teaspoon almond extract
1 tablespoon unsalted margarine

Heat oven to 425°. Prepare pastry. Stir together sugar and flour. Mix lightly with cherries. Pour into pastry-lined pie pan. Sprinkle fruit with extract and dot with margarine. Cover with Lattice Top (page 209). Cover edge with 2- to 3-inch strip of aluminum foil to prevent excessive browning; remove foil last 15 minutes of baking. Bake 35 to 45 minutes, or until crust is brown and filling begins to bubble.

8 servings.

1 serving = 322 calories
0 cholesterol
15 gm fat

DEEP-DISH FRUIT PIE

1 cup sugar
½ cup all-purpose flour
1 teaspoon nutmeg
1 teaspoon cinnamon
12 cups thinly sliced, pared apples
  (about 10)
½ recipe Pastry for 8- or 9-inch One-Crust
  Pie (page 209)

Stir together sugar, flour, nutmeg, and cinnamon. Mix with apples. Pour into baking pan, 9 x 9 x 2 inches. Dot fruit with margarine.

Heat oven to 425°. Prepare pastry as directed, but use only one half the amounts of ingredients and roll pastry into circle. Cut into ½-inch strips. Place strips lengthwise and crosswise on fruit. Fold edges of strips under just inside edge of pan. Bake 1 hour, or until juice begins to bubble. Serve warm.

9 servings.
1 serving
  (apples) = 246 calories
                0 cholesterol
                5 gm fat
1 serving
  (peaches) = 273 calories
                0 cholesterol
                5 gm fat

Note: Sliced peeled peaches can be substituted for the apples.

ALL-AMERICAN APPLE PIE

8-inch Pie
Pastry for 8- or 9-inch Lattice-Topped Pie
  (page 209)
¼ cup sugar
3 tablespoons flour
¼ teaspoon nutmeg
¼ teaspoon cinnamon
5 cups thinly sliced, pared tart apples
  (about 5 medium)
2 teaspoons unsalted margarine

9-inch Pie
Pastry for 8- or 9-inch Lattice-Topped Pie
  (page 209)
⅓ cup sugar
¼ cup all-purpose flour
½ teaspoon nutmeg
½ teaspoon cinnamon
6 cups thinly sliced, pared tart apples
  (about 6 medium)
1 tablespoon unsalted margarine

Heat oven to 425°. Prepare pastry. Stir together sugar, flour, nutmeg, and cinnamon. Mix lightly with apples. Pour into pastry-lined pie pan. Dot with margarine. Cover with Lattice Top (page 209). Cover edge with 2- to 3-inch strip of aluminum foil to prevent excessive browning; remove foil last 15 minutes of baking. Bake 40 to 50 minutes, or until crust is brown and filling begins to bubble. Serve warm.

8 servings.
1 serving
  (8-inch) = 294 calories
                0 cholesterol
                15 gm fat
1 serving
  (9-inch) = 321 calories
                0 cholesterol
                16 gm fat

BROWNIES

2 ounces unsweetened chocolate
⅓ cup unsalted margarine
1 cup sugar
½ cup egg substitute
1 teaspoon vanilla
⅔ cup all-purpose flour
½ teaspoon baking powder
½ cup chopped nuts

Heat oven to 350°. Spray baking pan, 8 x 8 x 2 inches, with vegetable spray. Melt chocolate and margarine in saucepan over low heat. Remove from heat. Add sugar, egg substitute, and vanilla and beat until smooth. Stir in remaining ingredients. Spread in pan. Bake 25 minutes or until brownies start to pull away from sides of pan. Cool slightly. Cut into bars, about 1½ x 1½ inches.

20 brownies.

> 1 brownie = 128 calories
> 0 cholesterol
> 7 gm fat

MERINGUE KISSES

2 egg whites
1 cup sugar
⅛ teaspoon salt
½ teaspoon almond extract or vanilla
1 teaspoon grated lemon or lime peel

Heat oven to 275°. Spray baking sheet with vegetable spray. Beat egg whites until foamy. Beat in sugar, 1 tablespoon at a time; beat until stiff and glossy. Do not underbeat. Stir in salt, almond extract, and lemon peel.

Drop mixture by rounded teaspoonfuls onto baking sheet. Bake 25 to 30 minutes. Remove from baking sheet immediately.

About 2 dozen cookies.

> 1 cookie = 18 calories
> 0 cholesterol
> 0 fat

PRUNE BARS

¼ cup unsalted margarine, softened
½ cup sugar
1¾ cups all-purpose flour
1 teaspoon baking soda
½ teaspoon salt
½ teaspoon cinnamon
¼ teaspoon nutmeg
¼ teaspoon ground cloves
½ cup unsweetened prune juice
½ cup water
1 cup chopped cooked prunes
½ cup egg substitute

Heat oven to 350°. Spray baking pan, 13 x 9 x 2 inches, with vegetable spray. Cream margarine and sugar thoroughly. Mix in flour, soda, salt, cinnamon, nutmeg, and cloves alternately with prune juice and water. Stir in prunes.

Beat egg substitute with rotary beater 2 minutes. Fold into batter. Spread in pan.

Bake 35 to 40 minutes, or until wooden pick inserted in center comes out clean. Cool 30 minutes. Cut into bars, 2½ x 1½ inches.

36 bars.

> 1 bar = 59 calories
> 0 cholesterol
> 1 gm fat

COOKIE MIX

2 cups all-purpose flour
2 cups whole-wheat flour
1¼ cups granulated sugar
1¼ cups brown sugar (packed)
3 teaspoons baking powder
1½ cups unsalted margarine

Mix flours, sugars, and baking powder in large bowl. Cut in margarine with pastry blender until mixture is like coarse meal. Do not overmix.

Measure desired amounts of Cookie Mix into jars or plastic containers: 2 cups for about 3 dozen Chocolate Chip Cookies; 2½ cups each for 3 dozen Banana Cookies, Spice Cookies, and Chocolate-Nut Cookies. (Can be baked immediately.) Seal tightly, label, and refrigerate.

9 to 10 cups mix.

CHOCOLATE CHIP COOKIES

2 cups Cookie Mix
¼ cup egg substitute
1 cup mini semisweet chocolate pieces
1 cup chopped walnuts

Heat oven to 375°. Mix all ingredients. Drop dough by rounded teaspoonfuls 2 inches apart onto ungreased baking sheet. Bake 12 to 15 minutes or until light brown.

3 dozen cookies

    1 cookie = 87 calories
               0 cholesterol
               5 gm fat

CHOCOLATE-NUT COOKIES

2½ cups Cookie Mix
¼ cup cocoa
¼ cup egg substitute
1 teaspoon vanilla
1 teaspoon water
1 cup chopped walnuts

Heat oven to 375°. Mix all ingredients. Drop dough by rounded teaspoonfuls 2 inches apart onto ungreased baking sheet. Bake 12 to 15 minutes, or until almost no imprint remains when touched lightly.

3 dozen cookies.

    1 cookie = 71 calories
               0 cholesterol
               4 gm fat

BANANA COOKIES

2½ cups Cookie Mix
½ cup mashed ripe banana
1 teaspoon vanilla
3 tablespoons egg substitute
½ cup chopped walnuts

Heat oven to 375°. Mix all ingredients. Drop dough by rounded teaspoonfuls 2 inches apart onto ungreased baking sheet. Bake 12 to 15 minutes or until light brown.

3 dozen cookies.

    1 cookie = 59 calories
               0 cholesterol
               3 gm fat

CINNAMON-RAISIN COOKIES

2½ cups Cookie Mix
3 tablespoons egg substitute
½ teaspoon cinnamon
½ teaspoon lemon extract
½ cup raisins
½ cup chopped walnuts

Heat oven to 375°. Mix all ingredients. Drop dough by rounded teaspoonfuls 2 inches apart onto ungreased baking sheet. Bake 12 to 15 minutes or until light brown.

3 dozen cookies.

    1 cookie = 62 calories
               0 cholesterol
               3 gm fat

NUTTY ORANGE OATMEAL COOKIES

⅓ cup unsalted margarine, softened
⅓ cup low-fat yogurt
¼ cup brown sugar (packed)
1 teaspoon vanilla
1⅓ cups all-purpose flour
1 cup oats (quick cooking or regular)
¼ teaspoon soda
2 tablespoons finely chopped walnuts
¾ teaspoon grated orange peel

Heat oven to 325°. Blend margarine, yogurt, sugar, and vanilla. Mix in remaining ingredients. Shape dough by rounded teaspoonfuls into 1-inch balls. Place about 2 inches apart on ungreased baking sheet; flatten slightly with fork.

Bake 12 to 15 minutes. Immediately remove from baking sheet.

4½ dozen cookies.

1 cookie = 34 calories
trace cholesterol
1 gm fat

Nutty Orange Oatmeal Balls: Place 1-inch balls 1 inch apart on baking sheet. (Do not flatten.) Bake 15 to 20 minutes.

SODA CRACKER PIE

4 egg whites
1 teaspoon baking powder
¾ cup sugar
1 teaspoon vanilla
½ cup cut-up dates
½ cup chopped pecans
2 tablespoons wheat germ
¾ cup soda-cracker crumbs (see *Note*)

Heat oven to 350°. Beat egg whites until foamy in small mixer bowl. Add baking powder and beat until stiff. Beat in sugar, 1 tablespoon at a time; continue beating until stiff and glossy. Fold in vanilla, dates, nuts, wheat germ, and cracker crumbs. Turn into 8-inch pie pan that has been sprayed with vegetable spray. Bake 25 minutes.

8 servings.

1 serving = 192 calories
0 cholesterol
6 gm fat

Note: Use crackers with unsalted tops.

RAISIN OATMEAL COOKIES

½ cup all-purpose flour
½ cup whole-wheat flour
½ teaspoon soda
½ teaspoon salt
1½ cups quick-cooking oats
¼ teaspoon cinnamon
2 egg whites
1 cup brown sugar (packed)
⅓ cup vegetable oil
½ cup skim milk
1 teaspoon vanilla
1 cup raisins

Heat oven to 375°. Stir together flours, soda, salt, oats, and cinnamon in large mixing bowl. Beat egg whites slightly; mix in remaining ingredients and mix into flour mixture.

Drop dough by teaspoonfuls onto sprayed baking sheet. Bake 12 minutes for chewy soft cookies; 15 minutes for crisp cookies.

3 dozen cookies.
  1 cookie = 81 calories
              trace cholesterol
              2 gm fat

CUT-OUT COOKIES

¾ cup unsalted margarine, softened
1 cup sugar
¼ cup egg substitute
1 teaspoon vanilla or ½ teaspoon lemon extract
2½ cups all-purpose flour
1 teaspoon baking powder

Mix thoroughly margarine, sugar, egg substitute, and flavoring. Blend in flour and baking powder. Cover dough and chill at least 1 hour.

Heat oven to 400°. Roll dough ⅛ inch thick on lightly floured cloth-covered board. Cut into desired shapes with cookie cutters. Place on ungreased baking sheet. Bake 6 to 8 minutes, or until very light brown.

About 4 dozen 3-inch cookies.
  1 cookie = 68 calories
              0 cholesterol
              3 gm fat

DATE-NUT BARS

¼ cup egg substitute
½ cup sugar
½ teaspoon vanilla
½ cup all-purpose flour
½ teaspoon baking powder
2 cups cut-up dates
1 cup chopped walnuts

Heat oven to 350°. Spray baking pan, 9 x 9 x 2 inches, with vegetable spray. Beat egg substitute, sugar, and vanilla thoroughly. Mix in flour and baking powder; stir in dates and nuts. Spread in pan. Bake 25 to 30 minutes. Cool; cut into bars, about 2 x 1½ inches.

20 bars.
  1 bar = 127 calories
            0 cholesterol
            4 gm fat

ZUCCHINI SPICE COOKIES

¼ cup unsalted margarine, softened
1 teaspoon grated orange peel
¾ teaspoon cinnamon
¼ teaspoon nutmeg
¼ teaspoon cloves
½ cup brown sugar (packed)
¼ cup egg substitute
1¾ cups all-purpose flour
2 teaspoons baking powder
¼ teaspoon salt
¼ cup skim milk
1½ cups shredded unpared zucchini
½ cup chopped nuts
½ cup raisins

Heat oven to 375°. Mix margarine, orange peel, cinnamon, nutmeg, cloves, and sugar thoroughly. Blend in egg substitute. Mix in flour, baking powder, and salt alternately with the milk. Stir in nuts and raisins.

Drop dough by teaspoonfuls 2 inches apart onto baking sheet sprayed with vegetable spray. Bake 15 minutes or until edges are dark brown.

4 dozen cookies.

1 cookie = 50 calories
0 cholesterol
2 gm fat

Carrot Spice Cookies: Substitute 1½ cups shredded carrots for the zucchini.

ANNE'S OATMEAL BARS

¼ cup unsalted margarine, softened
¼ cup sugar
¼ cup molasses
¼ cup egg substitute
1 can (6 ounces) frozen orange juice
  concentrate, thawed
½ cup oats
¼ cup raisins
¼ cup chopped walnuts
2 cups all-purpose flour
1 teaspoon soda
½ teaspoon ginger
½ teaspoon cinnamon
¼ teaspoon salt
¼ teaspoon cloves
¼ teaspoon nutmeg

Heat oven to 325°. Spray baking pan, 13 x 9 x 2 inches, with vegetable spray.

Cream margarine and sugar until fluffy. Stir in molasses, egg substitute, and orange juice concentrate. Mix in remaining ingredients. Spread in pan.

Bake 25 to 30 minutes. Cool; cut into bars, about 2 x 1½ inches.

32 bars.

1 bar = 78 calories
0 cholesterol
2 gm fat

Nutritive Values of Recipes

Recipes		Calories	Protein gm	Carbohy-drate gm	Total Fat gm	Poly-unsat-urated Fat gm	Sat-urated Fat gm	Choles-terol mg	Sodium mg
All American Apple Pie 8-Inch Pie	8 servings	2356.4	23.57	296.83	120.77	42.57	21.86	0.0	12.77
	1 serving	294.5	2.95	37.10	15.10	5.32	2.73	0.0	1.60
All-American Apple Pie 9-Inch Pie	8 servings	2565.8	24.66	337.14	125.62	44.04	22.62	0.0	14.49
	1 serving	320.7	3.08	42.14	15.70	5.50	2.83	0.0	1.81
Aloha Dip	6 servings	816.7	14.86	180.11	4.09	0.07	1.27	11.0	150.70
	1 serving	136.1	2.48	30.02	0.68	0.01	0.21	1.8	25.12
Angel Food Cake	16 servings	1829.3	46.45	402.62	0.77	0.32	0.14	0.0	968.76
	1 serving	114.3	2.90	25.16	0.05	0.02	0.01	0.0	60.55
Anne's Oatmeal Bars	32 servings	2511.5	47.32	410.18	76.17	33.19	12.34	0.0	1901.25
	1 serving	78.5	1.48	12.82	2.38	1.04	0.39	0.0	59.41
Apple Omelet	2 servings	353.6	23.81	18.41	20.48	9.27	3.64	0.0	547.36
	1 serving	176.8	11.91	9.21	10.24	4.63	1.82	0.0	273.68
Apple Snow	4 servings	318.2	7.99	68.87	1.20	0.00	0.00	0.0	100.48
	1 serving	79.6	2.00	17.22	0.30	0.00	0.00	0.0	25.12
Apricot Coffee Cake	24 servings	2090.0	76.50	363.04	36.54	11.29	9.45	26.8	1476.30
	1 serving	87.1	3.19	15.13	1.52	0.47	0.39	1.1	61.51
Artichokes	1 servings	52.6	2.80	9.90	0.20	0.00	0.00	0.0	30.00
	1 serving	52.6	2.80	9.90	0.20	0.00	0.00	0.0	30.00
Asparagus	4 servings	119.2	12.80	15.20	0.80	0.00	0.00	0.0	4.00
	1 serving	29.8	3.20	3.80	0.20	0.00	0.00	0.0	1.00
Babka	20 servings	3629.2	70.10	530.83	137.15	59.45	22.77	0.0	240.63
	1 serving	181.5	3.51	26.54	6.86	2.97	1.14	0.0	12.03

Source: Figures are based on information from the National Nutrition Coding Center. Computer analysis of the recipes was done at the Mayo Clinic.

NUTRITIVE VALUES OF RECIPES—Continued

Recipes		Calories	Protein gm	Carbohy-drate gm	Total Fat gm	Poly-unsat-urated Fat gm	Sat-urated Fat gm	Choles-terol mg	Sodium mg
Bagels	8 servings	1347.5	39.22	289.73	3.52	1.79	0.65	0.0	404.39
	1 serving	168.4	4.90	36.22	0.44	0.22	0.08	0.0	50.55
Baked Apple Rice Pudding	6 servings	1170.3	22.96	203.33	28.16	10.00	5.00	0.0	1355.26
	1 serving	195.1	3.83	33.89	4.69	1.67	0.83	0.0	225.88
Baked Apple Surprise	1 servings	108.1	0.29	22.40	1.93	0.72	0.30	0.0	21.61
	1 serving	108.1	0.29	22.40	1.93	0.72	0.30	0.0	21.61
Baked Clams Bretonne	6 servings	819.8	40.49	38.86	55.56	22.80	10.05	113.9	796.41
	1 serving	136.6	6.75	6.48	9.26	3.80	1.68	19.0	132.73
Baked Fish Fillets	4 servings	1076.5	69.81	2.76	87.36	37.87	17.24	237.6	1276.18
	1 serving	269.1	17.45	0.69	21.84	9.47	4.31	59.4	319.04
Baked Lasagne	8 servings	4320.7	331.18	203.43	242.21	38.90	99.47	825.7	3590.17
	1 serving	540.1	41.40	25.43	30.28	4.86	12.43	103.2	448.77
Baked Stuffed Acorn Squash	4 servings	1087.2	79.36	105.75	38.59	1.70	15.47	200.5	562.92
	1 serving	271.8	19.84	26.44	9.65	0.42	3.87	50.1	140.73
Baked Stuffed Fish	6 servings	1330.6	212.57	21.75	43.98	16.74	11.66	712.8	880.27
	1 serving	221.8	35.43	3.63	7.33	2.79	1.94	118.8	146.71
Baked Stuffed Summer Squash	4 servings	583.5	17.21	89.59	17.37	6.74	3.22	1.5	901.93
	1 serving	145.9	4.30	22.40	4.34	1.69	0.80	0.4	225.48
Baked Tomatoes Provençal	6 servings	1054.7	15.86	72.39	78.49	7.12	10.95	0.4	264.40
	1 serving	175.8	2.64	12.07	13.08	1.19	1.82	0.1	44.07
Baking Powder Biscuits	16 servings	1588.1	32.02	201.42	72.66	42.05	9.46	2.9	1675.78
	1 serving	99.3	2.00	12.59	4.54	2.63	0.59	0.2	104.74
Banana Bread	16 servings	3285.0	46.29	471.20	136.55	49.05	24.88	0.0	2348.60
	1 serving	205.3	2.89	29.45	8.53	3.07	1.55	0.0	146.79
Banana Citrus Shake	2 servings	225.6	3.00	52.32	0.48	0.00	0.00	0.0	3.60
	1 serving	112.8	1.50	26.16	0.24	0.00	0.00	0.0	1.80

NUTRITIVE VALUES OF RECIPES–Continued

Recipes		Calories	Protein gm	Carbohy-drate gm	Total Fat gm	Poly-unsat-urated Fat gm	Sat-urated Fat gm	Choles-terol mg	Sodium mg
Banana Cookies	36 servings	2124.6	29.66	246.56	114.32	51.88	17.87	0.0	301.42
	1 serving	59.0	0.82	6.85	3.18	1.44	0.50	0.0	8.37
Banana Freeze	16 servings	1389.5	91.58	247.32	2.32	0.07	1.00	41.0	1203.38
	1 serving	86.8	5.72	15.46	0.15	0.00	0.06	2.6	75.21
Banana Yogurt Cake	20 servings	3262.2	67.55	467.54	123.58	62.47	19.46	16.8	2112.57
	1 serving	163.1	3.38	23.38	6.18	3.12	0.97	0.8	105.63
Basic Meringue Topping 8-Inch Pie	8 servings	133.8	7.19	25.59	0.00	0.00	0.00	0.0	169.61
	1 serving	16.7	0.90	3.20	0.00	0.00	0.00	0.0	21.20
Basic Meringue Topping 9-Inch Pie	8 servings	203.6	10.79	38.79	0.00	0.00	0.00	0.0	217.92
	1 serving	25.4	1.35	4.85	0.00	0.00	0.00	0.0	27.24
Basic Salad Dressing	¼ cup	515.5	0.15	1.93	56.65	33.12	6.61	0.0	117.15
	1 tablespoon	128.9	0.04	0.48	14.16	8.28	1.65	0.0	29.29
Bean Sprout Spread	12 servings	146.6	8.24	5.32	10.26	4.56	1.84	0.0	589.98
	1 serving	12.2	0.69	0.44	0.86	0.38	0.15	0.0	49.16
Beef or Lamb Shish Kebabs	4 servings	896.9	49.43	19.14	69.28	35.62	11.51	131.0	29.54
	1 serving	224.2	12.36	4.78	17.32	8.91	2.88	32.8	7.38
Beef Kebabs (Appetizer)	55 servings	1172.5	137.43	35.36	53.48	17.40	14.86	382.6	1173.53
	1 meatball	21.3	2.50	0.64	0.97	0.32	0.27	7.0	21.34
Bengal Sausages	8 servings	1721.4	249.27	20.14	71.63	6.30	27.73	764.2	795.65
	1 serving	215.2	31.16	2.52	8.95	0.79	3.47	95.5	99.46
Blueberry Crumb Cake	12 servings	1953.2	33.53	281.37	77.86	27.77	14.13	2.2	1358.43
	1 serving	162.8	2.79	23.45	6.49	2.31	1.18	0.2	113.20
Blueberry Muffins	12 servings	1793.6	41.76	277.27	57.46	32.55	7.58	4.3	2012.67
	1 serving	149.5	3.48	23.11	4.79	2.71	0.63	0.4	167.72

NUTRITIVE VALUES OF RECIPES-Continued

Recipes		Calories	Protein gm	Carbohy-drate gm	Total Fat gm	Poly-unsat-urated Fat gm	Sat-urated Fat gm	Choles-terol mg	Sodium mg
Blueberry Pie 8-Inch Pie	8 servings	2272.2	26.36	272.80	120.81	42.62	21.88	0.0	11.09
	1 serving	284.0	3.30	34.10	15.10	5.33	2.74	0.0	1.39
Blueberry Pie 9-Inch Pie	8 servings	2480.0	28.13	312.28	125.61	44.09	22.64	0.0	12.92
	1 serving	310.0	3.52	39.04	15.70	5.51	2.83	0.0	1.61
Blueberry Winner Coffee Cake	18 servings	1943.7	42.26	363.33	35.76	19.92	4.74	1.1	149.14
	1 serving	108.0	2.35	20.18	1.99	1.11	0.26	0.1	8.29
Bohemian Mushrooms	6 servings	595.8	18.26	34.01	42.97	23.08	7.09	12.6	1161.97
	1 serving	99.3	3.04	5.67	7.16	3.85	1.18	2.1	193.66
Bouillabaisse	8 servings	3338.4	507.13	28.83	132.95	34.36	27.29	1641.1	3347.86
	1 serving	417.3	63.39	3.60	16.62	4.30	3.41	205.1	418.48
Bran Date Nut Bread	16 servings	3124.0	61.16	495.09	99.84	59.63	12.28	0.0	2577.98
	1 serving	195.3	3.82	30.94	6.24	3.73	0.77	0.0	161.12
Bran Muffins	12 servings	1347.5	38.24	197.26	45.03	25.62	6.09	4.3	1917.55
	1 serving	112.3	3.19	16.44	3.75	2.14	0.51	0.4	159.80
Bran Muffins (Variation of Muffins)	12 servings	1582.3	37.80	229.47	56.98	32.66	7.59	4.3	2113.04
	1 serving	131.9	3.15	19.12	4.75	2.72	0.63	0.4	176.09
Broccoli in Chervil Margarine	6 servings	518.3	24.23	44.37	27.04	10.76	4.45	0.0	417.10
	1 serving	86.4	4.04	7.39	4.51	1.79	0.74	0.0	69.52
Broccoli Polonaise	4 servings	747.4	21.31	49.56	51.78	21.85	9.14	0.4	871.49
	1 serving	186.8	5.33	12.39	12.95	5.46	2.29	0.1	217.87
Broccoli Vinaigrette	6 servings	905.6	19.33	42.45	73.16	40.75	8.89	0.0	101.00
	1 serving	150.9	3.22	7.08	12.19	6.79	1.48	0.0	16.83
Broccoli with Lemon	6 servings	415.8	17.47	28.80	25.92	8.58	4.44	0.0	90.54
	1 serving	69.3	2.91	4.80	4.32	1.43	0.74	0.0	15.09

NUTRITIVE VALUES OF RECIPES—Continued

Recipes		Calories	Protein gm	Carbohy-drate gm	Total Fat gm	Poly-unsat-urated Fat gm	Sat-urated Fat gm	Choles-terol mg	Sodium mg
Broiled Grapefruit	2 servings	130.7	1.03	31.20	0.21	0.00	0.00	0.0	3.37
	1 serving	65.4	0.51	15.60	0.10	0.00	0.00	0.0	1.68
Broiled Herbed Eggplant	6 servings	947.2	12.09	50.96	77.17	28.12	11.50	0.7	1346.20
	1 serving	157.9	2.02	8.49	12.86	4.69	1.92	0.1	224.37
Broiled Lemon Chicken	4 servings	1002.4	171.25	14.68	28.75	6.60	7.20	280.0	811.26
	1 serving	250.6	42.81	3.67	7.19	1.65	1.80	70.0	202.81
Broiled Scallops (Appetizer)	32 servings	2026.6	167.37	1.07	150.26	61.71	18.18	381.6	2683.64
	1 serving	63.3	5.23	0.03	4.70	1.93	0.57	11.9	83.86
Broiled Scallops (Main Course)	8 servings	2026.6	167.37	1.07	150.26	61.71	18.18	381.6	2683.64
	1 serving	253.3	20.92	0.13	18.78	7.71	2.27	47.7	335.45
Broiled Shad	6 servings	1237.8	138.82	3.78	74.06	37.36	13.49	475.2	1552.07
	1 serving	206.3	23.14	0.63	12.34	6.23	2.25	79.2	258.68
Broiled Stuffed Mushrooms	65 servings	947.5	29.51	49.32	70.44	27.44	15.46	26.8	1231.06
	1 mushroom	14.6	0.45	0.76	1.08	0.42	0.24	0.4	18.94
Broiled Turbot	4 servings	823.3	69.99	3.79	58.85	27.99	10.88	237.6	690.73
	1 serving	205.8	17.50	0.95	14.71	7.00	2.72	59.4	172.68
Brown Sauce	1½ cups	56.1	5.84	7.99	0.09	0.00	0.00	0.0	807.23
	¼ cup	9.3	0.97	1.33	0.01	0.00	0.00	0.0	134.54
Browned Margarine Frosting	15 servings	2092.6	1.08	374.65	64.27	22.88	11.86	0.5	20.39
	1 serving	139.5	0.07	24.98	4.28	1.53	0.79	0.0	1.36
Brownies	20 servings	2565.7	35.78	290.68	139.30	52.33	36.75	0.0	407.50
	1 serving	128.3	1.79	14.53	6.97	2.62	1.84	0.0	20.37
Brussels Sprouts Medley	6 servings	382.9	15.10	39.39	18.32	9.36	2.39	0.0	119.40
	1 serving	63.8	2.52	6.57	3.05	1.56	0.40	0.0	19.90

NUTRITIVE VALUES OF RECIPES–Continued

Recipes		Calories	Protein gm	Carbohy-drate gm	Total Fat gm	Poly-unsat-urated Fat gm	Sat-urated Fat gm	Choles-terol mg	Sodium mg
Cabbage and Carrot Slaw	12 servings	885.6	13.09	121.65	39.53	22.80	0.06	0.0	1110.74
	1 serving	73.8	1.09	10.14	3.29	1.90	0.00	0.0	92.56
Caesar Salad	8 servings	772.1	18.40	39.82	60.46	5.34	9.08	252.0	143.25
	1 serving	96.5	2.30	4.98	7.56	0.67	1.14	31.5	17.91
Cafe Diable Mold	8 servings	633.2	13.05	106.36	0.35	0.00	0.00	0.0	12.58
	1 serving	79.2	1.63	13.29	0.04	0.00	0.00	0.0	1.57
Calcutta Vegetable Dip	2 cups	354.4	10.28	28.79	22.41	8.79	5.30	31.7	495.19
	¼ cup	44.3	1.28	3.60	2.80	1.10	0.66	4.0	61.90
Calico Scrambled Eggs	4 servings	476.3	26.63	14.16	34.65	19.03	4.72	0.0	409.46
	1 serving	119.1	6.66	3.54	8.66	4.76	1.18	0.0	102.36
Cantaloupe Cups	6 servings	782.0	13.48	176.16	2.60	0.00	0.00	0.0	170.80
	1 serving	130.3	2.25	29.36	0.43	0.00	0.00	0.0	28.47
Carousel Kebabs	6 servings	220.2	3.51	48.19	1.49	0.00	0.00	0.0	24.64
	1 serving	36.7	0.59	8.03	0.25	0.00	0.00	0.0	4.11
Carrot-Raisin Bread	32 servings	4254.1	115.31	839.18	48.77	21.50	8.78	4.3	2381.20
	1 serving	132.9	3.60	26.22	1.52	0.67	0.27	0.1	74.41
Carrot Spice Cookies	48 servings	2437.3	43.89	359.52	91.93	44.36	13.85	1.1	1455.06
	1 serving	50.8	0.91	7.49	1.92	0.92	0.29	0.0	30.31
Carrot Tea Cake	16 servings	4433.3	47.11	621.52	194.81	111.34	24.90	0.0	3132.34
	1 serving	277.1	2.94	38.84	12.18	6.96	1.56	0.0	195.77
Carrots and Green Beans	6 servings	256.5	4.55	30.60	12.85	5.38	2.23	0.0	1041.77
	1 serving	42.8	0.76	5.10	2.14	0.90	0.37	0.0	173.63
Challah	12 servings	1919.5	45.10	315.21	53.72	19.92	9.89	0.0	505.02
	1 serving	160.0	3.76	26.27	4.48	1.66	0.82	0.0	42.08

NUTRITIVE VALUES OF RECIPES–Continued

Recipes		Calories	Protein gm	Carbohy-drate gm	Total Fat gm	Poly-unsat-urated Fat gm	Sat-urated Fat gm	Choles-terol mg	Sodium mg
Cheese-Filled Shells	6 servings	2377.7	128.65	208.49	114.23	17.61	47.41	242.6	2097.05
	1 serving	396.3	21.44	34.75	19.04	2.94	7.90	40.4	349.51
Cheese Omelet	2 servings	423.5	37.91	3.84	28.66	9.51	8.74	33.0	818.25
	1 serving	211.8	18.96	1.92	14.33	4.75	4.37	16.5	409.12
Cheese Omelet Roll	1 servings	103.0	10.16	1.10	6.47	2.41	1.73	5.3	206.40
	1 serving	103.0	10.16	1.10	6.47	2.41	1.73	5.3	206.40
Cherry Frosting	15 servings	2116.6	1.12	380.53	64.31	22.88	11.86	0.5	20.39
	1 serving	141.1	0.07	25.37	4.29	1.53	0.79	0.0	1.36
Cherry Pie	8 servings	2576.0	25.58	343.26	123.45	43.96	22.59	0.0	13.76
	1 serving	322.0	3.20	42.91	15.43	5.50	2.82	0.0	1.72
Cherry Tomatoes with Garlic	6 servings	273.5	8.67	34.69	11.47	5.82	1.27	0.0	40.04
	1 serving	45.6	1.44	5.78	1.91	0.97	0.21	0.0	6.67
Chick-Pea Salad	8 servings	1808.1	102.87	245.58	47.34	3.13	5.02	0.0	498.24
	1 serving	226.0	12.86	30.70	5.92	0.39	0.63	0.0	62.28
Chicken Beef Kebabs	8 servings	917.1	125.70	57.16	20.67	2.21	7.73	299.4	761.35
	1 serving	114.6	15.71	7.15	2.58	0.28	0.97	37.4	95.17
Chicken Brochette	4 servings	874.3	57.46	27.27	59.43	32.07	8.14	124.8	141.75
	1 serving	218.6	14.37	6.82	14.86	8.02	2.03	31.2	35.44
Chicken Cacciatora	8 servings	2421.0	150.51	186.20	119.40	46.56	20.61	513.0	1902.07
	1 serving	302.6	18.81	23.27	14.93	5.82	2.58	64.1	237.76
Chicken Gourmet	6 servings	1140.9	171.90	7.44	47.03	16.70	9.96	421.2	691.37
	1 serving	190.2	28.65	1.24	7.84	2.78	1.66	70.2	115.23
Chicken Paprika	4 servings	1005.8	82.08	25.56	63.51	27.90	12.85	339.8	1683.13
	1 serving	251.5	20.52	6.39	15.88	6.98	3.21	84.9	420.78

NUTRITIVE VALUES OF RECIPES–Continued

Recipes		Calories	Protein gm	Carbohy-drate gm	Total Fat gm	Poly-unsat-urated Fat gm	Sat-urated Fat gm	Choles-terol mg	Sodium mg
Chicken Rollups	6 servings	1438.9	122.25	136.11	45.51	16.46	9.44	224.9	2125.43
	1 serving	239.8	20.37	22.68	7.59	2.74	1.57	37.5	354.24
Chicken Salad Plate	2 servings	305.6	33.38	16.18	11.99	4.31	1.60	101.4	170.76
	1 serving	152.8	16.69	8.09	5.99	2.15	0.80	50.7	85.38
Chicken Scaloppine	4 servings	1127.6	119.02	11.69	67.32	16.18	11.88	280.8	556.54
	1 serving	281.9	29.75	2.92	16.83	4.05	2.97	70.2	139.13
Chicken with Yogurt	4 servings	1229.2	103.73	85.97	52.50	21.03	10.09	410.4	899.33
	1 serving	307.3	25.93	21.49	13.12	5.26	2.52	102.6	224.83
Chive Muffins	12 servings	1704.4	41.21	257.24	56.83	32.55	7.58	4.3	2019.67
	1 serving	142.0	3.43	21.44	4.74	2.71	0.63	0.4	168.31
Chocolate Chip Cookies	36 servings	3146.0	43.73	294.15	201.35	73.90	58.92	0.0	380.95
	1 serving	87.4	1.21	8.17	5.59	2.05	1.64	0.0	10.58
Chocolate-Nut Cookies	36 servings	2582.8	43.50	245.30	159.64	77.40	26.37	0.0	328.10
	1 serving	71.7	1.21	6.81	4.43	2.15	0.73	0.0	9.11
Chuckwagon Egg Sandwich	2 servings	484.4	23.41	54.26	19.30	8.46	3.57	1.4	883.19
	1 serving	242.2	11.70	27.13	9.65	4.23	1.79	0.7	441.59
Cinnamon Fruit Mold	8 servings	621.8	10.27	140.73	1.86	0.00	0.00	0.0	10.47
	1 serving	77.7	1.28	17.59	0.23	0.00	0.00	0.0	1.31
Cinnamon-Raisin Bread	32 servings	3940.6	95.05	802.15	38.75	20.79	5.58	0.0	2400.25
	1 serving	123.1	2.97	25.07	1.21	0.65	0.17	0.0	75.01
Cinnamon-Raisin Cookies	36 servings	2250.8	30.33	279.26	114.29	51.88	17.87	0.0	319.90
	1 serving	62.5	0.84	7.76	3.17	1.44	0.50	0.0	8.89
Cinnamon Rolls	12 servings	2718.1	47.03	405.46	101.91	36.91	18.76	1.6	200.10
	1 roll	226.5	3.92	33.79	8.49	3.08	1.56	0.1	16.68

NUTRITIVE VALUES OF RECIPES–Continued

Recipes		Calories	Protein gm	Carbohy-drate gm	Total Fat gm	Poly-unsat-urated Fat gm	Sat-urated Fat gm	Choles-terol mg	Sodium mg
Citrus Slaw	12 servings	828.3	9.94	71.26	57.53	34.20	0.09	0.0	1501.50
	1 serving	69.0	0.83	5.94	4.79	2.85	0.01	0.0	125.12
Citrus Slimmer Salad	1 serving	209.9	17.10	31.86	1.59	0.05	0.74	3.5	495.99
	1 serving	209.9	17.10	31.86	1.59	0.05	0.74	3.5	495.99
Citrus Surprise Pops	12 servings	438.2	5.88	101.52	0.96	0.00	0.00	0.0	8.40
	1 serving	36.5	0.49	8.46	0.08	0.00	0.00	0.0	0.70
Combination Vegetable Gels— Combination 1	6 servings	338.9	9.99	73.37	0.59	0.00	0.00	0.0	91.01
	1 serving	56.5	1.66	12.23	0.10	0.00	0.00	0.0	15.17
Combination Vegetable Gels— Combination 2	6 servings	462.4	17.32	96.11	1.12	0.00	0.00	0.0	171.72
	1 serving	77.1	2.89	16.02	0.19	0.00	0.00	0.0	28.62
Combination Vegetable Gels— Combination 3	6 servings	299.5	9.10	64.82	0.42	0.00	0.00	0.0	31.90
	1 serving	49.9	1.52	10.80	0.07	0.00	0.00	0.0	5.32
Confetti Burgers	4 servings	815.4	130.12	12.11	27.43	2.58	10.99	364.0	651.23
	1 serving	203.9	32.53	3.03	6.86	0.64	2.75	91.0	162.81
Connoisseur French Dressing	¾ cup	1004.6	1.89	11.75	105.84	61.13	13.33	0.0	6.60
	1 tablespoon	83.7	0.16	0.98	8.82	5.09	1.11	0.0	0.55
Coquilles Saint Jacques	8 servings	2011.1	189.65	58.45	113.09	47.24	21.81	394.1	3494.89
	1 serving	251.4	23.71	7.31	14.14	5.90	2.73	49.3	436.86
Corn Bread	12 servings	1634.6	38.32	241.69	57.13	32.75	7.53	4.3	1816.08
	1 serving	136.2	3.19	20.14	4.76	2.73	0.63	0.4	151.34
Corn Bread Muffins	12 servings	1634.6	38.32	241.69	57.13	32.75	7.53	4.3	1816.08
	1 serving	136.2	3.19	20.14	4.76	2.73	0.63	0.4	151.34
Cottage Cheese– Dill Batter Bread	20 servings	2429.0	110.88	429.60	29.18	11.38	7.23	28.6	3113.40
	1 serving	121.5	5.54	21.48	1.46	0.57	0.36	1.4	155.67

NUTRITIVE VALUES OF RECIPES–Continued

Recipes		Calories	Protein gm	Carbohydrate gm	Total Fat gm	Poly-unsaturated Fat gm	Saturated Fat gm	Cholesterol mg	Sodium mg
Country-Style Rolls	16 servings	1401.7	38.49	242.39	30.91	17.57	4.19	0.0	890.31
	1 serving	87.6	2.41	15.15	1.93	1.10	0.26	0.0	55.64
Country Tuna	4 servings	1505.5	116.65	89.83	76.48	26.58	14.31	216.5	700.48
	1 serving	376.4	29.16	22.46	19.12	6.65	3.58	54.1	175.12
Crabmeat Salad Plate	2 servings	250.7	24.68	17.50	9.17	4.07	0.45	121.2	1332.36
	1 serving	125.3	12.34	8.75	4.58	2.04	0.23	60.6	666.18
Cranberry Apple Gelatin	6 servings	955.2	6.90	228.35	1.57	0.00	0.00	0.0	6.55
	1 serving	159.2	1.15	38.06	0.26	0.00	0.00	0.0	1.09
Cranberry Tea Cooler	6 servings	333.3	1.23	81.15	0.42	0.00	0.00	0.0	4.15
	1 serving	55.6	0.20	13.53	0.07	0.00	0.00	0.0	0.69
Creamed Fresh Beans and Celery	5 servings	459.7	12.02	40.60	27.70	10.76	4.45	0.0	458.20
	1 serving	91.9	2.40	8.12	5.54	2.15	0.89	0.0	91.64
Creamy Cooked Dressing	½ cup	202.0	9.39	25.15	7.43	2.56	1.07	1.4	166.47
	1 tablespoon	25.3	1.17	3.14	0.93	0.32	0.13	0.2	20.81
Creamy Garden Salad	8 servings	259.1	16.95	38.49	4.46	0.10	2.40	16.8	156.44
	1 serving	32.4	2.12	4.81	0.56	0.01	0.30	2.1	19.55
Crepes	14 servings	792.0	28.30	107.84	27.49	15.79	3.68	4.3	602.48
	1 serving	56.6	2.02	7.70	1.96	1.13	0.26	0.3	43.03
Crunchy Vegetable Curls	1 serving	7.0	0.22	1.44	0.04	0.00	0.00	0.0	5.00
	1 serving	7.0	0.22	1.44	0.04	0.00	0.00	0.0	5.00
Cuban Eggplant	4 servings	598.1	10.31	45.61	41.10	3.49	5.54	0.0	23.12
	1 serving	149.5	2.58	11.40	10.28	0.87	1.38	0.0	5.78
Cucumber Sauce (Variation of Med. White Sauce)	2 servings	382.6	11.25	28.54	24.82	10.85	4.63	4.3	428.72
	1 serving	191.3	5.62	14.27	12.41	5.42	2.31	2.2	214.36

NUTRITIVE VALUES OF RECIPES—Continued

Recipes		Calories	Protein gm	Carbohy-drate gm	Total Fat gm	Poly-unsat-urated Fat gm	Sat-urated Fat gm	Choles-terol mg	Sodium mg
Cucumbers in Yogurt	6 servings	175.7	10.21	23.86	4.44	0.10	2.40	16.8	144.05
	1 serving	29.3	1.70	3.98	0.74	0.02	0.40	2.8	24.01
Curried Fruit Salad Dressing	1 cup	303.1	7.07	20.57	21.92	11.47	1.83	12.6	560.58
	1 tablespoon	18.9	0.44	1.29	1.37	0.72	0.11	0.8	35.04
Curried Tuna Dip	2 cups	583.6	80.95	23.80	18.43	4.79	5.52	124.1	1085.04
	1 tablespoon	18.2	2.53	0.74	0.58	0.15	0.17	3.9	33.91
Curry Dill Dip	1 cup	443.2	6.12	16.35	40.29	22.85	1.26	8.4	997.94
	1 tablespoon	27.7	0.38	1.02	2.52	1.43	0.08	0.5	62.37
Curry Sauce (Variation of Med. White Sauce)	2 servings	362.4	10.50	24.54	24.70	10.85	4.63	4.3	711.90
	1 serving	181.2	5.25	12.27	12.35	5.42	2.31	2.2	355.95
Cut-Out Cookies	48 servings	3251.3	38.64	438.04	149.68	54.07	27.59	0.0	510.18
	1 serving	67.7	0.81	9.13	3.12	1.13	0.57	0.0	10.63
Date-Nut Bars	20 servings	2544.4	37.63	414.60	81.14	51.47	8.80	0.0	307.64
	1 serving	127.2	1.88	20.73	4.06	2.57	0.44	0.0	15.38
Deep-Dish Fruit Pie (with Apples)	9 servings	2211.8	15.58	439.72	43.63	14.09	7.19	0.0	15.69
	1 serving	245.8	1.73	48.86	4.85	1.57	0.80	0.0	1.74
Deep Dish Fruit Pie (with Peaches)	9 servings	2454.8	25.58	492.72	42.63	14.09	7.19	0.0	25.69
	1 serving	272.8	2.84	54.75	4.74	1.57	0.80	0.0	2.85
Dessert Crêpes	14 servings	1160.4	44.65	179.27	29.12	10.84	5.55	8.6	586.63
	1 serving	82.9	3.19	12.80	2.08	0.77	0.40	0.6	41.90
Devils Food Cake	16 servings	4552.9	70.76	674.67	173.68	71.69	44.88	6.5	1237.56
	1 serving	284.6	4.42	42.17	10.86	4.48	2.80	0.4	77.35
Dijon-Type Mustard	2 cups	2418.2	93.12	113.91	181.04	4.65	7.38	0.0	26.75
	1 tablespoon	75.6	2.91	3.56	5.66	0.15	0.23	0.0	0.84

NUTRITIVE VALUES OF RECIPES–Continued

Recipes		Calories	Protein gm	Carbohy-drate gm	Total Fat gm	Poly-unsat-urated Fat gm	Sat-urated Fat gm	Choles-terol mg	Sodium mg
Dill Sauce (Variation of Med. White Sauce)	2 servings	380.0	11.01	26.43	25.42	10.85	4.63	4.3	421.52
	1 serving	190.0	5.51	13.22	12.71	5.42	2.31	2.2	210.76
Dilled Onions	8 servings	37.7	1.33	7.43	0.26	0.00	0.00	0.0	8.07
	1 serving	4.7	0.17	0.93	0.03	0.00	0.00	0.0	1.01
Dilled Zucchini	6 servings	187.4	3.78	12.98	13.43	7.57	1.65	0.0	7.50
	1 serving	31.2	0.63	2.16	2.24	1.26	0.28	0.0	1.25
Dinner Rolls	16 servings	2357.4	61.45	395.92	58.66	33.52	7.90	3.2	212.14
	1 roll	147.3	3.84	24.74	3.67	2.10	0.49	0.2	13.26
Doughnut Balls	30 servings	2110.3	39.08	356.63	58.34	32.55	7.54	3.2	1300.28
	1 serving	70.3	1.30	11.89	1.94	1.08	0.25	0.1	43.34
Downhome Vegetable Soup	10 servings	722.0	64.89	90.59	11.12	0.78	4.03	127.4	5974.46
	1 serving	72.2	6.49	9.06	1.11	0.08	0.40	12.7	597.45
Drop Biscuits	16 servings	1616.7	34.90	205.50	72.74	42.05	9.51	4.3	1717.38
	1 serving	101.0	2.18	12.84	4.55	2.63	0.59	0.3	107.34
Dumplings	10 servings	1092.8	26.23	154.51	41.06	23.68	5.42	3.2	997.36
	1 serving	109.3	2.62	15.45	4.11	2.37	0.54	0.3	99.74
Eastern Shore Clam Bake	6 servings	2033.4	217.68	211.50	35.18	9.23	5.18	873.6	4224.00
	1 serving	338.9	36.28	35.25	5.86	1.54	0.86	145.6	704.00
Easy Skillet Dinner	4 servings	1488.7	156.52	91.99	54.78	17.30	15.45	409.5	1094.40
	1 serving	372.2	39.13	23.00	13.69	4.32	3.86	102.4	273.60
Easy Zucchini	4 servings	317.8	4.48	18.64	24.99	10.76	4.45	0.0	302.72
	1 serving	79.4	1.12	4.66	6.25	2.69	1.11	0.0	75.68
Egg Salad	4 servings	493.7	25.73	13.88	37.74	19.91	3.67	0.0	1067.40
	1 serving	123.4	6.43	3.47	9.44	4.98	0.92	0.0	266.85

NUTRITIVE VALUES OF RECIPES–Continued

Recipes		Calories	Protein gm	Carbohy-drate gm	Total Fat gm	Poly-unsat-urated Fat gm	Sat-urated Fat gm	Choles-terol mg	Sodium mg
Eggnog	2 servings	182.7	14.52	24.78	2.26	0.97	0.50	4.3	224.52
	1 serving	91.4	7.26	12.39	1.13	0.49	0.25	2.2	112.26
Eggplant and Tomato Casserole	8 servings	1585.2	101.40	123.47	76.14	19.19	29.27	159.7	2900.21
	1 serving	198.1	12.68	15.43	9.52	2.40	3.66	20.0	362.53
Elegant But Easy Tea Ring	17 servings	2712.0	43.60	499.82	59.43	28.50	9.19	1.3	204.67
	1 serving	159.5	2.56	29.40	3.50	1.68	0.54	0.1	12.04
Endive Salad	8 servings	979.7	16.69	39.02	84.49	33.08	9.44	0.0	892.66
	1 serving	122.5	2.09	4.88	10.56	4.14	1.18	0.0	111.58
English Muffins	11 servings	1906.2	43.90	306.54	56.05	32.34	7.34	0.0	792.56
	1 serving	173.3	3.99	27.87	5.10	2.94	0.67	0.0	72.05
Epicurian Trout	6 servings	2439.6	166.59	55.12	172.69	73.95	31.21	534.6	1972.05
	1 serving	406.6	27.76	9.19	28.78	12.33	5.20	89.1	328.67
Escalopes de Veau au Citron	6 servings	1943.5	207.28	15.90	116.75	19.52	24.11	594.0	692.87
	1 serving	323.9	34.55	2.65	19.46	3.25	4.02	99.0	115.48
Fiesta Yellow Squash	6 servings	560.6	9.88	70.43	26.54	10.76	4.45	0.0	717.68
	1 serving	93.4	1.65	11.74	4.42	1.79	0.74	0.0	119.61
Fillets of Sole Meunière	6 servings	1827.7	126.00	30.55	133.60	51.70	23.50	453.6	746.26
	1 serving	304.6	21.00	5.09	22.27	8.62	3.92	75.6	124.38
Fish Fillets	6 servings	1079.3	115.47	18.37	60.44	21.66	11.36	356.4	335.62
	1 serving	179.9	19.25	3.06	10.07	3.61	1.89	59.4	55.94
Fish Poached in Court Bouillon	6 servings	947.5	161.28	0.00	33.60	13.02	9.07	554.4	387.58
	1 serving	157.9	26.88	0.00	5.60	2.17	1.51	92.4	64.60
Fish Salad	4 servings	1446.5	93.93	18.32	111.09	48.53	20.16	336.0	47.46
	1 serving	361.6	23.48	4.58	27.77	12.13	5.04	84.0	11.86

NUTRITIVE VALUES OF RECIPES–Continued

Recipes		Calories	Protein gm	Carbohy-drate gm	Total Fat gm	Poly-unsat-urated Fat gm	Sat-urated Fat gm	Choles-terol mg	Sodium mg
Fish Salad Plate	2 servings	270.2	26.84	16.18	10.97	4.71	1.30	79.2	132.36
	1 serving	135.1	13.42	8.09	5.48	2.35	0.65	39.6	66.18
Fish Steak Broil	4 servings	1154.0	108.16	1.97	79.23	33.80	16.44	396.6	1466.37
	1 serving	288.5	27.04	0.49	19.81	8.45	4.11	92.4	366.59
Fish Steaks	8 servings	2571.7	226.02	5.89	182.78	67.13	31.70	840.0	984.88
	1 serving	321.5	28.25	0.74	22.85	8.39	3.96	105.0	123.11
Fish Stock	8 servings	589.9	5.39	23.73	52.83	4.65	7.38	0.0	1565.36
	1 serving	73.7	0.67	2.97	6.60	0.58	0.92	0.0	195.67
Florida Health Salad	8 servings	661.9	27.70	125.72	5.35	0.10	2.40	16.8	271.00
	1 serving	82.7	3.46	15.71	0.67	0.01	0.30	2.1	33.87
Fluffy Meringue Pie Shell	16 servings	858.6	14.39	200.24	0.00	0.00	0.00	0.0	267.72
	1 serving	53.7	0.90	12.52	0.00	0.00	0.00	0.0	16.73
Fourth-of-July Cooked Dressing	8 servings	195.2	9.05	24.93	6.96	2.20	1.07	1.4	117.12
	1 serving	24.4	1.13	3.12	0.87	0.28	0.13	0.2	14.64
Fourth-of-July Potato Salad	8 servings	365.0	16.15	54.56	9.23	1.64	2.16	252.7	147.31
	1 serving	45.6	2.02	6.82	1.15	0.20	0.27	31.6	18.41
French Bread	15 servings	1856.7	56.66	367.30	17.88	10.06	2.55	0.0	1230.07
	1 serving	123.8	3.78	24.49	1.19	0.67	0.17	0.0	82.00
French Dressing	1½ cups	1989.1	1.47	23.01	211.29	122.26	26.67	0.0	2.91
	1 tablespoon	82.9	0.06	0.96	8.80	5.09	1.11	0.0	0.12
French Toast	6 servings	1573.3	64.24	230.12	44.27	18.35	8.29	7.8	2781.19
	1 serving	262.2	10.71	38.35	7.38	3.06	1.38	1.3	463.53
Fresh Corn Vinaigrette	8 servings	1326.6	30.09	164.83	61.63	34.42	7.50	0.0	34.23
	1 serving	165.8	3.76	20.60	7.70	4.30	0.94	0.0	4.28

NUTRITIVE VALUES OF RECIPES–Continued

Recipes		Calories	Protein gm	Carbohy- drate gm	Total Fat gm	Poly- unsat- urated Fat gm	Sat- urated Fat gm	Choles- terol mg	Sodium mg
Fresh Fruit Cup	4 servings	480.8	5.84	111.84	1.12	0.00	0.00	0.0	7.20
	1 serving	120.2	1.46	27.96	0.28	0.00	0.00	0.0	1.80
Fresh Melon Sherbet	12 servings	460.2	10.77	102.55	0.77	0.00	0.00	0.0	77.90
	1 serving	38.3	0.90	8.55	0.06	0.00	0.00	0.0	6.49
Fresh Vegetable Souffle	4 servings	671.5	25.17	48.96	41.59	22.66	7.80	40.3	1054.65
	1 serving	167.9	6.29	12.24	10.40	5.67	1.95	10.1	263.66
Frozen Grapefruit Medley	4 servings	450.9	8.64	99.64	1.97	0.00	0.00	0.0	68.80
	1 serving	112.7	2.16	24.91	0.49	0.00	0.00	0.0	17.20
Fruit Boats	4 servings	634.4	5.20	132.38	2.16	0.00	0.00	0.0	29.94
	1 serving	158.6	1.30	33.09	0.54	0.00	0.00	0.0	7.48
Fruit Clouds (with Straw- berries)	8 servings	889.5	14.99	200.63	3.00	0.00	0.00	0.0	612.62
	1 serving	111.2	1.87	25.08	0.37	0.00	0.00	0.0	76.58
Fruit Cornucopia	6 servings	425.8	3.61	98.72	1.24	0.00	0.00	0.0	24.38
	1 serving	71.0	0.60	16.45	0.21	0.00	0.00	0.0	4.06
Fruit Jewelled Melon	4 servings	639.4	14.67	139.89	2.35	0.00	0.00	0.0	101.85
	1 serving	159.8	3.67	34.97	0.59	0.00	0.00	0.0	25.46
Fruit Kebabs Grand Marnier	8 servings	558.6	4.50	106.51	9.28	3.59	1.48	0.0	107.09
	1 serving	69.8	0.56	13.31	1.16	0.45	0.19	0.0	13.39
Fruit Salad Dressing	1½ cups	1160.4	2.12	50.76	105.43	9.40	14.91	0.0	3.95
	1 tablespoon	48.3	0.09	2.11	4.39	0.39	0.62	0.0	0.16
Fruit Syrup, Apricot	1⅔ cups	1045.2	2.50	258.25	0.25	0.00	0.00	0.0	217.00
	2 tablespoons	80.4	0.19	19.87	0.02	0.00	0.00	0.0	16.69
Fruit Syrup, Blackberry	2 cups	1041.9	2.64	253.38	1.98	0.00	0.00	0.0	206.20
	2 tablespoons	65.1	0.16	15.84	0.12	0.00	0.00	0.0	12.89

NUTRITIVE VALUES OF RECIPES–Continued

Recipes		Calories	Protein gm	Carbohy-drate gm	Total Fat gm	Poly-unsat-urated Fat gm	Sat-urated Fat gm	Choles-terol mg	Sodium mg
Fruit Syrup, Cherry	2 cups	1086.0	3.12	266.76	0.72	0.00	0.00	0.0	208.80
	2 tablespoons	67.9	0.19	16.67	0.04	0.00	0.00	0.0	13.05
Fruit Syrup, Peach	2 cups	1020.0	1.71	252.64	0.28	0.00	0.00	0.0	206.85
	2 tablespoons	63.7	0.11	15.79	0.02	0.00	0.00	0.0	12.93
Fruit Syrup, Pineapple	1¾ cups	1051.0	0.96	261.24	0.24	0.00	0.00	0.0	206.40
	2 tablespoons	75.1	0.07	18.66	0.02	0.00	0.00	0.0	14.74
Fruit Syrup, Raspberry	2 cups	1027.4	2.40	252.20	1.00	0.00	0.00	0.0	206.00
	2 tablespoons	64.2	0.15	15.76	0.06	0.00	0.00	0.0	12.87
Fruit Syrup, Strawberry	2 cups	992.0	1.57	243.90	1.12	0.00	0.00	0.0	206.25
	2 tablespoons	62.0	0.10	15.24	0.07	0.00	0.00	0.0	12.89
Fruit Whip	8 servings	569.4	8.11	131.56	1.21	0.00	0.00	0.0	14.94
	1 serving	71.2	1.01	16.45	0.15	0.00	0.00	0.0	1.87
Garlic Bread	32 servings	3365.2	91.74	663.43	38.31	20.79	5.58	0.0	2360.86
	1 serving	105.2	2.87	20.73	1.20	0.65	0.17	0.0	73.78
Garlic French Bread	26 servings	2143.0	41.11	250.03	109.87	40.93	20.41	6.3	2611.70
	1 serving	82.4	1.58	9.62	4.23	1.57	0.79	0.2	100.45
Garlic-Wine Pasta Sauce	6 servings	923.2	4.11	7.90	97.42	43.06	17.81	0.0	2327.44
	1 serving	153.9	0.68	1.32	16.24	7.18	2.97	0.0	387.91
Gazpacho Gelatin Salad	6 servings	784.5	14.17	44.11	63.95	37.94	3.36	0.0	985.03
	1 serving	130.8	2.36	7.35	10.66	6.32	0.56	0.0	164.17
Gazpacho Relish	2¾ cups	178.0	5.03	39.03	1.00	0.00	0.00	0.0	411.37
	¼ cup	16.2	0.46	3.55	0.09	0.00	0.00	0.0	37.40
Glazed Pineapple Almond Coffee Crescent	18 servings	3269.5	58.43	539.98	97.61	35.75	12.26	1.1	207.99
	1 serving	181.6	3.25	30.00	5.42	1.99	0.68	0.1	11.55

NUTRITIVE VALUES OF RECIPES–Continued

Recipes		Calories	Protein gm	Carbohy- drate gm	Total Fat gm	Poly- unsat- urated Fat gm	Sat- urated Fat gm	Choles- terol mg	Sodium mg
Gourmet Dressing	1½ cups	1710.6	5.36	30.37	173.94	93.15	21.91	0.0	408.75
	1 tablespoon	71.3	0.22	1.27	7.25	3.88	0.91	0.0	17.03
Grandmother's White Bread	32 servings	3350.5	91.08	660.51	38.28	20.79	5.58	0.0	2360.30
	1 serving	104.7	2.85	20.64	1.20	0.65	0.17	0.0	73.76
Grapefruit Sizzle	2 servings	203.4	1.17	30.73	8.37	3.59	1.48	0.0	100.95
	1 serving	101.7	0.59	15.37	4.19	1.79	0.74	0.0	50.47
Grapes and Yogurt	8 servings	970.0	11.76	217.50	5.88	0.10	2.40	16.8	171.90
	1 serving	121.2	1.47	27.19	0.73	0.01	0.30	2.1	21.49
Green and Red Cabbage Slaw	4 servings	154.7	2.92	14.66	9.64	5.70	0.01	0.0	335.70
	1 serving	38.7	0.73	3.66	2.41	1.42	0.00	0.0	83.92
Green Pepper Omelet	2 servings	301.0	24.21	5.40	20.28	9.27	3.64	0.0	551.70
	1 serving	150.5	12.10	2.70	10.14	4.63	1.82	0.0	275.85
Grilled Melon	6 servings	412.0	4.17	42.87	24.87	10.76	4.45	0.0	364.50
	1 serving	68.7	0.69	7.14	4.14	1.79	0.74	0.0	60.75
Grilled Whole Salmon	8 servings	2133.6	288.38	0.64	108.61	44.78	25.10	990.0	1367.41
	1 serving	266.7	36.05	0.08	13.58	5.60	3.14	123.7	170.93
Hamburger Toppers, Eggplant	4 servings	176.9	6.45	11.27	11.78	1.40	2.97	9.5	213.10
	1 serving	44.2	1.61	2.82	2.94	0.35	0.74	2.4	53.27
Hamburger Toppers, Horse- radish and Onions	4 servings	119.1	3.00	17.40	4.21	1.43	0.74	0.0	20.06
	1 serving	29.8	0.75	4.35	1.05	0.36	0.18	0.0	5.02
Hamburger Toppers, Mashed Potato	4 servings	70.2	5.39	11.54	0.28	0.01	0.10	0.9	240.60
	1 serving	17.6	1.35	2.88	0.07	0.00	0.02	0.2	60.15
Hamburger Toppers, Pepper and Onion	4 servings	103.5	2.70	13.50	4.30	2.33	0.51	0.0	23.00
	1 serving	25.9	0.67	3.37	1.07	0.58	0.13	0.0	5.75

NUTRITIVE VALUES OF RECIPES–Continued

Recipes		Calories	Protein gm	Carbohy-drate gm	Total Fat gm	Poly-unsat-urated Fat gm	Sat-urated Fat gm	Choles-terol mg	Sodium mg
Hamburger Toppers, Smothered Onion	4 servings	119.1	3.00	17.40	4.21	1.43	0.74	0.0	20.06
	1 serving	29.8	0.75	4.35	1.05	0.36	0.18	0.0	5.02
Hamburgers	4 servings	893.5	144.75	6.68	31.96	2.16	12.15	409.5	662.30
	1 serving	223.4	36.19	1.67	7.99	0.54	3.04	102.4	165.58
Hamburgers Deluxe	4 servings	879.2	132.52	5.80	36.25	6.68	13.27	382.2	404.40
	1 serving	219.8	33.13	1.45	9.06	1.67	3.32	95.5	101.10
Herb Bread	32 servings	3388.7	92.26	664.40	40.27	20.79	5.58	0.0	2361.45
	1 serving	105.9	2.88	20.76	1.26	0.65	0.17	0.0	73.80
Herb Cheese Dip	2 cups	342.3	60.72	13.22	5.29	0.19	2.98	13.9	1968.81
	1 tablespoon	21.4	3.80	0.83	0.33	0.01	0.19	0.9	123.05
Herb Omelet	2 servings	293.1	24.11	3.84	20.30	9.27	3.64	0.0	554.25
	1 serving	146.5	12.06	1.92	10.15	4.63	1.82	0.0	277.12
Herb Omelet Roll	1 servings	80.7	7.86	0.81	5.12	2.37	0.92	0.0	162.41
	1 serving	80.7	7.86	0.81	5.12	2.37	0.92	0.0	162.41
Herbed Asparagus with Lemon	4 servings	409.1	19.42	26.40	25.38	8.58	4.44	0.0	6.84
	1 serving	102.3	4.86	6.60	6.34	2.14	1.11	0.0	1.71
Herbed Scrambled Eggs	4 servings	427.6	25.91	1.92	35.15	8.14	9.03	1008.0	392.40
	1 serving	106.9	6.48	0.48	8.79	2.04	2.26	252.0	98.10
Herbed Tomatoes	6 servings	151.4	5.82	29.84	1.18	0.00	0.00	0.0	16.60
	1 serving	25.2	0.97	4.97	0.20	0.00	0.00	0.0	2.77
Hollandaise Sauce	1 cup	917.0	6.10	4.20	98.47	35.29	18.11	0.0	101.61
	¼ cup	229.2	1.53	1.05	24.62	8.82	4.53	0.0	25.40
Honey Cake	14 servings	2160.5	49.81	303.04	83.22	52.46	9.72	0.0	1478.46
	1 serving	154.3	3.56	21.65	5.94	3.75	0.69	0.0	105.60

NUTRITIVE VALUES OF RECIPES—Continued

Recipes		Calories	Protein gm	Carbohy-drate gm	Total Fat gm	Poly-unsat-urated Fat gm	Sat-urated Fat gm	Choles-terol mg	Sodium mg
Honey Dressing	½ cup	506.3	0.60	125.85	0.06	0.00	0.00	0.0	7.80
	1 tablespoon	63.3	0.07	15.73	0.01	0.00	0.00	0.0	0.97
Honey Lemon Cake	12 servings	2646.6	44.34	388.08	103.11	37.56	19.04	2.9	1495.65
	1 serving	220.6	3.69	32.34	8.59	3.13	1.59	0.2	124.64
Honey Lemon Tea	6 servings	489.4	1.06	120.44	0.28	0.00	0.00	0.0	7.64
	1 serving	81.6	0.18	20.07	0.05	0.00	0.00	0.0	1.27
Honey Orange Cake	12 servings	2648.2	44.37	388.49	103.10	37.56	19.04	2.9	1495.65
	1 serving	220.7	3.70	32.37	8.59	3.13	1.59	0.2	124.64
Honeyed Grapefruit	1 servings	82.4	0.60	19.67	0.15	0.00	0.00	0.0	1.60
	1 serving	82.4	0.60	19.67	0.15	0.00	0.00	0.0	1.60
Horseradish Sauce	32 servings	667.2	16.41	40.97	49.42	21.61	9.15	6.5	1263.36
	1 tablespoon	20.8	0.51	1.28	1.54	0.68	0.29	0.2	39.48
Horseradish Stuffed Rib Roast	11 servings	3275.6	564.68	8.22	109.94	8.64	48.60	1638.0	1139.12
	1 serving	297.8	51.33	0.75	9.99	0.79	4.42	148.9	103.56
Hot Cabbage Slaw	4 servings	272.9	7.21	29.37	14.38	5.38	2.23	0.0	233.41
	1 serving	68.2	1.80	7.34	3.59	1.35	0.56	0.0	58.35
Hot Grapefruit Toddy	6 servings	596.9	6.90	139.22	1.38	0.00	0.00	0.0	13.84
	1 serving	99.5	1.15	23.20	0.23	0.00	0.00	0.0	2.31
Hot Meatballs	48 servings	786.9	132.59	4.87	26.29	2.02	11.34	382.2	643.76
	1 Meatball	16.4	2.76	0.10	0.55	0.04	0.24	8.0	13.41
Hot Spicy Bread in Foil	32 servings	1489.2	23.92	132.71	99.98	34.32	20.18	2.4	1762.71
	1 serving	46.5	0.75	4.15	3.12	1.07	0.63	0.1	55.08
Iced Melon Morsels	4 servings	99.8	2.00	21.60	0.60	0.00	0.00	0.0	25.00
	1 serving	24.9	0.50	5.40	0.15	0.00	0.00	0.0	6.25

NUTRITIVE VALUES OF RECIPES—Continued

Recipes		Calories	Protein gm	Carbohy-drate gm	Total Fat gm	Poly-unsat-urated Fat gm	Sat-urated Fat gm	Choles-terol mg	Sodium mg
Iced Tea Lemonade	5 servings	236.6	0.40	58.39	0.16	0.00	0.00	0.0	1.30
	1 serving	47.3	0.08	11.68	0.03	0.00	0.00	0.0	0.26
Indian-Style String Beans	6 servings	458.5	8.78	36.59	30.73	17.47	3.81	0.0	792.30
	1 serving	76.4	1.46	6.10	5.12	2.91	0.63	0.0	132.05
Irish Omelet	1 servings	218.9	8.36	14.71	14.11	8.05	1.83	0.0	103.18
	1 serving	218.9	8.36	14.71	14.11	8.05	1.83	0.0	103.18
Island Chicken	4 servings	824.6	74.78	42.34	39.43	14.47	8.41	288.0	321.60
	1 serving	206.1	18.70	10.58	9.86	3.62	2.10	72.0	80.40
Italian Omelet	2 servings	418.7	14.80	7.30	36.94	15.93	6.57	504.0	145.10
	1 serving	209.4	7.40	3.65	18.47	7.97	3.29	252.0	72.55
Jellied Cranberry Relish Mold	10 servings	931.1	19.40	209.99	2.14	0.00	0.00	0.0	875.06
	1 serving	93.1	1.94	21.00	0.21	0.00	0.00	0.0	87.51
Jelly Omelet	4 servings	442.2	28.05	12.35	31.17	6.35	8.32	1009.1	393.28
	1 serving	110.5	7.01	3.09	7.79	1.59	2.08	252.3	98.32
Jelly Omelet Roll	1 servings	94.9	7.86	4.34	5.12	2.37	0.92	0.0	163.26
	1 serving	94.9	7.86	4.34	5.12	2.37	0.92	0.0	163.26
Jubilation Salad	4 servings	257.6	3.77	31.03	13.63	7.57	1.65	0.0	45.40
	1 serving	64.4	0.94	7.76	3.41	1.89	0.41	0.0	11.35
Lamb Chops L'Orange	6 servings	1211.4	159.34	52.81	40.38	2.27	15.93	540.0	8.29
	1 serving	201.9	26.56	8.80	6.73	0.38	2.65	90.0	1.38
Layered Fruit Salad	10 servings	648.1	17.67	139.74	2.04	0.00	0.00	0.0	25.77
	1 serving	64.8	1.77	13.97	0.20	0.00	0.00	0.0	2.58
Layered Ice	6 servings	397.3	7.17	90.94	0.54	0.00	0.00	0.0	51.20
	1 serving	66.2	1.19	15.16	0.09	0.00	0.00	0.0	8.53

NUTRITIVE VALUES OF RECIPES–Continued

Recipes		Calories	Protein gm	Carbohy-drate gm	Total Fat gm	Poly-unsat-urated Fat gm	Sat-urated Fat gm	Choles-terol mg	Sodium mg
Layered Pecan Coffee Cake	16 servings	2364.6	35.39	361.17	86.26	34.27	13.77	3.2	1854.57
	1 serving	147.8	2.21	22.57	5.39	2.14	0.86	0.2	115.91
Lemon Dill Carrots	6 servings	422.0	6.79	59.48	17.43	7.18	2.97	0.0	867.13
	1 serving	70.3	1.13	9.91	2.90	1.20	0.49	0.0	144.52
Lemon Filling	15 servings	823.3	0.62	177.55	12.32	5.38	2.23	0.0	150.53
	1 serving	54.9	0.04	11.84	0.82	0.36	0.15	0.0	10.04
Lemon-Margarine Sauce	4 servings	867.5	0.15	2.40	96.42	34.32	17.76	0.0	1.86
	1 serving	216.9	0.04	0.60	24.10	8.58	4.44	0.0	0.46
Lemon Meringue Pie	8 servings	1949.9	26.76	256.07	91.77	33.08	16.87	0.0	275.12
	1 serving	243.7	3.34	32.01	11.47	4.14	2.11	0.0	34.39
Lemon-Mint Cucumbers	6 servings	127.8	0.72	3.66	12.26	5.38	2.23	0.0	541.68
	1 serving	21.3	0.12	0.61	2.04	0.90	0.37	0.0	90.28
Lemon Parsley Sauce	8 servings	905.5	1.38	6.13	97.38	43.06	17.81	0.0	1577.08
	1 serving	113.2	0.17	0.77	12.17	5.38	2.23	0.0	197.13
Lemon Pound Cake	16 servings	3201.0	61.68	497.18	107.08	39.19	19.61	2.2	974.20
	1 serving	200.1	3.86	31.07	6.69	2.45	1.23	0.1	60.89
Lemon Relish	1½ cups	219.6	5.46	46.25	1.72	0.00	0.00	0.0	562.64
	¼ cup	36.6	0.91	7.71	0.29	0.00	0.00	0.0	93.77
Lemon Salmon Steaks	6 servings	1266.2	139.04	3.32	77.51	32.69	16.68	475.2	596.10
	1 serving	211.0	23.17	0.55	12.92	5.45	2.78	79.2	99.35
Lemon Sesame Dressing	½ cup	665.4	0.10	8.77	70.01	40.75	8.89	0.0	0.78
	1 tablespoon	83.2	0.01	1.10	8.75	5.09	1.11	0.0	0.10
Lentil Soup	12 servings	1385.1	91.78	226.77	12.52	1.02	1.10	64.6	2765.80
	1 serving	115.4	7.65	18.90	1.04	0.08	0.09	5.4	230.48

NUTRITIVE VALUES OF RECIPES–Continued

Recipes		Calories	Protein gm	Carbohy- drate gm	Total Fat gm	Poly- unsat- urated Fat gm	Sat- urated Fat gm	Choles- terol mg	Sodium mg
Lentils and Rice	6 servings	1623.5	57.55	281.76	29.56	15.98	3.63	0.0	1655.13
	1 serving	270.6	9.59	46.96	4.93	2.66	0.61	0.0	275.85
Lime Snow	8 servings	689.1	26.33	143.49	1.09	0.00	0.00	0.0	150.94
	1 serving	86.1	3.29	17.94	0.14	0.00	0.00	0.0	18.87
Linguine with White Clam Sauce	6 servings	2647.9	111.44	371.46	80.31	44.09	10.59	240.0	1017.68
	1 serving	441.3	18.57	61.91	13.39	7.35	1.76	40.0	169.61
Lobster Salad	4 servings	887.6	75.31	60.42	39.33	18.85	0.71	306.5	1485.83
	1 serving	221.9	18.83	15.10	9.83	4.71	0.18	76.6	371.46
Low-Calorie Salad Dressing	1¼ cups	425.6	16.44	58.80	14.21	7.57	1.65	0.0	119.48
	1 tablespoon	21.3	0.82	2.94	0.71	0.38	0.08	0.0	5.97
Luau Cottage Cheese and Pineapple	8 servings	890.2	73.77	123.11	10.83	0.34	5.95	39.8	2119.28
	1 serving	111.3	9.22	15.39	1.35	0.04	0.74	5.0	264.91
Macaroni Vegetable Soup	8 servings	490.5	52.70	46.19	9.67	0.67	3.78	127.4	161.18
	1 serving	61.3	6.59	5.77	1.21	0.08	0.47	15.9	20.15
Manicotti	8 servings	4408.1	323.02	248.37	237.47	67.81	63.58	624.9	8426.05
	1 serving	551.0	40.38	31.05	29.68	8.48	7.95	78.1	1053.26
Maple Nut Frosting	15 servings	2742.3	3.70	503.07	80.24	33.33	13.57	0.0	119.53
	1 serving	182.8	0.25	33.54	5.35	2.22	0.90	0.0	7.97
Margarine Frosting	15 servings	2092.6	1.08	374.65	64.27	22.88	11.86	0.5	20.39
	1 serving	139.5	0.07	24.98	4.28	1.53	0.79	0.0	1.36
Marinated Fruit	8 servings	877.8	10.32	203.36	2.56	0.00	0.00	0.0	12.80
	1 serving	109.7	1.29	25.42	0.32	0.00	0.00	0.0	1.60
Marinated Leg of Lamb	6 servings	1861.6	198.74	16.29	111.12	24.55	33.46	720.0	2071.17
	1 serving	310.3	33.12	2.72	18.52	4.09	5.58	120.0	343.20

NUTRITIVE VALUES OF RECIPES–Continued

Recipes		Calories	Protein gm	Carbohy-drate gm	Total Fat gm	Poly-unsat-urated Fat gm	Sat-urated Fat gm	Choles-terol mg	Sodium mg
Marinated Mushroom Salad	6 servings	868.6	14.32	43.07	71.96	40.75	8.89	0.0	117.64
	1 serving	144.8	2.39	7.18	11.99	6.79	1.48	0.0	19.61
Mayonnaise	1½ cups	1969.8	5.64	7.70	213.22	122.99	26.94	0.0	75.24
	1 tablespoon	82.1	0.23	0.32	8.88	5.12	1.12	0.0	3.13
Meat Loaf	6 servings	1166.3	158.53	58.38	33.26	4.57	10.71	389.1	2107.58
	1 serving	194.5	26.42	9.73	5.54	0.76	1.79	64.8	351.26
Medium White Sauce	2 servings	362.4	10.50	24.54	24.70	10.85	4.63	4.3	711.90
	1 serving	181.2	5.25	12.27	12.35	5.42	2.31	2.2	355.95
Meringue Kisses	24 servings	438.2	7.27	101.05	0.01	0.00	0.00	0.0	97.58
	1 serving	18.3	0.30	4.21	0.00	0.00	0.00	0.0	4.07
Minestrone	8 servings	1952.1	86.74	270.98	56.90	26.63	8.14	81.9	5232.35
	1 serving	244.0	10.84	33.87	7.11	3.33	1.02	10.2	654.04
Minted Cucumbers	6 servings	166.2	10.02	21.80	4.30	0.10	2.40	16.8	134.96
	1 serving	27.7	1.67	3.63	0.72	0.02	0.40	2.8	22.49
Mixed Melon Cooler	8 servings	567.9	9.10	113.22	4.07	0.08	1.29	6.6	144.16
	1 serving	71.0	1.14	14.15	0.51	0.01	0.16	0.8	18.02
Mock Sour Cream	1 cup	173.1	30.51	6.78	2.65	0.10	1.64	8.0	989.25
	1 tablespoon	10.8	1.91	0.42	0.17	0.01	0.10	0.5	61.83
Molded Tuna Supper	8 servings	1189.7	204.37	46.65	21.08	1.31	11.49	319.1	2422.28
	1 serving	148.7	25.55	5.83	2.63	0.16	1.44	39.9	302.78
Molded Vegetable Salad	4 servings	184.7	8.14	37.26	0.34	0.00	0.00	0.0	97.45
	1 serving	46.2	2.03	9.32	0.09	0.00	0.00	0.0	24.36
Moules à la Marinière	6 servings	972.4	174.07	44.89	10.89	4.03	1.74	381.6	2314.50
	1 serving	162.1	29.01	7.48	1.82	0.67	0.29	63.6	385.75

NUTRITIVE VALUES OF RECIPES–Continued

Recipes		Calories	Protein gm	Carbohy-drate gm	Total Fat gm	Poly-unsat-urated Fat gm	Sat-urated Fat gm	Choles-terol mg	Sodium mg
Muffins	12 servings	1697.7	40.78	255.85	56.76	32.55	7.58	4.3	2011.27
	1 serving	141.5	3.40	21.32	4.73	2.71	0.63	0.4	167.61
Mulligatawny Soup	4 servings	1094.5	64.48	74.05	60.01	23.70	11.24	156.6	1849.10
	1 serving	273.6	16.12	18.51	15.00	5.92	2.81	39.1	462.27
Mushroom Omelet	4 servings	488.5	33.17	19.70	30.78	17.08	4.01	0.0	434.47
	1 serving	122.1	8.29	4.92	7.70	4.27	1.00	0.0	108.62
Mushroom Omelet (with Egg Substitute)	2 servings	295.3	24.38	3.93	20.32	9.27	3.64	0.0	552.75
	1 serving	147.7	12.19	1.97	10.16	4.63	1.82	0.0	276.37
Mustard Sauce	8 servings	501.6	11.44	18.72	42.44	0.21	35.45	0.0	0.44
	1 serving	62.7	1.43	2.34	5.30	0.03	4.43	0.0	0.05
New England Mulled Cider	9 servings	1219.0	3.52	300.25	0.44	0.00	0.00	0.0	25.00
	1 serving	135.4	0.39	33.36	0.05	0.00	0.00	0.0	2.78
Noodle-Cheese Bake	8 servings	1811.5	98.11	238.88	51.44	17.68	14.06	46.9	3196.82
	1 serving	226.4	12.26	29.86	6.43	2.21	1.76	5.9	399.60
Nut and Raisin Loaf	16 servings	2377.8	52.27	335.23	91.94	48.89	14.04	4.3	2047.60
	1 serving	148.6	3.27	20.95	5.75	3.06	0.88	0.3	127.97
Nutty Orange Oatmeal Cookies	54 servings	1842.2	33.88	238.92	82.80	32.48	15.09	5.6	402.81
	1 serving	34.1	0.63	4.42	1.53	0.60	0.28	0.1	7.46
Oil-and-Vinegar Dressing	1 cup	1537.6	5.00	19.22	160.98	82.37	17.68	0.0	22.24
	1 tablespoon	96.1	0.31	1.20	10.06	5.15	1.10	0.0	1.39
Oil Pastry, 8 or 9-in. Lattice-Top or 10-in. One-Crust Pie	8 servings	1212.9	17.22	124.80	71.64	41.61	9.20	0.0	3.28
	1 serving	151.6	2.15	15.60	8.95	5.20	1.15	0.0	0.41
Oil Pastry, 8 or 9-in. One-Crust Pie	8 servings	1102.7	13.96	101.21	71.33	41.45	9.14	0.0	2.66
	1 serving	137.8	1.75	12.65	8.92	5.18	1.14	0.0	0.33

NUTRITIVE VALUES OF RECIPES—Continued

Recipes		Calories	Protein gm	Carbohy-drate gm	Total Fat gm	Poly-unsat-urated Fat gm	Sat-urated Fat gm	Choles-terol mg	Sodium mg
Okra Stir-Fry	6 servings	413.1	8.86	38.13	24.96	10.76	4.45	0.0	308.00
	1 serving	68.8	1.48	6.36	4.16	1.79	0.74	0.0	51.33
Old-Fashioned Poppy Seed Cake	16 servings	3339.1	70.79	537.23	99.41	35.78	18.44	4.3	1736.50
	1 serving	208.7	4.42	33.58	6.21	2.24	1.15	0.3	108.53
Omelet	2 servings	286.2	23.61	2.46	20.21	9.27	3.64	0.0	546.45
	1 serving	143.1	11.80	1.23	10.11	4.63	1.82	0.0	273.22
Omelet Française	3 servings	368.7	20.58	4.90	29.70	7.45	7.33	756.0	339.84
	1 serving	122.9	6.86	1.63	9.90	2.48	2.44	252.0	113.28
Omelet Roll	1 roll	80.7	7.86	0.81	5.12	2.37	0.92	0.0	162.41
Omelet Roll with Creole Sauce	3 servings	465.1	27.97	21.91	28.50	12.50	4.98	0.0	655.16
	1 roll	155.0	9.32	7.30	9.50	4.17	1.66	0.0	218.39
Omelet Roll with Mushroom Filling	4 servings	524.4	35.18	12.53	37.12	18.49	5.91	0.0	712.97
	1 serving	131.1	8.79	3.13	9.28	4.62	1.48	0.0	178.24
Omelet Souffle	4 servings	354.0	25.83	1.82	27.05	4.55	7.54	1008.0	293.35
	1 serving	88.5	6.46	0.45	6.76	1.14	1.89	252.0	73.34
Onion Bread	32 servings	3371.3	91.83	664.86	38.33	20.79	5.58	0.0	2365.30
	1 serving	105.4	2.87	20.78	1.20	0.65	0.17	0.0	73.92
Orange Gel	6 servings	474.1	9.77	107.53	0.55	0.00	0.00	0.0	5.90
	1 serving	79.0	1.63	17.92	0.09	0.00	0.00	0.0	0.98
Orange or Lemon Frosting	15 servings	2084.2	0.33	377.97	64.29	22.88	11.84	0.0	5.45
	1 serving	138.9	0.02	25.20	4.29	1.53	0.79	0.0	0.36
Orange Petite Cake	12 servings	2767.3	40.06	410.60	106.61	49.75	16.76	3.2	825.40
	1 serving	230.6	3.34	34.22	8.88	4.15	1.40	0.3	68.78
Orange Snow	8 servings	435.2	17.94	88.88	0.88	0.00	0.00	0.0	102.16
	1 serving	54.4	2.24	11.11	0.11	0.00	0.00	0.0	12.77

NUTRITIVE VALUES OF RECIPES—Continued

Recipes		Calories	Protein gm	Carbohy-drate gm	Total Fat gm	Poly-unsat-urated Fat gm	Sat-urated Fat gm	Choles-terol mg	Sodium mg
Pancakes	16 servings	1815.8	50.99	263.58	61.89	35.26	8.38	6.5	1991.90
	1 serving	113.5	3.19	16.47	3.87	2.20	0.52	0.4	124.49
Pancakes (Pancake and Waffle Mix)	20 servings	579.7	27.96	111.16	3.95	1.27	0.61	4.3	1386.25
	1 serving	29.0	1.40	5.56	0.20	0.06	0.03	0.2	69.31
Panned Red Cabbage	6 servings	381.7	6.32	32.02	25.35	10.76	4.45	0.0	769.08
	1 serving	63.6	1.05	5.34	4.23	1.79	0.74	0.0	128.18
Parfaits: Orange Parfait	1 serving	151.2	5.78	29.50	1.12	0.04	0.64	5.5	67.70
Parfaits: Peach Parfait	1 serving	144.9	5.58	28.25	1.07	0.04	0.64	5.5	67.70
Parfaits: Raspberry Parfait	1 serving	133.5	5.46	25.44	1.09	0.04	0.64	5.5	67.35
Parfaits: Strawberry Parfait	1 serving	138.6	5.53	26.42	1.20	0.04	0.64	5.5	67.56
Parsleyed New Potatoes	4 servings	457.2	6.92	53.30	24.50	8.58	4.44	0.0	16.67
	1 serving	114.3	1.73	13.32	6.13	2.14	1.11	0.0	4.17
Parsleyed Potatoes	4 servings	567.5	11.38	76.92	24.98	8.58	4.44	0.0	49.04
	1 serving	141.9	2.85	19.23	6.24	2.14	1.11	0.0	12.26
Perfect Apricot Pie	8 servings	2502.5	30.08	328.29	120.14	42.57	21.86	0.0	14.66
	1 serving	312.8	3.76	41.04	15.02	5.32	2.73	0.0	1.83
Perfect Peach Pie 8-Inch Pie	8 servings	2355.5	26.53	296.99	119.29	42.57	21.86	0.0	13.91
	1 serving	294.4	3.32	37.12	14.91	5.32	2.73	0.0	1.74
Perfect Peach Pie 9-Inch Pie	8 servings	2621.1	28.31	352.13	123.55	44.04	22.62	0.0	16.20
	1 serving	327.6	3.54	44.02	15.44	5.50	2.83	0.0	2.02
Pesto (Basil, Garlic, and Cheese Sauce)	9 servings	2446.1	28.61	33.59	245.44	28.71	43.36	61.4	498.31
	1 serving	271.8	3.18	3.73	27.27	3.19	4.82	6.8	55.37

NUTRITIVE VALUES OF RECIPES–Continued

Recipes		Calories	Protein gm	Carbohy-drate gm	Total Fat gm	Poly-unsat-urated Fat gm	Sat-urated Fat gm	Choles-terol mg	Sodium mg
Petits Fours	35 servings	9109.0	49.29	1999.68	99.10	35.62	18.38	4.3	1855.07
	1 serving	260.3	1.41	57.13	2.83	1.02	0.53	0.1	53.00
Pineapple Almond Coffee Crescent	18 servings	2853.3	58.35	436.06	97.59	35.75	12.26	1.1	176.29
	1 serving	158.5	3.24	24.23	5.42	1.99	0.68	0.1	9.79
Pineapple Frosting	15 servings	2114.0	0.32	385.20	64.32	22.88	11.84	0.0	5.59
	1 serving	140.9	0.02	25.68	4.29	1.53	0.79	0.0	0.37
Piquant Flank Steak	6 servings	1749.7	229.63	20.69	83.27	6.95	24.98	655.2	828.30
	1 serving	291.6	38.27	3.45	13.88	1.16	4.16	109.2	138.05
Pizza Muffin	1 serving	204.1	7.19	32.27	5.16	1.90	0.98	0.5	390.89
Poached Bass	6 servings	1460.1	187.47	95.37	37.24	5.45	5.61	595.2	2081.00
	1 serving	243.4	31.24	15.89	6.21	0.91	0.94	99.2	346.83
Poached Chicken and Vegetables	6 servings	1713.2	105.98	160.98	71.64	26.93	14.66	342.0	2812.66
	1 serving	285.5	17.66	26.83	11.94	4.49	2.44	57.0	468.78
Poached Egg	1 servings	183.8	8.65	13.68	10.60	2.73	2.66	252.4	237.20
	1 serving	183.8	8.65	13.68	10.60	2.73	2.66	252.4	237.20
Poached Fish	4 servings	410.2	69.27	0.87	14.41	5.58	3.89	237.6	1.00
	1 serving	102.6	17.32	0.22	3.60	1.39	0.97	59.4	0.25
Poached Fish with Caper Sauce	4 servings	585.9	82.82	17.12	20.81	6.32	6.89	282.4	292.97
	1 serving	146.5	20.70	4.28	5.20	1.58	1.72	70.6	73.24
Poteca	60 servings	5418.9	124.28	631.32	266.72	140.98	39.30	16.2	1234.82
	1 serving	90.3	2.07	10.52	4.45	2.35	0.66	0.3	20.58
Pound Cake	16 servings	2719.2	44.50	402.64	103.07	37.56	19.05	3.2	1501.36
	1 serving	169.9	2.78	25.17	6.44	2.35	1.19	0.2	93.83
Prune Bars	36 servings	2134.9	37.96	371.13	55.85	20.24	10.00	0.0	2354.23
	1 serving	59.3	1.05	10.31	1.55	0.56	0.28	0.0	65.40

NUTRITIVE VALUES OF RECIPES–Continued

Recipes		Calories	Protein gm	Carbohy-drate gm	Total Fat gm	Poly-unsat-urated Fat gm	Sat-urated Fat gm	Choles-terol mg	Sodium mg
Pumpkin Pie	8 servings	1877.0	55.18	232.23	80.17	27.86	14.70	2.2	1403.72
	1 serving	234.6	6.90	29.03	10.02	3.48	1.84	0.3	175.47
Quick Concentrate Gels	4 servings	322.9	9.77	69.72	0.55	0.00	0.00	0.0	5.52
	1 serving	80.7	2.44	17.43	0.14	0.00	0.00	0.0	1.38
Raisin Muffins	12 servings	1922.7	42.53	310.03	56.90	32.55	7.58	4.3	2030.17
	1 serving	160.2	3.54	25.84	4.74	2.71	0.63	0.4	169.18
Raisin Oatmeal Cookies	36 servings	2911.9	47.48	497.94	81.24	44.72	10.73	2.2	1721.75
	1 serving	80.9	1.32	13.83	2.26	1.24	0.30	0.1	47.83
Raisin-Stuffed Eggplant	4 servings	1256.3	12.65	153.90	65.46	33.53	9.45	0.0	889.66
	1 serving	314.1	3.16	38.48	16.37	8.38	2.36	0.0	222.42
Ratatouille	6 servings	681.5	10.01	40.55	53.55	4.65	7.38	0.0	816.08
	1 serving	113.6	1.67	6.76	8.93	0.78	1.23	0.0	136.01
Ratatouille Omelet	2 servings	507.4	26.83	15.44	37.69	10.79	6.06	0.0	559.75
	1 serving	253.7	13.42	7.72	18.84	5.40	3.03	0.0	279.87
Ratatouille Omelet Roll	12 servings	1296.2	98.88	29.43	87.14	43.02	14.18	0.0	1966.26
	1 roll	108.0	8.24	2.45	7.26	3.59	1.18	0.0	163.85
Refrigerator Rolls	18 servings	2041.0	48.72	339.04	54.45	24.45	9.97	0.0	709.48
	1 roll	113.4	2.71	18.84	3.02	1.36	0.55	0.0	39.42
Rhubarb-Strawberry Pie 8-Inch Pie	8 servings	2189.0	25.90	255.07	119.75	42.61	21.88	0.0	15.83
	1 serving	273.6	3.24	31.88	14.97	5.33	2.73	0.0	1.98
Rhubarb-Strawberry Pie 9-Inch Pie	8 servings	2567.2	28.04	337.49	124.25	44.10	22.64	0.0	19.78
	1 serving	320.9	3.50	42.19	15.53	5.51	2.83	0.0	2.47
Rich Holiday Fruitcake	12 servings	3924.0	70.61	554.75	156.33	59.28	39.52	0.0	537.98
	1 serving	327.0	5.88	46.23	13.03	4.94	3.29	0.0	44.83

Recipes		Calories	Protein gm	Carbohy- drate gm	Total Fat gm	Poly- unsat- urated Fat gm	Sat- urated Fat gm	Choles- terol mg	Sodium mg
Rosemary Chicken	6 servings	843.3	107.75	0.71	45.46	16.33	10.39	432.0	1458.90
	1 serving	140.5	17.96	0.12	7.58	2.72	1.73	72.0	243.15
Rye Bread	42 servings	3157.1	90.30	683.45	9.71	2.76	1.01	0.0	1585.59
	1 serving	75.2	2.15	16.27	0.23	0.07	0.02	0.0	37.75
Rye Bread (Variation of Grandmother's White Bread)	32 servings	3692.4	103.83	733.36	41.03	20.01	5.30	0.0	2359.80
	1 serving	115.4	3.24	22.92	1.28	0.63	0.17	0.0	73.74
Salmon Burgers	6 servings	1566.2	124.49	72.68	86.73	37.37	15.14	169.2	3669.20
	1 serving	261.0	20.75	12.11	14.46	6.23	2.52	28.2	611.53
Salmon Salad Plate	2 servings	297.0	28.40	16.18	13.25	6.04	1.18	42.0	596.76
	1 serving	148.5	14.20	8.09	6.62	3.02	0.59	21.0	298.38
Salmon Salad Sandwich	2 servings	435.0	26.73	35.50	20.76	10.61	2.86	35.0	734.59
	1 serving	217.5	13.37	17.75	10.38	5.30	1.43	17.5	367.29
Salsa Fria (Cold Sauce)	2 cups	522.1	11.74	54.79	28.12	15.14	3.30	0.0	1203.44
	1 tablespoon	16.3	0.37	1.71	0.88	0.47	0.10	0.0	37.61
Sauteed Veal Scallop à la Dillon	4 servings	1229.3	105.34	23.92	78.77	20.85	22.95	356.4	1089.21
	1 serving	307.3	26.33	5.98	19.69	5.21	5.74	89.1	272.30
Savory Beef Stew	6 servings	1971.1	186.18	120.19	83.10	24.29	23.54	491.4	3531.95
	1 serving	328.5	31.03	20.03	13.85	4.05	3.92	81.9	588.66
Scrambled Eggs	4 servings	433.2	26.20	2.06	35.58	8.14	9.03	1008.0	392.11
	1 serving	108.3	6.55	0.52	8.89	2.04	2.26	252.0	98.03
Scrambled Eggs (Egg Substitute)	4 servings	442.5	47.04	4.80	26.13	13.60	4.10	0.0	796.80
	1 serving	110.6	11.76	1.20	6.53	3.40	1.03	0.0	199.20
Scrambled Eggs (Egg Substitute) Variation 1	4 servings	450.7	47.69	6.39	26.24	13.60	4.10	0.0	805.40
	1 serving	112.7	11.92	1.60	6.56	3.40	1.03	0.0	201.35

NUTRITIVE VALUES OF RECIPES—Continued

Recipes		Calories	Protein gm	Carbohydrate gm	Total Fat gm	Poly-unsaturated Fat gm	Saturated Fat gm	Cholesterol mg	Sodium mg
Scrambled Eggs (Egg Substitute) Variation 2	4 servings	703.4	74.64	4.80	42.85	14.08	14.30	66.0	1324.80
	1 serving	175.8	18.66	1.20	10.71	3.52	3.58	16.5	331.20
Seafood Shish Kebab	4 servings	1550.7	168.33	19.04	89.10	38.70	13.48	493.2	986.03
	1 serving	387.7	42.08	4.76	22.27	9.68	3.37	123.3	246.51
Seasoned Croutons	4 cups	1192.2	10.86	63.32	100.18	35.32	18.65	1.5	522.06
	¼ cup	74.5	0.68	3.96	6.26	2.21	1.17	0.1	32.63
Sesame Rainbow Trout	6 servings	1443.9	162.95	9.44	83.82	38.67	15.81	534.6	775.46
	1 serving	240.7	27.16	1.57	13.97	6.45	2.63	89.1	129.24
Shiny Vichy Carrots	6 servings	424.6	5.31	44.19	25.23	10.76	4.45	0.0	1285.01
	1 serving	70.8	0.88	7.37	4.20	1.79	0.74	0.0	214.17
Shish Kebabs Appetizer	12 servings	2382.0	210.32	53.36	147.48	44.93	37.91	720.0	592.80
	1 serving	198.5	17.53	4.45	12.29	3.74	3.16	60.0	49.40
Shish Kebabs Main Dish	6 servings	2382.0	210.32	53.36	147.48	44.93	37.91	720.0	592.80
	1 serving	397.0	35.05	8.89	24.58	7.49	6.32	120.0	98.80
Snow Pudding	6 servings	874.3	17.27	197.84	1.66	0.00	0.00	0.0	102.00
	1 serving	145.7	2.88	32.97	0.28	0.00	0.00	0.0	17.00
Soda Cracker Pie	8 servings	1538.6	25.63	248.36	47.67	11.49	4.62	0.0	763.90
	1 serving	192.3	3.20	31.04	5.96	1.44	0.58	0.0	95.49
Souffléed Hollandaise	1 cup	474.1	6.65	2.40	49.23	17.65	9.06	0.0	98.99
	¼ cup	118.5	1.66	0.60	12.31	4.41	2.26	0.0	24.75
Spanish Rice	5 servings	871.4	11.17	94.38	49.77	21.65	9.00	0.0	926.76
	1 serving	174.3	2.23	18.88	9.95	4.33	1.80	0.0	185.35
Spiced Citrus Sections	6 servings	519.8	6.27	118.45	2.27	0.00	0.00	0.0	18.15
	1 serving	86.6	1.05	19.74	0.38	0.00	0.00	0.0	3.02

NUTRITIVE VALUES OF RECIPES–Continued

Recipes		Calories	Protein gm	Carbohy-drate gm	Total Fat gm	Poly-unsat-urated Fat gm	Sat-urated Fat gm	Choles-terol mg	Sodium mg
Spiced Lamb Burgers	8 servings	1449.9	209.59	29.79	54.82	3.82	21.09	700.3	2233.94
	1 serving	181.2	26.20	3.72	6.85	0.48	2.64	87.5	279.24
Spiced Minted Pears	6 servings	393.6	3.99	87.27	2.50	0.00	0.00	0.0	12.98
	1 serving	65.6	0.66	14.55	0.42	0.00	0.00	0.0	2.16
Spiced Oven-Fried Chicken	4 servings	792.1	98.53	37.38	27.56	7.09	7.38	411.9	743.10
	1 serving	198.0	24.63	9.35	6.89	1.77	1.85	103.0	185.78
Spicy Iced Tea	5 servings	97.0	0.35	23.12	0.27	0.00	0.00	0.0	2.50
	1 serving	19.4	0.07	4.62	0.05	0.00	0.00	0.0	0.50
Spicy Orange Chicken	4 servings	1387.7	87.81	155.76	46.00	16.07	10.09	323.0	2286.38
	1 serving	346.9	21.95	38.94	11.50	4.02	2.52	80.7	571.59
Spicy Vegetable Combo	4 servings	524.6	4.29	16.80	48.91	21.53	8.90	0.0	606.92
	1 serving	131.2	1.07	4.20	12.23	5.38	2.23	0.0	151.73
Spinach	4 servings	556.9	25.50	40.95	32.35	17.47	3.81	0.0	542.50
	1 serving	139.2	6.37	10.24	8.09	4.37	0.95	0.0	135.62
Spinach and Cauliflower Salad	6 servings	954.4	20.03	38.49	80.77	45.41	9.91	0.0	277.16
	1 serving	159.1	3.34	6.42	13.46	7.57	1.65	0.0	46.19
Spinach Salad Provençal	8 servings	655.8	12.16	30.64	53.66	30.27	6.60	0.0	519.09
	1 serving	82.0	1.52	3.83	6.71	3.78	0.83	0.0	64.89
Spinach with Yogurt	4 servings	617.1	18.41	30.26	46.89	25.31	7.98	16.8	1285.52
	1 serving	154.3	4.60	7.57	11.72	6.33	1.99	4.2	321.38
Spoon Bread	6 servings	766.6	38.31	92.67	27.26	9.84	5.22	10.8	896.64
	1 serving	127.8	6.38	15.44	4.54	1.64	0.87	1.8	149.44
Spring Salad	1 servings	156.8	16.03	17.55	2.50	0.08	1.36	9.1	460.00
	1 serving	156.8	16.03	17.55	2.50	0.08	1.36	9.1	460.00

NUTRITIVE VALUES OF RECIPES—Continued

Recipes		Calories	Protein gm	Carbohy- drate gm	Total Fat gm	Poly- unsat- urated Fat gm	Sat- urated Fat gm	Choles- terol mg	Sodium mg
Standard Pie Pastry 10-Inch One-Crust Pie	8 servings	1450.3	17.53	127.09	98.03	35.19	18.08	0.0	4.90
	1 serving	181.3	2.19	15.89	12.25	4.40	2.26	0.0	0.61
Standard Pie Pastry 8 or 9-Inch Lat- tice-Topped Pie	8 servings	1632.1	19.74	143.07	110.28	39.59	20.34	0.0	5.51
	1 serving	204.0	2.47	17.88	13.79	4.95	2.54	0.0	0.69
Standard Pie Pastry 8 or 9-Inch One-Crust Pie	8 servings	1122.5	13.12	95.12	77.53	27.82	14.30	0.0	3.73
	1 serving	140.3	1.64	11.89	9.69	3.48	1.79	0.0	0.47
Steamed Carrots	6 servings	180.0	3.80	30.56	4.81	1.79	0.74	0.0	582.49
	1 serving	30.0	0.63	5.09	0.80	0.30	0.12	0.0	97.08
Steamed New Potatoes	6 servings	538.5	9.96	78.21	20.76	8.97	3.71	0.0	267.25
	1 serving	89.7	1.66	13.03	3.46	1.49	0.62	0.0	44.54
Steamed Sugar Peas	6 servings	331.9	21.45	49.58	5.31	1.79	0.74	0.0	532.35
	1 serving	55.3	3.57	8.26	0.88	0.30	0.12	0.0	88.72
Steamed Vegetable Combo	4 servings	106.0	3.88	21.52	0.49	0.00	0.00	0.0	95.50
	1 serving	26.5	0.97	5.38	0.12	0.00	0.00	0.0	23.87
Steamed Zucchini and Yellow Squash	6 servings	449.9	19.82	42.14	22.40	5.57	7.77	31.3	769.63
	1 serving	75.0	3.30	7.02	3.73	0.93	1.29	5.2	128.27
Stewed Fruit Compote	8 servings	1706.8	28.50	390.45	3.45	0.00	0.00	0.0	125.00
	1 serving	213.4	3.56	48.81	0.43	0.00	0.00	0.0	15.62
Stewed Tomatoes	6 servings	377.7	12.72	74.77	3.06	0.50	0.44	0.7	672.20
	1 serving	63.0	2.12	12.46	0.51	0.08	0.07	0.1	112.03
Stollen	32 servings	5351.5	90.52	726.41	233.67	75.37	37.29	0.1	784.02
	1 serving	167.2	2.83	22.70	7.30	2.36	1.17	0.0	24.50
Strawberry Ice	6 servings	614.9	6.00	140.30	3.30	0.00	0.00	0.0	12.40
	1 serving	102.5	1.00	23.38	0.55	0.00	0.00	0.0	2.07

NUTRITIVE VALUES OF RECIPES–Continued

Recipes		Calories	Protein gm	Carbohy- drate gm	Total Fat gm	Poly- unsat- urated Fat gm	Sat- urated Fat gm	Choles- terol mg	Sodium mg
Strawberry Tart	10 servings	2299.6	30.76	337.10	93.96	33.32	23.33	31.5	1515.86
	1 serving	230.0	3.08	33.71	9.40	3.33	2.33	3.2	151.59
Stuffed Rock Cornish Hens	4 servings	1554.6	105.98	151.26	58.39	16.43	10.92	411.4	1411.84
	1 serving	388.6	26.49	37.81	14.60	4.11	2.73	102.9	352.96
Summer Slush	2 servings	361.6	1.98	83.02	2.40	0.08	1.50	7.0	21.80
	1 serving	180.8	0.99	41.51	1.20	0.04	0.75	3.5	10.90
Swedish Orange Rye Bread	32 servings	3712.1	104.19	738.28	41.09	20.01	5.30	0.0	2360.88
	1 serving	116.0	3.26	23.07	1.28	0.63	0.17	0.0	73.78
Syrian Meatballs	8 servings	1625.5	173.34	9.32	99.98	6.89	28.71	600.0	515.00
	1 serving	203.2	21.67	1.16	12.50	0.86	3.59	75.0	64.38
Thick White Sauce	2 servings	635.7	12.25	36.07	49.15	21.69	9.11	4.3	1008.30
	1 serving	317.8	6.13	18.04	24.57	10.84	4.55	2.2	504.15
Thin White Sauce	2 servings	217.0	9.36	16.87	12.45	5.41	2.38	4.3	563.65
	1 serving	108.5	4.68	8.43	6.22	2.71	1.19	2.2	281.83
Three Green Salad	4 servings	172.5	11.50	29.50	0.95	0.00	0.00	0.0	118.00
	1 serving	43.1	2.87	7.37	0.24	0.00	0.00	0.0	29.50
Toast Cups	6 servings	618.3	13.23	75.87	29.10	12.26	5.79	2.2	1056.60
	1 serving	103.0	2.20	12.64	4.85	2.04	0.96	0.4	176.10
Toasted Chicken and Tomato Sandwich	1 serving	296.1	11.10	19.74	18.94	7.87	3.65	25.8	379.33
Tomato-Cucumber Marinade	6 servings	604.7	4.95	26.45	53.44	30.27	6.60	0.0	18.96
	1 serving	100.8	0.83	4.41	8.91	5.05	1.10	0.0	3.16
Tomato Salad	6 servings	633.3	7.51	41.87	48.64	27.36	5.97	0.0	38.18
	1 serving	105.6	1.25	6.98	8.11	4.56	0.99	0.0	6.36

NUTRITIVE VALUES OF RECIPES—Continued

Recipes		Calories	Protein gm	Carbohy-drate gm	Total Fat gm	Poly-unsat-urated Fat gm	Sat-urated Fat gm	Choles-terol mg	Sodium mg
Tomato Sauce for Pasta	8 servings	1467.4	21.98	108.68	104.54	26.18	16.29	0.0	1141.10
	1 serving	183.4	2.75	13.58	13.07	3.27	2.04	0.0	142.64
Tomato-Zucchini Pie	6 servings	1744.7	56.13	136.39	109.17	38.32	23.51	47.2	1415.15
	1 serving	290.8	9.35	22.73	18.19	6.39	3.92	7.9	235.86
Topping for Baked Potatoes	4 servings	214.8	33.33	9.37	4.96	0.17	2.98	19.9	1005.51
	1 serving	53.7	8.33	2.34	1.24	0.04	0.74	5.0	251.38
Tropical Cooler	6 servings	496.7	4.56	117.72	0.84	0.00	0.00	0.0	44.40
	1 serving	82.8	0.76	19.62	0.14	0.00	0.00	0.0	7.40
Tuna Casserole	6 servings	887.7	74.81	108.90	16.24	6.29	2.91	108.5	956.35
	1 serving	147.9	12.47	18.15	2.71	1.05	0.48	18.1	159.39
Tuna-Chutney Dip	2½ cups	1112.0	136.01	31.31	55.19	12.18	17.08	325.6	2526.0
	2 tablespoons	55.6	6.80	1.57	2.76	0.61	0.85	16.3	126.30
Tuna Salad	6 servings	1050.9	122.63	53.72	39.38	22.08	0.82	252.0	1157.30
	1 serving	175.1	20.44	8.95	6.56	3.68	0.14	42.0	192.88
Tuna Salad Plate	2 servings	277.9	37.40	16.18	7.13	3.09	0.24	75.6	181.56
	1 serving	139.0	18.70	8.09	3.56	1.54	0.12	37.8	90.78
Turkey Salad Surprise	6 servings	1269.3	95.72	65.44	70.47	29.59	5.15	243.6	1312.70
	1 serving	211.6	15.95	10.91	11.74	4.93	0.86	40.6	218.78
Turkish Baked Fish	4 servings	1154.9	78.26	58.51	67.61	35.85	10.49	237.6	224.61
	1 serving	288.7	19.56	14.63	16.90	8.96	2.62	59.4	56.15
Vanilla Custard	6 servings	554.5	22.50	105.01	3.21	1.38	0.72	6.5	320.99
	1 serving	92.4	3.75	17.50	0.53	0.23	0.12	1.1	53.50
Veal Chops Italian Style	6 servings	2237.8	247.61	63.01	110.62	36.19	26.08	682.3	1117.88
	1 serving	373.0	41.27	10.50	18.44	6.03	4.35	113.7	186.31

NUTRITIVE VALUES OF RECIPES—Continued

Recipes		Calories	Protein gm	Carbohy- drate gm	Total Fat gm	Poly- unsat- urated Fat gm	Sat- urated Fat gm	Choles- terol mg	Sodium mg
Veal Marsala	4 servings	941.0	102.08	14.66	52.76	7.90	19.07	356.4	405.64
	1 serving	235.2	25.52	3.67	13.19	1.98	4.77	89.1	101.41
Veal Piccata	6 servings	1508.2	164.83	6.12	91.57	14.96	32.53	594.0	702.03
	1 serving	251.4	27.47	1.02	15.26	2.49	5.42	99.0	117.00
Veal Rollups	6 servings	2114.9	227.13	136.11	74.01	18.11	18.56	566.9	2319.23
	1 serving	352.5	37.85	22.68	12.34	3.02	3.09	94.5	386.54
Veal Stew with Dill	6 servings	1638.8	199.23	28.92	80.64	5.08	33.71	712.8	1375.03
	1 serving	273.1	33.21	4.82	13.44	0.85	5.62	118.8	229.17
Veal with Fines Herbes	4 servings	1198.9	130.96	1.73	74.24	24.07	16.66	376.2	846.79
	1 serving	299.7	32.74	0.43	18.56	6.02	4.16	94.0	211.70
Vegetable and Brown Rice Casserole	4 servings	927.4	53.58	149.26	12.89	0.66	6.40	39.6	1219.16
	1 serving	231.8	13.39	37.31	3.22	0.17	1.60	9.9	304.79
Vegetable Curry	8 servings	1341.4	42.72	152.85	62.12	21.72	13.70	33.6	2126.98
	1 serving	167.7	5.34	19.11	7.76	2.71	1.71	4.2	265.87
Vegetable Salad	6 servings	623.4	13.18	99.67	19.73	11.40	0.03	0.0	595.78
	1 serving	103.9	2.20	16.61	3.29	1.90	0.00	0.0	99.30
Vegetarian Casserole	4 servings	132.2	6.44	23.30	1.17	0.00	0.00	0.0	792.43
	1 serving	33.1	1.61	5.83	0.29	0.00	0.00	0.0	198.11
Vegetarian Pasta Sauce	6 servings	1199.2	20.77	92.97	81.96	32.60	10.30	0.0	1894.77
	1 serving	199.9	3.46	15.50	13.66	5.43	1.72	0.0	315.79
Vegetarian's Fancy	4 servings	1062.3	35.48	149.87	35.26	16.57	5.61	0.0	338.41
	1 serving	265.6	8.87	37.47	8.81	4.14	1.40	0.0	84.60
Vinaigrette Dressing	1 cup	1421.4	0.00	3.54	157.00	115.80	14.76	0.0	0.60
	1 tablespoon	88.8	0.00	0.22	9.81	7.24	0.92	0.0	0.04

NUTRITIVE VALUES OF RECIPES–Continued

Recipes		Calories	Protein gm	Carbohy-drate gm	Total Fat gm	Poly-unsat-urated Fat gm	Sat-urated Fat gm	Choles-terol mg	Sodium mg
Vinaigrette Dressing Variation 1	1 cup	1287.0	0.55	6.03	140.13	103.26	13.16	0.0	1.36
	1 tablespoon	80.4	0.03	0.38	8.76	6.45	0.82	0.0	0.08
Vinaigrette Dressing Variation 2	1 cup	1924.0	4.18	6.32	210.13	154.90	19.75	0.0	68.25
	1 tablespoon	120.3	0.26	0.40	13.13	9.68	1.23	0.0	4.27
Vinaigrette Dressing Variation 3	1 cup	1499.6	4.23	14.59	158.33	115.80	14.76	0.0	9.96
	1 tablespoon	93.7	0.26	0.91	9.90	7.24	0.92	0.0	0.62
Vinaigrette Dressing Variation 4	1 cup	1495.6	4.88	12.06	158.47	115.81	14.81	0.3	59.43
	1 tablespoon	93.5	0.30	0.75	9.90	7.24	0.93	0.0	3.71
Waffles	7 servings	696.7	27.96	111.16	16.95	8.84	2.26	4.3	1386.25
	1 serving	99.5	3.99	15.88	2.42	1.26	0.32	0.6	198.04
Walnut Coffee Cake	12 servings	2632.3	38.42	332.71	128.80	51.17	22.58	2.9	1206.18
	1 serving	219.4	3.20	27.73	10.73	4.26	1.88	0.2	100.52
Watercress and Orange Salad	6 servings	336.8	12.50	67.86	1.71	0.00	0.00	0.0	110.30
	1 serving	56.1	2.08	11.31	0.28	0.00	0.00	0.0	18.38
Watermelon Basket	24 servings	2176.1	30.90	486.76	11.72	0.00	0.00	0.0	144.10
	1 serving	90.7	1.29	20.28	0.49	0.00	0.00	0.0	6.00
Wheat Germ Casserole Bread	12 servings	1891.1	63.22	328.30	36.40	15.65	6.60	0.0	3142.89
	1 serving	157.6	5.27	27.36	3.03	1.30	0.55	0.0	261.91
Whipped Topping	12 servings	259.2	14.62	46.13	0.35	0.02	0.21	1.2	251.80
	2 tablespoons	21.6	1.22	3.84	0.03	0.00	0.02	0.1	20.98
White Cake	16 servings	3114.3	49.29	505.56	99.10	35.62	18.38	4.3	1727.08
	1 serving	194.6	3.08	31.60	6.19	2.23	1.15	0.3	107.94
White Swirl Frosting	15 servings	666.9	7.19	156.28	0.00	0.00	0.00	0.0	148.36
	1 serving	44.5	0.48	10.42	0.00	0.00	0.00	0.0	9.89

NUTRITIVE VALUES OF RECIPES—Continued

Recipes		Calories	Protein gm	Carbohy-drate gm	Total Fat gm	Poly-unsat-urated Fat gm	Sat-urated Fat gm	Choles-terol mg	Sodium mg
Wholesome Whole Wheat Bread	32 servings	4428.4	116.39	644.44	160.37	57.32	28.91	4.3	465.23
	1 serving	138.4	3.64	20.14	5.01	1.79	0.90	0.1	14.54
Wholesome Whole Wheat Buns	12 servings	4428.4	116.39	644.44	160.37	57.32	28.91	4.3	468.23
	1 bun	369.0	9.70	53.70	13.36	4.78	2.4	0.4	38.76
Wholesome Whole Wheat Cloverleaf Rolls	16 servings	4428.4	116.39	644.44	160.37	57.32	28.91	4.3	465.23
	1 roll	276.8	7.27	40.28	10.02	3.58	1.80	0.2	29.08
Wholesome Whole Wheat Pan Rolls	24 servings	4428.4	116.39	644.44	160.37	57.32	28.91	4.3	465.23
	1 roll	184.5	4.85	26.85	6.68	2.39	1.20	0.2	19.38
Whole Wheat Bread	16 servings	2003.5	69.42	369.10	32.82	10.85	5.41	4.3	1019.52
	1 serving	125.2	4.34	23.07	2.05	0.68	0.34	0.3	63.72
Whole Wheat Muffins	12 servings	1665.6	44.28	248.47	58.01	31.90	7.34	4.3	1612.52
	1 serving	138.8	3.69	20.71	4.83	2.66	0.61	0.4	134.38
Whole Wheat Yogurt Bread	18 servings	4054.4	156.91	692.25	86.53	29.05	17.10	33.6	1854.61
	1 serving	225.2	8.72	38.46	4.81	1.61	0.95	1.9	103.03
Wonderful Wings	30 servings	1243.3	80.55	8.86	98.53	48.27	16.90	409.5	2.32
	1 wing	41.4	2.68	0.30	3.28	1.61	0.56	13.6	0.08
Yellow Cake	15 servings	3958.0	58.58	627.78	136.24	49.49	25.22	5.4	1167.64
	1 serving	263.9	3.91	41.85	9.08	3.30	1.68	0.4	77.84
Yogurt Vegetable Mold (Main Dish)	6 servings	484.7	32.01	72.29	7.82	0.17	4.20	29.4	233.61
	1 serving	80.8	5.33	12.05	1.30	0.03	0.70	4.9	38.93
Yogurt Vegetable Mold (Salad)	10 servings	484.7	32.01	72.29	7.82	0.17	4.20	29.4	233.61
	1 serving	48.5	3.20	7.23	0.78	0.02	0.42	2.9	23.36
Zabaglione	8 servings	397.7	17.76	35.91	6.05	2.92	1.06	0.0	303.85
	1 serving	49.7	2.22	4.49	0.76	0.36	0.13	0.0	37.98

NUTRITIVE VALUES OF RECIPES—Continued

Recipes		Calories	Protein gm	Carbohy-drate gm	Total Fat gm	Poly-unsat-urated Fat gm	Sat-urated Fat gm	Choles-terol mg	Sodium mg
Zesty French Dressing	1 cup	1335.9	2.22	11.15	142.28	81.51	17.78	0.0	23.82
	1 tablespoon	83.5	0.14	0.70	8.89	5.09	1.11	0.0	1.49
Zucchini and Cherry Tomatoes	4 servings	285.3	5.06	19.86	20.71	11.64	2.54	0.0	396.62
	1 serving	71.3	1.26	4.96	5.18	2.91	0.63	0.0	99.15
Zucchini Salad	6 servings	423.7	9.64	35.45	27.23	15.14	3.30	0.0	435.89
	1 serving	70.6	1.61	5.91	4.54	2.52	0.55	0.0	72.65
Zucchini Spice Cookies	48 servings	2401.1	44.10	350.49	91.83	44.36	13.85	1.1	1379.76
	1 serving	50.0	0.92	7.30	1.91	0.92	0.29	0.0	28.75
Zucchini Spread	12 servings	142.3	7.23	4.79	10.47	4.57	1.99	1.0	594.78
	1 serving	11.9	0.60	0.40	0.87	0.38	0.17	0.1	49.56

Nutritive Values of Some Common Foods

Recipes		Calories	Protein gm	Carbohy- drate gm	Total Fat gm	Poly- unsat- urated Fat gm	Sat- urated Fat gm	Choles- terol mg	Sodium mg
Bacon	1 strip	48.2	2.43	0.26	4.16	0.44	1.45	6.3	81.68
Baking Powder	1 teaspoon	4.2	0.00	1.00					400.00
Baking Soda	1 teaspoon								1360.00
Beef, Ground, 15% Fat	3 ounces	227.7	25.74	0.00	13.86	0.69	5.67	81.9	
Beef, Ground, 20% Fat	3 ounces	253.1	24.39	0.00	17.28	0.84	7.20	84.6	54.00
Beef, Ground, 25% Fat	3 ounces	287.2	23.40	0.00	21.51	0.96	8.55	84.6	
Beef, Ground, 30% Fat	3 ounces	342.0	20.70	0.00	28.80	1.20	11.97	84.6	
Beef, Prime Ribs, High Fat	3 ounces	342.0	20.70	0.00	28.80	1.20	11.97	84.6	
Beer	12 ounces	149.8	1.08	13.68	0.00	0.00	0.00	0.0	25.20
Bouillon	8 ounces	30.7	5.04	2.64	0.00	0.00	0.00	0.0	782.40
Cake, Commercial, White Frosted	1 piece	201.6	2.60	43.30	2.00	0.19	0.88	45.3	113.00
Cake, Homemade, Mix, Chocolate Frosted	1 piece	264.5	3.60	45.30	7.66	0.64	3.64	45.2	117.00
Cake, Homemade, Mix, Plain Frosted	1 piece	268.4	3.20	49.20	6.53	0.56	2.93	46.3	115.00

Source: Figures are based on information from the National Nutrition Coding Center and supplemented with figures from the nutrient composition of foods data base at the Mayo Clinic.

NUTRITIVE VALUES OF SOME COMMON FOODS–Continued

Recipes		Calories	Protein gm	Carbohy-drate gm	Total Fat gm	Poly-unsat-urated Fat gm	Sat-urated Fat gm	Choles-terol mg	Sodium mg
Catsup	1 tablespoon	19.2	0.34	4.32	0.07	0.00	0.00	0.0	177.14
Cheese, American, Brick, Camembert, Cheddar	1 ounce	119.5	7.50	0.63	9.66	0.36	6.01	30.7	210.00
Cheese, Cottage, Creamed	¼ cup	62.3	8.16	1.74	2.52	0.07	1.56	8.8	137.40
Cheese, Cottage, Uncreamed	¼ cup	48.9	10.20	1.62	0.18	0.01	0.12	4.0	174.00
Cheese, Cream	1 ounce	69.9	2.13	1.05	6.35	0.23	3.95	22.8	210.00
Cheese, Limburger	1 ounce	119.5	7.50	0.63	9.66	0.36	6.01	30.7	210.00
Cheese, Parmesan	1 ounce	119.5	7.50	0.63	9.66	0.36	6.01	30.7	210.00
Cheese, Pasturized Process, American	1 ounce	97.1	5.94	2.13	7.20	0.27	4.48	20.4	341.00
Cheese, Pasturized Process, Cheese Spreads	1 ounce	97.1	5.94	2.13	7.20	0.27	4.48	20.4	488.00
Cheese, Roquefort	1 ounce	119.5	7.50	0.63	9.66	0.36	6.01	30.7	210.00
Cheese, Swiss	1 ounce	119.5	7.50	0.63	9.66	0.36	6.01	30.7	210.00
Cheeseburger, Fast Food	1 serving, with bun	320.00			50.0				690.00
Chocolate Candy Bar, Plain	1	192.2	2.69	19.91	11.30	0.34	6.63	6.3	32.90
Chocolate Cream Candy	1 piece	67.5	0.57	10.54	2.56	0.19	1.45	2.2	27.30
Chow Mein, Vegetable, No Noodles	1 cup	53.2	4.00	8.90	0.18	0.00	0.00	0.0	292.00
Cocoa, Mixes	1 tablespoon	63.5	0.72	13.56	0.71	0.13	0.31	0.0	27.00
Coconut, Shredded, Unsweetened	2 tablespoons	105.7	1.08	3.45	9.73	0.18	8.56	0.0	3.00
Cold Cuts	1 ounce	90.1	3.63	0.33	8.25	0.64	3.16	27.4	390.00
Cookie, Average	1	83.7	1.80	16.50	1.17	0.09	0.63	11.7	60.00

NUTRITIVE VALUES OF SOME COMMON FOODS–Continued

Recipes		Calories	Protein gm	Carbohydrate gm	Total Fat gm	Polyunsaturated Fat gm	Saturated Fat gm	Cholesterol mg	Sodium mg
Corn Chips	1 ounce	172.0	2.04	15.99	11.10	2.66	2.66	0.0	168.90
Crackers, Graham	2	57.4	1.12	10.26	1.32	0.21	0.49	1.3	93.80
Crackers, Saltine	5	73.1	1.53	12.15	2.04	0.24	0.81	0.8	187.00
Crackers, Soda	2	61.5	1.29	9.88	1.83		0.42	0.0	154.00
Doughnut, Commercial, Cake	1	112.5	2.50	21.40	1.88	0.36	0.61	21.4	175.00
Doughnut, Commercial, Yeast	1	98.0	2.40	15.70	2.84	0.55	0.96	11.5	80.00
Dried Beef	1 ounce	58.2	10.29	0.00	1.89	0.07	0.78	27.3	1290.00
Fats, Butter	1 teaspoon	36.6	0.03	0.02	4.05	0.15	2.49	11.4	49.35
Fats, Lard	1 tablespoon	36.0	0.00	0.00	4.00	0.47	1.58	3.8	0.00
Fats, Margarine, Diet	1 teaspoon	18.0	0.00	0.00	2.00	0.62	0.40	0.0	39.50
Fats, Margarine	1 teaspoon	36.6	0.03	0.02	4.05	0.52	0.80	0.0	49.35
Fats, Margarine, Whipped	1 teaspoon	22.0	0.02	0.01	2.43	0.34	0.49	0.0	29.61
Fats, Oil, Coconut	1 tablespoon	126.0	0.00	0.00	14.00	0.26	12.08	0.0	0.00
Fats, Oil, Corn	1 tablespoon	126.0	0.00	0.00	14.00	7.80	1.70	0.0	0.00
Fats, Oil, Olive	1 tablespoon	126.0	0.00	0.00	14.00	1.25	1.99	0.0	0.00
Fats, Oil, Peanut	1 tablespoon	126.0	0.00	0.00	14.00	4.20	2.67	0.0	0.00
Fats, Oil, Safflower	1 tablespoon	126.0	0.00	0.00	14.00	10.33	1.32	0.0	0.00
Fats, Oil, Sunflower	1 tablespoon	126.0	0.00	0.00	14.00	8.93	1.44	0.0	0.00
Fats, Shortening, Vegetable	1 tablespoon	117.0	0.00	0.00	13.00	3.08	3.76	0.0	0.00
Fats, Shortening, Vegetable-Animal	1 tablespoon	117.0	0.00	0.00	13.00	1.20	5.55	6.2	0.00
Fish Sticks, Breaded	1 ounce	51.3	3.18	5.67	1.77	0.52	0.31	22.5	53.00

NUTRITIVE VALUES OF SOME COMMON FOODS—Continued

Recipes		Calories	Protein gm	Carbohy-drate gm	Total Fat gm	Poly-unsat-urated Fat gm	Sat-urated Fat gm	Choles-terol mg	Sodium mg
Fishwich, Fast Food	1 serving	400.0			15.0				690.00
Frankfurters	1	165.4	6.82	0.88	14.96	1.74	5.53	34.1	550.00
French Fries, Fast Food	1 serving	220.0			12.00				345.00
Fried Crispy Chicken Dinner, Fast Food	3 pieces chicken, potato, coleslaw, roll	1070.0			62.00				2300.00
Fruit Ice	1 cup	250.8	0.76	61.94	0.00	0.00	0.00	0.0	0.00
Ham	1 ounce	84.7	6.27	0.00	6.63	0.74	2.32	26.7	330.00
Hamburger, Fast Food		250.0			18.00				391.00
Hamburger Meal, Fast Food	Double burger or house special, french fries, milk shake	1200.0			55.0				1171.00
Heinz 57 Sauce	1 tablespoon	17.0	0.30	3.81	0.06	0.00	0.00	0.0	156.30
Ice Cream	½ cup	127.8	2.92	13.52	6.89	0.25	4.28	26.0	40.95
Ice Milk	½ cup	134.6	4.18	19.49	4.44	0.17	2.78	12.5	59.16
Jello	½ cup	74.9	1.80	16.92	0.00	0.00	0.00	0.0	61.20
Meat, Canned	1 ounce	90.1	3.63	0.33	8.25	0.98	2.92	26.7	390.00
Milk Shake	1 cup	278.6	9.60	26.30	15.00	0.55	9.36	57.1	136.00
Milk Shake, Malted	1 cup	270.4	10.40	30.50	11.87	0.44	7.42	41.0	191.00
Milk, Whole	1 cup	156.2	8.40	11.76	8.40	0.31	5.28	32.4	120.00
Mustard, Prepared	1 tablespoon	11.2	0.70	0.96	0.66		0.15		187.80
Olives, Green	3	10.0	0.11	0.10	1.02	0.09	0.14	0.0	192.00
Pickle, Dill	1 large	6.7	0.35	1.10	0.10	0.00	0.00	0.0	714.00
Pickle, Sweet	1	45.7	0.21	10.95	0.12	0.00	0.00	0.0	71.00
Pickle Relish	2 teaspoons	14.3	0.05	3.40	0.06	0.00	0.00	0.0	71.20

NUTRITIVE VALUES OF SOME COMMON FOODS–Continued

Recipes		Calories	Protein gm	Carbohy-drate gm	Total Fat gm	Poly-unsat-urated Fat gm	Sat-urated Fat gm	Choles-terol mg	Sodium mg
Pizza, Cheese	⅛ of 14-inch	131.3	7.90	14.60	4.59	0.23	2.74	16.3	254.00
Potato Chips	1 ounce	173.8	1.59	15.00	11.94	6.05	3.12	0.0	102.00
Pretzels, Small	5	57.5	1.47	11.38	0.67	0.07	0.17	0.0	252.00
Pudding, Commercial	½ cup	354.8	9.00	59.30	9.07	0.57	5.37	32.4	522.00
Pudding, Home-made, Vanilla	½ cup	337.9	11.70	47.40	11.28	0.66	6.13	158.4	151.00
Pudding, Home-made, Chocolate	½ cup	535.00	9.80	84.50	17.53	1.06	10.35	105.6	102.00
Salad Dressing, French, Italian	1 tablespoon	85.3	0.03	1.03	9.00	5.18	1.36	0.0	313.80
Salad Dressing, Roquefort, 1000 Island	1 tablespoon	63.4	0.09	2.62	5.83	3.36	0.88	0.0	205.50
Salmon, Canned	1 ounce	40.5	6.15	0.00	1.77	0.80	0.29	10.5	116.10
Sardine, Canned	1 ounce	58.8	7.20	0.00	3.33	0.97	0.90	42.0	246.90
Sauerkraut	½ cup	25.5	1.17	4.68	0.23	0.00	0.00	0.0	873.99
Sausage	1 ounce	141.1	5.43	0.00	13.26	1.59	4.79	26.7	287.40
Sherbet	½ cup	119.7	0.78	26.80	1.04	0.03	0.65	3.0	8.70
Soup, Canned, Chicken Noodle	1 cup	67.0	3.84	6.96	2.64	1.20	0.60	2.4	916.80
Soup, Canned, Split Pea	1 cup	163.9	7.68	20.88	5.52	1.73	1.46	5.3	967.20
Soup, Canned, Vegetable Beef	1 cup	163.9	7.68	20.88	5.52	1.73	1.46	5.3	967.20
Soy Sauce	1 tablespoon	10.0							1099.00
Sweet Roll	1	185.9	4.70	38.80	1.32	0.27	0.44	32.5	195.00
Tomato Paste	½ cup	109.9	4.08	22.32	0.48	0.00	0.00	0.0	45.60
Tomato Juice, Canned	½ cup	26.0	1.08	5.16	0.12	0.00	0.00	0.0	240.00

NUTRITIVE VALUES OF SOME COMMON FOODS–Continued

Recipes		Calories	Protein gm	Carbohy-drate gm	Total Fat gm	Poly-unsat-urated Fat gm	Sat-urated Fat gm	Choles-terol mg	Sodium mg
Tuna, Canned In Oil	1 ounce	56.7	8.64	0.00	2.46	1.33	0.49	19.5	240.00
V-8 Juice	½ cup	26.0	1.08	5.16	0.12	0.00	0.00	0.0	240.00
Worcestershire Sauce	1 tablespoon	12.0							250.00
Yogurt, Part Skim Milk, Flavored	8 ounces	247.8	10.56	46.80	2.04	0.07	1.27	11.0	134.40
Yogurt, Part Skim Milk, Plain	8 ounces	119.3	8.16	12.48	4.08	0.10	2.40	16.8	122.40
Yogurt, Whole Milk, Flavored	8 ounces	289.4	7.20	46.80	8.16	0.24	5.28	31.7	112.80
Yogurt, Whole Milk, Plain	8 ounces	149.3	7.20	11.76	8.16	0.24	5.28	31.7	112.80

How to Calculate the Nutritive Value of Other Recipes

IF YOU want to eat a favorite food or make a favorite recipe, but the nutrient value has not been given in this book, you can consult one of the following sources:

1. *Agricultural Handbook #8: Composition of Foods,* Superintendent of Documents, U.S. Government Printing Office, Washington, D.C. 20402.

2. *Food Values of Portions Commonly Used,* 12th ed., by Charles F. Church and Helen N. Church (Philadelphia, PA: J.B. Lippincott, 1975).

3. *The Dictionary of Sodium, Fats, and Cholesterol,* by Barbara Kraus (New York: Grosset and Dunlap, 1977).

These sources give the exact figures for the ingredients in a particular recipe. The nutrient values are often given in milligrams or grams. Add the nutrient values for each food item and divide the total by the number of servings in the recipe.

If the data is given for a 100-gram portion, keep in mind that 1 ounce equals approximately 30 grams and calculate the nutrient content as shown at the bottom of this page.

Follow the same procedure for each ingredient in a favorite recipe. Then add up the nutrient values for each item for the overall value of the recipe. Divide this number by the number of servings or cups the recipe yields to arrive at the exact nutrient value of one serving.

A	B		C		D		E
Nutrient value for a specific item per 100 grams	÷	100 grams	=	Nutrient value for 1 gram	×	Gram weight of serving desired	=	Nutrient value for serving desired

For example, to calculate the sodium and caloric content of crackers, which weigh 15 grams (½ ounce), calculate:

	A		B		C		D		E
Sodium	407 mg	÷	100	=	4.07	×	15	=	61.05
Calories	475	÷	100	=	4.75	×	15	=	71 calories

Summary of Diets for Primary Hyperlipoproteinemia

Factor	Type I	Type II	Type III	Type IV	Type V
Dietary prescription	Low fat (25 to 35 gm)	Low cholesterol, polyunsaturated fat increased	Low cholesterol; caloric distribution about 20% protein, 40% fat, 40% carbohydrate	Controlled carbohydrate (about 40% to 45% of calories), moderately restricted cholesterol	Restricted fat (30% of calories), controlled carbohydrate (50%), moderately restricted cholesterol
Calories	Not restricted	Not restricted except in type IIb, where weight reduction is often indicated	Achieve and maintain "ideal" weight; reducing diet if necessary	Achieve and maintain "ideal" weight; reducing diet if necessary	Achieve and maintain "ideal" weight; reducing diet if necessary
Protein	Total intake not limited	Total intake not limited	High intake	Not limited other than for weight control	High intake
Fat	Restricted to 25 to 35 gm; kind of fat not important	Intake of saturated fat limited; intake of polyunsaturated fat increased	Controlled to 40% to 45% of calories (polyunsaturated fat recommended in preference to saturated fat)	Not limited other than for weight control (polyunsaturated fat recommended in preference to saturated fat)	Restricted to 30% of calories (polyunsaturated fat recommended in preference to saturated fat)
Cholesterol	Not restricted	Less than 300 mg or as low an intake as possible only source is meat	Less than 300 mg; only source is meat	Moderately restricted to 300 to 500 mg	Moderately restricted to 300 to 500 mg
Carbohydrate	Not restricted	Not restricted (may be controlled in type IIb)	Controlled; most concentrated sweets eliminated	Controlled; most concentrated sweets eliminated	Controlled; most concentrated sweets eliminated
Alcohol	Not recommended	May be used with discretion	Limited to two servings (substituted for carbohydrate)	Limited to two servings (substituted for carbohydrate)	Not recommended

Source: "The Dietary Management of Hyperlipoproteinemia," National Heart, Lung, and Blood Institute, National Institutes of Health, Publ. No. (NIH) 78–110.

Glossary

Aneurysm (an′u-rizm): A ballooning-out of the wall of a vein, an artery, or the heart as a result of weakening of the wall by disease, traumatic injury, or a congenital abnormality.

Angina Pectoris (an-ji′nah *or* an′ji-nah pek′-tor-is): An episode of chest pain due to a temporary discrepancy between the supply and demand of oxygen to the heart. Most often, angina pectoris is a chronic condition caused by a blood supply restriced by hardening and narrowing of the coronary arteries supplying the heart muscle (coronary atherosclerosis). It may also be caused by low oxygen levels in the blood (from smoking or respiratory disease), to a restricted blood flow to the heart (coronary insufficiency), or to an increase in heart work beyond normal levels.

An angina attack is not to be confused with a heart attack (myocardial infarction), which results from a severe and prolonged lack of oxygenated blood to a part of the heart.

Anticoagulant (an″ti-ko-ag′u-lant): A drug that delays clotting of the blood (coagulation). When given in cases of a blood vessel plugged up by a clot, it tends to prevent new clots from forming or existing clots from enlarging, but it does not dissolve an existing clot. Examples are heparin and coumarin derivatives.

Antihypertensive Drugs (an″ti-hi″per-ten′siv): Drugs that control high blood pressure (hypertension). Those most often given are the diuretics (primarily the thiazides), which promote the natural elimination of excess fluids and sodium in the tissues and circulation. Some of the other major antihypertensive drugs lower blood pressure by their direct or indirect dilating effect on the arteries. Hydralazine, for example, directly relaxes the tiny muscles in the artery walls. Other drugs, such as reserpine, methyldopa, and guanethidine, block or damper the nerves that signal the arteries to constrict. The drug propranolol slows the heartbeat, decreases the force of the heart's contraction, and thus lowers the blood pressure.

Aorta (a-or′tah): The main trunk artery that receives blood from the left ventricle of the heart. It originates from the base of the heart, arches up over the heart like a cane handle, and passes down through the chest and abdomen in front of the spine. Many lesser arteries branch off from it and conduct blood to all parts of the body except the lungs.

Arrhythmia (ar-rith′me-ah): Any variation from the normal rhythm of the heartbeat.

Arteriosclerosis (ar-te″re-o-skie-ro′sis): A group of diseases characterized by thickening and loss of elasticity of artery walls. This may be a result of an accumulation of fibrous tissue, fatty substances (lipids), and/or minerals. (*See* Atherosclerosis.)

Artery (ar′ter-e): Blood vessels that carry blood away from the heart to the various parts of the body. They usually carry oxygenated blood, except for the pulmonary artery, which carries unoxygenated blood from the heart to the lungs for oxygenation. (*See* Arteriosclerosis.)

Atherosclerosis (ath″er-o″skie-ro′sis): A kind of arteriosclerosis in which the inner layer of the artery wall is made thick and irregular by deposits of a fatty substance. These deposits (called atheromata or plaque) project above the surface of the inner layer of the artery and thus decrease the diameter of the internal channel of the vessel. (*See* Arteriosclerosis.)

Autonomic Nervous System (aw″to-nom′ik): Also called the involuntary nervous system. The nerves of this system regulate tissues and functions normally not under conscious control (heartbeat, blood pressure). It consists of two divisions, the sympathetic and parasympathetic, which usually have opposing effects on the cardiovascular system. The sympathetic nerves, when stimulated, tend to increase heart rate, constrict blood vessels, and raise blood pressure; the parasympathetic tend to slow the heart rate, relax blood vessels, and lower blood pressure.

Behavior, Type A and Type B: Two kinds of behavior patterns, as recognized in medicine. Type A behavior is characterized by high degrees of competitiveness, aggressiveness, and feelings of the pressure of time. This type of behavior is thought by some cardiologists to be a risk factor in the development of coronary heart disease. Individuals who exhibit the converse, Type B behavior, are more easygoing, contemplative, and more easily satisfied.

Blood Pressure: The force the flowing blood exerts against the artery walls. Two pressures are usually measured: (1) the upper, or *systolic,* pressure occurs each time the heart contracts (systole) and pumps blood into the aorta; and (2) the lower, or *diastolic,* pressure occurs when the heart relaxes (diastole) and refills with blood flowing in from the large veins, the venae cavae. The blood pressure is therefore expressed by two numbers, with the systolic over the diastolic; for example, 120/80, or "120 over 80."

Calorie (kal′o-re): Sometimes called large or kilocalorie. Unit used to express food energy. The amount of heat required to raise the temperature of 1 kilogram of water 1 degree Centigrade. A high caloric diet has a prescribed caloric value above the total daily energy requirement. A low caloric diet has a prescribed caloric value below the total energy requirement.

Cardiac (kar′de-ak): Pertaining to the heart. Sometimes refers to a person who has heart disease.

Cardiac Arrest: Cessation of the heartbeat. As a result, blood pressure drops abruptly and the circulation of the blood ceases. Until recently, this was always fatal. Today, the heart can be stimulated to start beating again and death averted under certain circumstances. (*See* Cardiopulmonary Resuscitation.)

Cardiopulmonary Resuscitation (CPR) (kar″de-o-pul′mon-ner-e re-sus″i-ta′shun): Also called Basic Life Support. An emergency measure used by one or two people to maintain another person's breathing and heartbeat artificially in the event these functions suddenly stop. CPR consists of keeping the airway open and performing rescue breathing and external cardiac compression (heart massage) to keep oxygenated blood circulating through the body. (*See* Heart Massage.)

Cardiovascular (kar″de-o-vas′ku-lar): Pertaining to the heart and blood vessels.

Cardiovascular-Renal Disease (kar″de-o-vas′ku-lar re′nal): Disease involving the heart, blood vessels, and kidneys.

Cerebrovascular (ser"e-bro-vas'ku-lar): Pertaining to the blood vessels in the brain.

Cholesterol (ko-les'ter-ol): A fatlike substance found in animal tissue. The normal level for Americans is assumed to be between 180 and 220 milligrams per 100 cc of blood. A higher level is often associated with high risk of coronary atherosclerosis.

Circulatory (ser'ku-lah-to"re): Pertaining to the heart, blood vessels, and the circulation of the blood.

Claudication (klaw"di-ka'shun): Pain and lameness or limping. Can be caused by defective circulation of the blood in the vessels of the limbs. (*See* Intermittent Claudication.)

Congestive Heart Failure (kon-jes'tiv): *Heart failure* is a condition in which the heart is unable to pump its required amount of blood.

Heart failure is often congestive because loss of pumping power by the heart leads to congestion in the body tissues; fluid accumulates (edema) in the abdomen and legs and/or in the lungs (pulmonary edema). Congestive heart failure often develops gradually over several years, although it can be acute (short and severe). It can be treated by drugs or in some cases by surgery. (*See* Heart Failure.)

Coronary Arteries (kor'o-na-re): Arteries, arising from the base of the aorta, that conduct blood to the heart muscle. These arteries, and the network of vessels branching off from them, come down over the top of the heart like a crown (corona).

Coronary Atherosclerosis (ath"er-o"skle-ro'sis): Commonly called *coronary heart disease*. An irregular thickening of the inner layer of the walls of the arteries that conduct blood to the heart muscle. The internal channel of these arteries (the coronaries) becomes narrowed, and the blood supply to the heart muscle is reduced. (*See* Atherosclerosis.)

Coronary Bypass Surgery: Surgery to improve the blood supply to the heart muscle when narrowed coronary arteries reduce flow of the oxygen-containing blood, which is vital to the pumping heart. This reduction in blood flow causes chest pain and leads to increased risk of heart attack. Thus coronary bypass surgery involves constructing detours through which blood can bypass narrowed portions of coronary arteries to keep the heart muscle supplied. Veins or arteries taken from other parts of the body where they are not essential are grafted onto the heart to construct these detours.

Coronary Heart Disease: Also called *coronary artery disease* and *ischemic heart disease*. Heart ailments caused by narrowing of the coronary arteries, which results in a decreased blood supply to the heart (ischemia).

Coronary Insufficiency: A condition that occurs whenever the coronary arteries (which supply the heart muscle with blood) do not provide oxygen adequate to the needs of the pumping heart. This may produce chest pain (angina pectoris) or a heart attack, or no pain may occur at all.

Acute coronary insufficiency describes chest pain that is more severe than that of angina pectoris, but in which no heart muscle damage is done (as there would be in a heart attack).

Diet: Daily allowance or intake of food and drink.

Digitalis (dij"e-tal'is): A drug prepared from leaves of the foxglove plant. Its main effect is cardiotonic, that is, it causes the heart muscle to pump more forcefully and effectively, thereby improving the circulation of the blood and promoting the normal elimination of excess fluid. Digitalis is often used to treat heart failure because it can relieve one of the early effects of the condition, buildup of fluid in the body tissue. Digitalis is the most frequently used cardiotonic drug; other examples are ouabain and strophanthidin.

Diuretic (di"u-ret′ik): A medicine that promotes the excretion of urine, often used to treat conditions involving excess body fluid, such as hypertension and congestive heart failure. One important class of diuretics is the thiazides.

Echocardiography (ek"o-kar"de-og′rah-fe): A diagnostic method by which pulses of sound (ultrasound) are transmitted into the body and the echoes returning from the surfaces of the heart and other structures are electronically plotted and recorded. Stop-action or real-time images of the heart can be made into a record of the heart's movements.

Edema (e-de′mah): Swelling resulting from abnormally large amounts of fluid in the tissues of the body.

Electrocardiogram (e-lek"tro-kar′de-o-gram"): Often referred to as ECG or EKG. A graphic record of the electric currents generated by the heart. The word *electrocardiogram* most often refers to a resting electrocardiogram, made while the patient is lying at rest. The recording can also be made while the patient is exercising. (*See* Stress Test.)

Embolism (em′bo-lizm): The blocking of a blood vessel by a clot or other substance carried in the bloodstream.

Embolus (em′bo-lus): A blood clot (or other substance, such as an air bubble, fat, or tumor) that drifts unattached in the blood-stream until it becomes lodged in a small vessel and obstructs circulation. (*See* Thrombus.)

Essential Hypertension (hi"per-ten′shun): Sometimes called primary hypertension and commonly known as high blood pressure. An elevated blood pressure of unknown cause.

Etiology (e"te-ol′o-je): The sum of knowledge about the causes of a disease.

Fibrillation (fi-bri-la′shun): A kind of cardiac arrhythmia. Uncoordinated contraction of the heart muscle occurring when the individual muscle fibers take up independent irregular contractions. *Atrial fibrillation* involves very rapid, irregular contractions of the atria, followed irregularly by contractions of the ventricles. This may occur suddenly and for a short time or, if there is an existing heart disease, can become chronic. Treatment is usually by drugs and sometimes by cardioversion (brief electric shock). *Ventricular fibrillation* involves contractions of the ventricles, which are irregular, haphazard, and ineffective, resulting in a rapid decline of blood circulation and death. Emergency treatment may include external cardiac massage (cardiopulmonary resuscitation, or CPR), electrical defibrillation (cardioversion), or drugs. (*See* Cardiopulmonary Resuscitation and Cardioversion.)

Genetics (je-net′iks): The study of heredity.

Heart Attack: The death of a portion of heart muscle, which may result in disability or death of the individual, depending on how much of the heart is damaged. A heart attack occurs when an obstruction in one of the coronary arteries prevents an adequate oxygen supply to the heart. Symptoms may be nonexistent, mild, or severe and may include chest pain (sometimes radiating to the shoulder, arm, neck, or jaw), nausea, cold sweat, and shortness of breath.

Doctors often refer to a heart attack in terms of the obstruction (i.e., coronary occlusion, coronary thrombosis, or simply *coronary*) or of the heart-muscle damage (myocardial infarction, infarct, or M.I.). In common usage, the term *heart attack* often incorrectly refers to irregular heartbeats or attacks of angina pectoris.

Heart Disease: A general term for ailments of the heart or blood vessels. Some are present at birth (congenital) and are either inherited or are the result of environmental influences on the embryo as it develops in the womb. The majority of cases of heart disease, however, are acquired later in life, through the development of atherosclerosis, for example.

Heart Failure: A condition in which the heart is unable to pump the amount of blood required to maintain a normal circulation. It can be isolated to either the left or the right side of the heart or can involve the whole heart. Heart failure can develop from many heart and circulatory disorders, especially high blood pressure (an increased resistance to blood flow in the arteries), heart attack, rheumatic heart disease, and birth defects.

Heart failure often leads to congestion in the body tissues; fluid accumulates (edema) in the abdomen and legs and/or in the lungs (pulmonary edema). Congestive heart failure often develops gradually over several years, although it can be acute (short and severe). It can be treated by drugs or in some cases by surgery.

Hemorrhage (hem´or-ij): Loss of blood from a blood vessel. In external hemorrhage, blood escapes from the body. In internal hemorrhage, blood passes into tissues surrounding the ruptured blood vessel.

High Blood Pressure: An unstable or persistent elevation of blood pressure above the normal range. Uncontrolled, chronic high blood pressure strains the heart, damages arteries, and creates a greater risk of heart attack, stroke, and kidney problems. Also known as hypertension.

Hydrogenated (hi´dro-jen-a˝tid): Combined with more hydrogen; more saturated.

Hypercholesteremia (hi˝per-ko-les˝ter-e´me-ah): An excess of cholesterol in the blood. Sometimes called hypercholesterolemia or hypercholesterinemia. (*See* Cholesterol.)

Hyperlipemia (hi˝per-li-pe´me-ah): An excess of fats or lipids in the blood. Also called hyperlipidemia.

Hyperlipoproteinemia (hi˝per-lip˝o-pro˝te-in-e´me-ah): The name for several types of blood-lipid disorders involving high blood levels of lipoproteins (complexes of lipids—either cholesterol or triglycerides—and certain kinds of proteins). Some types of hyperlipoproteinemia (Type II, Type III, Type IV) are associated with the premature development of atherosclerosis (hardening of the arteries) and therefore with increased risk of heart attack and stroke.

Hypertension: Commonly called high blood pressure. (*See* High Blood Pressure.)

Hyperuricemia (hi˝per-u-ri-se´me-ah): Elevated uric acid level in the blood.

Incidence: The number of new cases of a disease developing in a given population during a specified period of time, such as a year.

Infarct (in´farkt): The area of tissue that is damaged or dies as a result of receiving an insufficient blood supply. Frequently used in the phrase *myocardial infarct* to refer to the heart-muscle injury caused by an interrupted flow of blood through the coronary artery, which normally supplies it.

Infarction (in-fark'shun): The occurrence of an infarct.

Intermittent Claudication (klaw"di-ka'shun): Pain in the muscles of a limb that, similar to angina pectoris, occurs intermittently, during stress but not at rest. This condition frequently accompanies diseases of the peripheral blood vessels, such as thromboangitis obliterans. The resting muscle has an adequate blood supply, but when the need for blood increases (as during exercise), the disease impairs the circulation. An inadequate blood supply and the buildup of waste products of metabolism in the tissue cause pain. *Claudication* means lameness.

Ischemia (is-ke'me-ah): A local, usually temporary, deficiency of oxygen in part of the body, often caused by a constriction or obstruction in the blood vessel supplying that part.

Ischemic Heart Disease (is-kem'ik): Also called *coronary artery disease* and *coronary heart disease*. Heart ailments caused by narrowing of the coronary arteries and therefore a decreased blood supply to the heart (ischemia).

Lifestyle: An individual's typical way of life, including diet, kinds of recreation, job, home environment, location, temperament, and smoking, drinking, and sleeping habits.

Lipid (lip'id): A fatty substance.

Lipid-Lowering Drugs: Drugs used to treat the various types of hyperlipoproteinemia; that is, abnormally high concentrations of lipids (fats) in the blood. Also called *hypolipemic* and *hypolipidemic* drugs; those drugs that lower blood levels of the lipid cholesterol are called *hypocholesteremic*. The most common lipid-lowering drugs used are cholestyramine, clofibrate, and nicotinic acid.

Lipoprotein (lip"o-pro'te-in): A complex consisting of lipid (fat) and protein molecules bound together. Lipids do not dissolve in the blood but must circulate in the form of lipoproteins.

Metabolism (me-tab'o-lizm): A general term designating all chemical changes that occur to substances within the body.

Monounsaturated Fat (mon"o-un-sat'u-rated): A fat capable of absorbing some additional hydrogen, but not as much as polyunsaturated fats. In the diet, these fats have little effect on the amount of cholesterol in the blood. One example is olive oil. (*See* Polyunsaturated Fat.)

Morbidity Rate (mor-bid'i-te): The ratio of the number of cases of a disease to the number of well people in a given population during a specified period of time, such as a year. The term involves two separate concepts: (1) *incidence* is the number of new cases of a disease developing in a given population during a specific period of time, such as a year, and (2) *prevalence* is the number of cases of a given disease existing in a given population at a specified moment of time.

Mortality Rate, Cause-Specific (mor-tal'i-te): The ratio of deaths from a specific cause to total population during a given period of time.

Myocardial Infarction (mi"o-kar'de-al in-fark'shun): The damaging and death of an area of heart muscle (myocardium) resulting from an interruption in the blood supply reaching that area. (*See* Heart Attack.)

Myocardium (mi″o-kar′de-um): The muscular wall of the heart. The thickest of the three layers of the heart wall, it lies between the inner layer (endocardium) and the outer layer (epicardium).

Nitroglycerin (ni-tro-glis′er-in): A drug (one of the nitrites) that relaxes the muscles in the blood vessels. It is often prescribed to relieve attacks of angina pectoris and spasm of coronary arteries. It is one of the vasodilators.

Obesity (o-bees′i-te): An increase in body weight beyond physical and skeletal requirements because of an accumulation of excess fat. This puts a strain on the heart and increases the chance of developing two major heart attack risk factors: high blood pressure and diabetes.

Occlusive (o-kloo′siv): Closing or shutting off. A coronary occlusion is a closing off of a coronary artery (which supplies the heart muscle with blood).

Peripheral Vascular Disease (pe-rif′er-al vas′cu-lar): A term that, in its broadest sense, refers to diseases of any of the blood vessels outside of the heart and to diseases of the lymph vessels. These are circulation disorders caused by changes in the caliber of the vessels.

Phospholipids (fos″fo-lip′idz): One of the three major classes of lipids (fatty substances) in the blood. Unlike the other two classes— cholesterol and triglycerides—phospholipids are not known to be associated with atherosclerosis.

Platelets (plat′letz): One of the three kinds of formed elements found in the blood. Literally "little plates," they are small, colorless, disk-shaped bodies that are involved in the formation of blood clots. Also called thrombocytes.

Polyunsaturated Fat (pol″e-un-sat′u-rat-ed): A fat capable of absorbing additional hydrogen. Usually liquid oils of vegetable origin, such as corn oil or safflower oil, polyunsaturated fats tend to lower the amount of cholesterol in the blood. They are sometimes substituted for saturated fat in a diet in an effort to lessen the hazard of fatty deposits in the blood vessels. (*See* Monounsaturated Fat.)

Prevalence: The number of cases of a given disease existing in a given population at a specified moment of time.

Renal (re′nal): Pertaining to the kidney.

Risk Factors: In cardiology, characteristics associated with an increased risk of developing coronary heart disease. These include high blood pressure (hypertension), elevated blood levels of cholesterol and other lipids (hyperlipoproteinemia), cigarette smoking, obesity, diabetes, and a family history of heart disease. A competitive, aggressive lifestyle (Type A Behavior) is also thought to predispose a person to heart disease.

Saturated Fat: A fat incapable of absorbing any more hydrogen, usually a solid fat of animal origin, such as those in milk, butter, and meat. A diet high in saturated fat tends to increase the amount of cholesterol in the blood. Sometimes these fats are restricted in the diet in an effort to lessen the hazard of fatty deposits in the blood vessels.

Sodium (so′de-um): A mineral essential to life, found in nearly all plant and animal tissue. Table salt (sodium chloride) is nearly half sodium. In some types of heart disease, the body retains an excess of sodium and water, and therefore sodium intake is restricted.

Stress: Bodily or mental tension caused by physical, chemical, or emotional factors. Stress can refer to physical exertion as well as mental anxiety.

Stress Test: A diagnostic method used to determine the body's response to physical exertion (stress). Usually involves taking an ECG and other physiological measurements (such as breathing rate and blood pressure) while the patient is exercising, usually jogging on a treadmill, walking up and down a short set of stairs, or pedaling on a stationary bicycle.

Stroke: Also called cerebrovascular accident. An impeded blood supply to some part of the brain, generally caused by: (1) a blood clot forming in the vessel (cerebral thrombosis); (2) a rupture of the blood vessel wall (cerebral embolism); (3) a blood clot or other material from another part of the vascular system that flows to the brain and obstructs a cerebral vessel (cerebral embolism); and (4) pressure on a blood vessel, as by a tumor.

Triglyceride (tri-glis′er-id): The main type of lipid (fatty substance) found in the adipose (fat) tissue of the body and also the main dietary lipid. High levels of triglycerides in the blood may be associated with a greater risk of coronary atherosclerosis.

Unsaturated Fat: A fat whose molecules have one or more double bonds, so that it is capable of absorbing more hydrogen. *Monounsaturated fats*, such as olive oil, have only one double bond (the rest are single) and seem to have little effect on blood cholesterol. *Polyunsaturated fats*, such as corn oil and safflower oil, have two or more double bonds per molecule and tend to lower blood cholesterol. (*See* Saturated Fat.)

Vascular (vas′ku-lar): Pertaining to the blood vessels.

Vein: Any one of a series of vessels of the vascular system that carries blood from various parts of the body back to the heart. All veins in the body conduct unoxygenated blood except the pulmonary veins, which conduct freshly oxygenated blood from the lungs back to the heart.

Source: "A Handbook of Heart Terms," Public Health Service, U.S. Dept of Health, Education, and Welfare. Publ. No. (NIH) 78–131.

Selected Sources of Information

BEHAVIOR MODIFICATION

Directory of Behavioral Weight Control Programs (AABT). Harry S. Truman Memorial Veterans Hospital, 800 Stadium Road, Columbia, Mo. 65201

Ellis, A., and Harper, P. *Guide to Rational Living.* Englewood Cliffs, N.J.: Prentice-Hall, 1961.

Ferguson, J. *Habits Not Diets.* Palo Alto, Calif.: Bull Publishing Company, 1976.

Jordon, H.; Levitz, L.; and Kimbrell, G. *Eating is Okay.* New York: Rawson Associates, 1976.

Mahoney, M. *Cognition and Behavior Modification.* Cambridge, Mass.: Ballinger, 1974.

Mahoney, M., and Mahoney, K. *Permanent Weight Control.* New York: W.W. Norton, 1975.

Mahoney, M.J., and Thoresen, C.E. *Self-Control: Power to the Person.* Monterey, Calif.: Brooks/Cole Publishing Company, 1974.

Stuart, R.B., ed. *Behavior Self-Management: Strategies, Techniques, and Outcome.* New York: Brunner/Mazel, 1977.

Stuart, R.B. *Act Thin, Stay Thin.* New York: Norton, 1978.

Stuart, R.B., and Davis, B. *Slim Chance in a Fat World: Behavioral Control of Obesity.* Champaign, Ill.: Research Press, 1972.

HOW TO STOP SMOKING

American Cancer Society, 777 3rd Avenue, New York, New York 10017.

American Heart Association, 7320 Greenville Avenue, Dallas, Texas 75231.

American Lung Association, 1740 Broadway, New York, New York 10019.

National Interagency Council on Smoking and Health, 419 Park Avenue South, Suite 1301, New York, New York 10016.

Office on Smoking and Health, U.S. Department of Health, Education, and Welfare, 200 Independence Avenue, S.W., Room 622E, Washington, D.C. 20201.

Shick Laboratories, 1901 Avenue of the Stars, Suite 1530, Los Angeles, California 90067.

U.S. Department of Health and Human Services, Public Health Service, National Institute of Health, Bethesda, Maryland 20014.

Five-Day Plan to Stop Smoking, General Headquarters, Seventh Day Adventist Church, Narcotics Education Division, 6840 Eastern Avenue, N.W., Washington, D.C. 20012.

SmokeEnders, Memorial Parkway, Phillipsburg, New Jersey 08864. Call toll free (800) 631-7676. In New Jersey (800) 452-9773.

Pamphlets

Calling It Quits, National Cancer Institute, DEHW Publication No. (NIH) 79–1824.
How To Stop Smoking! American Heart Association, 7320 Greenville Avenue, Dallas, Texas 75231.
Me Quit Smoking? How? National Tuberculosis and Respiratory Disease Association. Available through local chapters.

EXERCISE

Cooper, K. *Aerobics.* New York: Bantam Books, 1972.
Cooper, K. *The New Aerobics.* New York: Bantam Books, 1970.
Fixx, S.F. *The Complete Book of Running.* New York: Random House, 1977.
Kuntzleman, C.T. *The Complete Book of Walking.* New York: Simon and Schuster, 1978.
The President's Course of Physical Fitness and Sports, 400 6th Street, S.W., Washington, D.C. 20024.
YMCA and YWCA.

FAT- AND CHOLESTEROL-CONTROLLED RECIPES

American Heart Association. *The American Heart Association Cookbook,* 3rd ed. New York: David McKay, 1979.
Bond, C.Y., et al. *The Low-Fat Low-Cholesterol Diet.* New York: Doubleday, 1971.
Cholesterol-Free Foods, Miles Laboratories, 7123 West 65th Street, Chicago, Illinois 60638.
Cutler, Carol. *Haute Cuisine for Your Heart's Delight.* New York: Clarkson W. Potter, 1975.
Dietary Control of Cholesterol, Standard Brands Educational Services, P.O. Box 2695, New York, New York 10017.
Jones, J. *Diet for a Happy Heart.* San Francisco: 101 Productions, 1975.
Page, H.C., and Shroeder, J.S. *The Whole Family Low-Cholesterol Cookbook.* New York: Grosset and Dunlap, 1976.
Rosenthal, S. *Live High on Low Fat.* Philadelphia: J.B. Lippincott, 1975.

SODIUM-CONTROLLED RECIPES

American Heart Association. *Cooking Without Your Salt Shaker.* New York: David McKay, 1980.
Bagg, Elma W. *Cooking Without a Grain of Salt.* New York: Doubleday, 1964.
Clairborne, Craig, and Franey, Pierre. *Craig Clairborne's Gourmet Diet.* New York: Times Books, 1980.
Delicious Low-Sodium Diets. Standard Brands Educational Services, P.O. Box 2695, New York, New York 10017.
Jones, Jeanne. *Secrets of Salt-Free Cooking.* San Francisco: 101 Productions, 1979.
Liebowitz, D.; Brown, W.J.; and Olness, M. *Cook to Your Heart's Content.* Menlo Park, Calif.: Pacific Coast Publishers, 1969.

SODIUM-CONTROLLED RECIPES—Continued

Margie, J.D., and Hunt, J.C. *Living with High Blood Pressure: The Hypertension Diet Cookbook.* Bloomfield, N.J.: HLS Press, 1978.

Conason, Emil B., and Ella, Mety. *The Salt-Free Diet Cookbook.* New York: Grosset and Dunlap, 1969.

Thorbuan, Anna H., with Turner, P. *Living Salt Free and Easy.* New York: Signet, 1976.

FOODS AND NUTRITION

Farquhar, J.W. *The American Way of Life Need Not Be Hazardous to Your Health.* New York: W.W. Norton, 1978. (Offers concrete methods to achieve permanent, life-enhancing changes to avert the risk of heart disease.)

Kraus, Barbara. *The Dictionary of Sodium, Fats, and Cholesterol.* New York: Grosset and Dunlap, 1977.

Nutrition Labeling: How It Can Work for You. National Nutrition Consortium Inc., 1975.

Food and Drug Administration. *We Want You to Know About Nutrition Labeling.* U.S. Government Printing Office, Washington, D.C. 20402. Stock No. 1712–00–190.

United States Department of Agriculture. *Composition of Foods: Raw, Processed, Prepared.* Revised. U.S.D.A. Agriculture Handbook. November 8, 1975.

United States Department of Agriculture. *Food.* U.S.D.A. Home and Garden Bulletin No. 228. U.S. Government Printing Office, Washington, D.C. 20402. Stock No. 001–000–03881–8.

United States Department of Agriculture. *Nutrition Value of American Foods in Common Units.* U.S.D.A. Agriculture Handbook. November 4, 5, 6, 1975.

United States Department of Health and Human Services. *Healthy People: The Surgeon General's Report on Health Promotion and Disease Prevention.* U.S. Government Printing Office, Washington, D.C. 20402. Stock No. 017–001–00416–2.

HYPERLIPOPROTEINEMIA DIETS

Request information from your physician. Publications specific to each type of hyperlipoproteinemia are available without charge to physicians and dieticians. Write:

Hyperlipoproteinemia Diets
Public Inquiries Branch
National Heart, Lung, and Blood Institute
National Institutes of Health
Bethesda, MD 20205

Index

General Index

Recipe Index